Essential Quick Review

OPERATIVE DENTISTRY AND ENDODONTICS

Essential Quick Review
OPERATIVE DENTISTRY AND ENDODONTICS

Editior-in-Chief

Priya Verma Gupta MDS FPFA
Professor
Department of Pedodontics and Preventive Dentistry
Divya Jyoti College of Dental Sciences and Research
Ghaziabad, Uttar Pradesh, India

Co-Author

Vivek Hedge BDS MDS
Vice Principal, Professor and Head of Department
Department of Operative Dentistry and Endodontics
M.A. Rangoonwala Dental College
Pune, Maharashtra, India

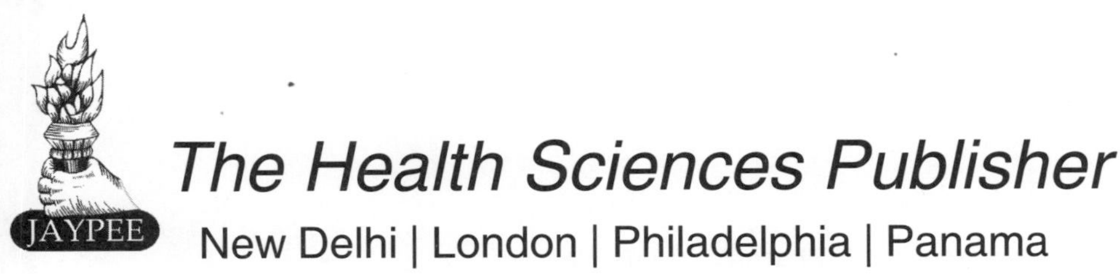

The Health Sciences Publisher
New Delhi | London | Philadelphia | Panama

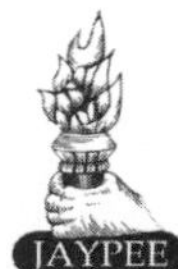 **Jaypee Brothers Medical Publishers (P) Ltd**

Headquarters

Jaypee Brothers Medical Publishers (P) Ltd
4838/24, Ansari Road, Daryaganj
New Delhi 110 002, India
Phone: +91-11-43574357
Fax: +91-11-43574314
Email: jaypee@jaypeebrothers.com

Overseas Offices

J.P. Medical Ltd
83 Victoria Street, London
SW1H 0HW (UK)
Phone: +44 20 3170 8910
Fax: +44 (0)20 3008 6180
Email: info@jpmedpub.com

Jaypee-Highlights Medical Publishers Inc.
City of Knowledge, Bld. 235, 2nd Floor, Clayton
Panama City, Panama
Phone: +1 507-301-0496
Fax: +1 507-301-0499
Email: cservice@jphmedical.com

Jaypee Medical Inc.
325 Chestnut Street
Suite 412, Philadelphia, PA 19106, USA
Phone: +1 267-519-9789
Email: support@jpmedus.com

Jaypee Brothers Medical Publishers (P) Ltd
17/1-B Babar Road, Block-B, Shaymali
Mohammadpur, Dhaka-1207
Bangladesh
Mobile: +08801912003485
Email: jaypeedhaka@gmail.com

Jaypee Brothers Medical Publishers (P) Ltd
Bhotahity, Kathmandu, Nepal
Phone: +977-9741283608
Email: kathmandu@jaypeebrothers.com

Website: www.jaypeebrothers.com
Website: www.jaypeedigital.com

© 2016, Jaypee Brothers Medical Publishers

The views and opinions expressed in this book are solely those of the original contributor(s)/author(s) and do not necessarily represent those of editor(s) of the book.

All rights reserved. No part of this publication may be reproduced, stored or transmitted in any form or by any means, electronic, mechanical, photocopying, recording or otherwise, without the prior permission in writing of the publishers.

All brand names and product names used in this book are trade names, service marks, trademarks or registered trademarks of their respective owners. The publisher is not associated with any product or vendor mentioned in this book.

Medical knowledge and practice change constantly. This book is designed to provide accurate, authoritative information about the subject matter in question. However, readers are advised to check the most current information available on procedures included and check information from the manufacturer of each product to be administered, to verify the recommended dose, formula, method and duration of administration, adverse effects and contraindications. It is the responsibility of the practitioner to take all appropriate safety precautions. Neither the publisher nor the author(s)/editor(s) assume any liability for any injury and/or damage to persons or property arising from or related to use of material in this book.

This book is sold on the understanding that the publisher is not engaged in providing professional medical services. If such advice or services are required, the services of a competent medical professional should be sought.

Every effort has been made where necessary to contact holders of copyright to obtain permission to reproduce copyright material. If any have been inadvertently overlooked, the publisher will be pleased to make the necessary arrangements at the first opportunity.

Inquiries for bulk sales may be solicited at: jaypee@jaypeebrothers.com

Essential Quick Review: Operative Dentistry and Endodontics

First Edition: **2016**

ISBN: 978-93-86056-22-1

Printed at Rajkamal Electric Press, Plot No. 2, Phase-IV, Kundli, Haryana.

Editorial Board

Priya Verma Gupta MDS FPFA
Professor, Department of Pedodontics and Preventive Dentistry
Divya Jyoti College of Dental Sciences and Research
Ghaziabad, Uttar Pradesh, India

Gunjan Gupta MDS
Assistant Professor
Department of Periodontics
Shree Bankey Bihari Dental College and Research Centre
Ghaziabad, Uttar Pradesh, India

Nishant Gupta MDS
Assistant Professor
Department of Orthodontics and Dentofacial Orthopedics
Shree Bankey Bihari Dental College and Research Centre
Ghaziabad, Uttar Pradesh, India

Rishab Malhotra MDS
Assistant Professor
Department of Pedodontics and Preventive Dentistry
Jaipur Dental College
Jaipur, Rajasthan, India

Preface

I am very pleased to introduce you to the first edition of Essential Quick Review; A series for final year undergraduate students.

The series will be available in eight subjects, i.e., Periodontics, Operative Dentistry and Endodontics, Pedodontics, Prosthodontics, Oral Surgery, Oral Medicine and Radiology, Orthodontics and Public Health Dentistry covering essential parts of each subject. This book will not only help the student to attain the knowledge, but will also give an idea how to attempt a question during the examination, covering entire syllabus in a limited period of time.

The book gives a complete outline for writing an essay type, a short answer type or a viva-voce type of question. The language used is very simple enabling a better understanding with well-illustrated diagrams wherever possible. Each book also carries a section that contains recently asked questions covering majority of the universities in India.

What makes it different from other books is, that it is supported with a supplementary booklet for each subject that contains three sections, i.e., definitions, classifications and viva-voce covering the entire syllabus enabling the student to undergo a quick revision.

The study material provided in this book is an attempt to provide an additional help to students for easy retention and reproduction of subject in the examination. This book is in no way a replacement to standard text books.

I thank all my subject matter experts for their valued suggestions and contributions. A very special word of thanks to my family for being the source of constant encouragement. I profusely thank Shri Jitendar P Vij (CEO), Mr Ankit Vij (Group President), and production team of M/S Jaypee Brothers Medical Publishers (P) Ltd, New Delhi for their enthusiasm and constant efforts in bringing out this book.

Dr Priya Verma Gupta

Contents

SECTION 1

OPERATIVE DENTISTRY

CHAPTER 1

Introduction to Operative Dentistry

Question 1

Define operative dentistry. Write in brief about the historical background of the operative dentistry?

Answer

Definition

According to Sturdevant, Operative dentistry is the art and science of the diagnosis, treatment, and prognosis of defects of teeth that do not require full coverage restorations for corrections. Such treatment should result in the restoration of proper tooth form, function and aesthetics, while maintaining the physiologic integrity of the teeth in harmonious relationship with the adjacent hard and soft tissues, all of which should enhance the general health and welfare of the patient.

According to Gilmore, Operative dentistry is a subject which includes diagnosis, prevention and treatment of problems and conditions of natural teeth, vital or non-vital so as to preserve natural dentition and restore it to the best state of health, function and aesthetics.

Historical Background

- 4000 BC: Egyptians, Assyrians and Babylonians were familiar with gold
- 460 BC: Hippocrates, the father of medicine, wrote about teeth, their formation and eruption
- 650 AD: Su Kung, a Chinese, first used dental amalgam
- 1400 AD: Joannes Arculanus used gold for filling teeth
- 1728 AD: Pierre Fauchard, the father of dentistry, used lead, tin and gold for filling
- 1746 AD: Claude Mouton used gold-post and crown in root canal treated tooth
- 1744 AD: Alexis Duchateau first used porcelain as restorative material
- 1790 AD: Joseph Flagg first made dental chair
- 1818 AD: Louis Regnart developed amalgam, is called father of dental amalgam
- 1819 AD: Charles Bell first introduced Bell's putty
- 1840 AD: Baltimore Dental College: World's first dental college
- 1845 AD: William Rogers made first dental drill
- 1855 AD: Robert Arthur introduced cohesive annealed gold
- 1861 AD: Zsigmondy developed Palmer notation
- 1864 AD: SC Barnum developed rubber dam
- 1871 AD: JB Morrison invented foot engine
- 1886 AD: Charles L first developed all ceramic crown, called it porcelain jacket crown
- 1896 AD: Dr GV Black established the principles of cavity preparation
- 1897 AD: William and Schroeder first developed diamond burs
- 1907 AD: William H Taggart gave lost wax technique for casting
- 1930 AD: Frederick S McKay established relationship of fluorides to brown stains on teeth
- 1937 AD: Walter Wright developed reversible hydrocolloids
- 1941 AD: Jasper invented silver cones or silver points
- 1951 AD: Ultrahigh speed air rotor hand pieces introduced
- 1955 AD: Michael Buonocore described the acid-etch technique
- 1958 AD: Miles Markley described the cemented pins
- 1959 AD: William Eames gave the Eames technique for minimal mercury alloy ratio
- 1960 AD: RL Bowen first developed composite
- 1963 AD: Innes and Youdelis developed the high copper alloy
- 1971 AD: Wilson and Kent gave the glass ionomer cement
- 1971 AD: Dental notation given by Fédération Dentaire Internationale (FDI)
- 1976 AD: Bauer and Eden developed the base metal alloys
- 1980 AD: Amalgapin given by Showell

- 1989 AD: Home bleach first marketed for commercial use
- 1990s AD: Advances in aesthetic and restorative dentistry, bleaching, veneers
- 2000s AD: Advances in nanotechnology, lasers, implants and computer-aided design/computer-aided manufacturing (CAD/CAM) restorations.

SHORT ESSAYS

Question 1

Write a short note on the purpose and objective of operative dentistry. Write in detail about scope and indications of operative dentistry?

Answer

Purpose of Operative Dentistry

Diagnosis

- It helps in better treatment planning
- Indicate the extent and location of the lesion
- Helps in choosing the type of restoration material to be used
- Helps in the tooth preparation.

Prevention

It prevents the disease to occur.

Interception

- It should be done by stabilising the active disease so as to prevent further loss of tooth structure
- To preserve the remaining tooth structure and its vitality
- This should be applied to all operative procedures.

Restoration

Restoration of the damaged tooth so that it maintains its form, function, aesthetics and occlusion.

Objectives of Operative Dentistry

- To avoid extensive tooth preparation
- To stabilise and strengthen the remaining tooth structure
- To increase the retention of restorative material into the tooth
- To reduce micro leakage and also recurrent caries

Scope of Operative Dentistry

- Providing proper knowledge of the oral environment that accepts the chosen materials
- Diagnosis of dental problems and its effect on other body tissues

- For understanding the importance of infection control in patients and health professionals.
- Can be comparatively examined for all the oral and systemic conditions and just not involved tooth
- Improving the overall health and well-being of the patient by proper treatment plan which helps in restoring the affected area
- Understanding the effects of operative procedures
- Knowledge and function of the tooth and supporting structures
- Understanding dental anatomy, physiology and histology.

Indications

- Dental caries
- Aesthetic corrections
- Restoration
- Replacement and repair
- Fractured teeth
- Restoring non-carious lesions.

Question 2

What are recent advances in operative dentistry?

Answer

There has been a major change in concept that was given by GV Black. The current concept of operative dentistry is based on conservation and prevention of disease.

Recent advances are required in diagnosis, treatment planning, tooth preparation, restorative material, armamentarium and in prevention:

- Recent advances in diagnosis:
  - Ultrasonic imaging
  - Digital radiography
  - Computerised image analysis
  - Fibre-optic transillumination
  - Caries detecting dyes
  - Electrical conduction measurements
  - Lasers in diagnosis
  - Magnetic resonance micro imaging
  - Tuned aperture computed tomography.

- Advances in treatment planning:
  - Ozone therapy
  - Minimal interventional therapy.
- Advances in tooth preparation:
  - Use of ultrasonic
  - Use of air abrasion technique
  - Use of lasers.
- Advances in restorative materials:
  - Mercury free alloys
  - Nano composites
  - Ceromers
  - RMGI (Resin modified glass ionomer)
  - Giomer and compomers
  - Tooth-coloured restorations for posterior tooth
  - Dentine bonding agents
  - Corrosion resistant amalgam alloys
  - CAD/CAM ceramics
  - Packable and flowable composites.
- Advances in rotary instruments:
  - Fibre-optic hand pieces
  - Chemical vapour deposition (CVD) diamond burs
  - Smart prep burs.
- Advances in preventive dentistry:
  - Fluoride application at multiple times to reduce caries incidence
  - Research in anti-caries vaccine
  - Dentrifrobots (nanotechnology)
  - Use of casein phosphopeptide-amorphous calcium phosphate (CCP-ACP) complex.

Isolation

Question 1

Discuss the importance of isolation of the operating field and various methods to achieve it in conservative dentistry?

Answer

Moisture Control

- To keep an ideal environment at the time of operative dentistry procedures, it requires a clean, dry field to avoid saliva and blood for the best results
- Proper isolation creates good working conditions of the working area and it improves the quality of the treatment.

Goals of Isolation

- Control of moisture
- Protection
- Retardation
- Good treatment quality.

Method of Isolation

Indirect Methods

- Relaxed position of the patient
- Local anaesthesia
- Drugs (antisialagogue, anxiety drugs, muscle relaxant).

Direct Methods

- Rubber dam
- Threat shields
- Gingival retraction
- Cotton rolls
- High volume evacuators and saliva ejectors.

Indirect Methods

Relaxed Position of the Patient

The patient is made to relax, so that there is no unnecessary excess salivation.

Local Anaesthesia(LA)

LA will eliminate the pain and also let the patient to relax and inturn help in less salivation.

Drugs

Drugs like atropine 0.3–1mg, 1 hour before the procedure will help in controlling the salivation.

Direct Methods

Rubber Dam

Rubber dam ensures complete moisture control in the mouth. It isolates the tooth or multiple teeth from rest of the mouth.

Indications

Rubber dam should be routinely used. It is used in:
- Endodontic procedures
- Excavation of deep caries
- Bleaching
- High risk patients e.g., HIV, hepatitis, infected
- Restorations.

Contraindications

- Not fully erupted teeth which are insufficient to supporter retainer
- Third molar
- Mal-positioned teeth
- Asthma and patients with breathing problems
- Latex allergy.

Throat Shields

- Used in recovering small objects
- Used when there are chances of aspirating and swallowing small objects
- A gauge sponge is unfolded with spread over the tongue and the posterior part of the mouth.

Gingival Tissue Retraction

During subgingival tooth preparation to get proper visibility and accessibility apical and lateral displacement of gingival tissue is done, which aids in proper flow of impression material into the area.

Methods

- Physicomechanical method
- Chemical method
- Electrosurgical method
- Surgical method.

- Physicomechanical Method: Mechanically forcing the gingival tissue away from tooth surface which can be both laterally and apically.

  Methods, such as:
  - Copper bands
  - Aluminium shell
  - Placement of extra-heavy weight rubber dam
  - Placement of cotton twigs with ZOE.

- Chemical Method: Various chemicals are carried into gingival sulcus. They coagulate blood and tissue fluids, e.g., epinephrine, norepinephrine and tannic acid.

- Electrosurgical Method: It is divided into four subtypes:
  - Cutting
  - Coagulating
  - Fulguration
  - Desiccation.
    - Cutting is mainly used for the gingival tissue retraction.

- Surgical Method: Gingivoplasty and rotary gingival curettage are used.

Cotton Roll Isolation

- Cotton rolls, absorbent waters and saliva ejectors provide fast and instant control in operating field
- Medium sized cotton roll is placed on the facial vestibule and larger one between tongue and teeth is placed.

High Volume Evacuators and Saliva Ejectors

- They are used to suck out the water discharged from elevator water spray
- It is high speed suction and the tip is usually made of plastic.

Discuss methods of sterilisation. Elaborate the methods of sterilisation of operative instrument?

Sterilisation

It is defined as the process by which an article, surface or medium is freed of all microorganisms either in the vegetative or spore state.

Methods of Sterilisation

- Mechanical or physical
- Chemical.

Mechanical Sterilisation

Sunlight

Eliminates appreciable bacterial activity.

Drying

Only kills bacteria as virus and spores are more resistant.

Heat

Dry heat

- It is the use of heat without moisture content. Various form of dry heat are:

Flaming

- Bunsen flame are exposed to loops or wires, spatulas, point of forceps till they become red hot for sterilisation
- Scalpel, needles, glass sides, cover strips mouth of culture tubes can be treated by flaming.

Incineration

- It is a method for rapidly destroying materials, such as bedding, seated dressing and pathological materials
- PVC, plastic and polythene can also be incinerated.

Conventional Dry Heat Hot Air Ovens

- It is the most commonly used form of dry heat. It is rapidly achieved at a temperature above 320°F (160°C). Conventional hot air ovens have chambers which are heated that allow air circulation by gravity flow
- Packs of instruments are placed apart for 2 hours at 160°C. The main advantage is safe sterilisation of metal instruments no corrosion of carbon steel instruments and burns. Disadvantage is long cycle, poor penetration and heavy wrapping.

High Heat Operated by Heat Transfer Devices

- It consists of a metal cup containing table salt or glass beads at 425°F (218°C)–475°F (246°C)
- Advantages include the sterilization of files, reamers and broaches in 5 seconds and absorbent points and cotton pellets in 10 seconds.

Moist Heat

Temperature below 100°C / Pasteurisation

It is a process of moist heat of less than the boiling temperature to prevent various heat liable pathogens and organisms.

Temperature at 100°C / Boiling

- Boiling water at 100°C for 10–30 minutes promotes sterilisation
- Spore-forming bacteria needs much more time
- Advantage being easy, economical and good penetration
- Disadvantage is that it dulls the cutting edges and corrodes.

Steam at Atmosphere Pressure (100°C)

- The sterilisation in this is done with steaming for few minutes at 100°C, 3–4 times successively at 24 hours interval, at room temperature
- It works on the principle that 1st exposure kills vegetative bacteria, and spores will be killed over the subsequent occasions, e.g., Koch and Arnold steamer
- Temperature above 100°C/autoclave:
  - Saturated steam under pressure is the most effective sterilisation method
  - Apparatus used is called autoclave
  - It works on the principle that steam under pressure is hotter. The higher the pressure that higher the temperature (Pressure Cooker effect).
- Autoclave has:
  - Inlet valves: for steam
  - Pressure gauges
  - Temperature regulators
  - Indicator
  - Safety valves
  - Exhaust
  - Chamber.
- Advantages: Excellent penetration, short cycle, wide material range and economical
- Disadvantage: Corrosion and dulling of instruments.

Unsaturated Chemical Vapour Sterilisation

- It works on heat, water and chemical synergism
- It reduces the corrosion of metal items

- Temperature and pressure is more hot than autoclave
- The unit is called chemiclave. It operates at 27°F (131°C) with pressure of 20 pounds and 20–40 cycles/minute.

Hot Oil Bath

- It is done by instruments kept at 175°C for 15 minutes
- The disadvantage being poor sporicidal activity.

Radiations

- Ionizing radiations:
  - High electromagnetic wave, X-rays, gaming rays, cosmic rays are used because they have high penetration power.
- Non-ionizing radiations:
  - It includes infrared and ultraviolet rays.
- Lasers:
  - Carbon dioxide (CO_2), argon, neodymium-doped yttrium aluminium garnet (Nd: YAG) are used.
- Ultrasonic and sonic vibrations:
  - It is done by magnetostrictive oscillation or piezoelectric crystals.
- Freezing:
  - Supercoiling to –100° to 15°C decreases disruptive to cell function.
- Filtration:
  - Used in case of heat liable liquids and solutions, e.g., candle filters, asbestos filters, membrane filters, etc.

Chemical Sterilisation

Ethylene Oxide

- It is a sterilant and not a disinfectant
- It is gas with temperature of 10.8°C which is highly toxic which destroys by alkylation
- Used in complex instrument as well as in delicate materials
- It is virucidal and sporicidal which evaporates without residue and not damages the material
- Advantages: High penetration, no damage to heat sensitivity and it evaporates with no residue
- Disadvantages: Slowness, toxicity, and instruments have to be dried.

Aldehydes

Formaldehyde

- Highly irritating gas
- It contains strong reducing agent
- Inactivates enzymes and amino group of protein.

Glutaraldehyde

- ❏ It is same as formaldehyde
- ❏ Most active against tubercle bacilli, fungi and viruses
- ❏ Less toxic than formaldehyde.
- ❏ Advantages:
  - ○ They do not harm rubber and plastic
  - ○ So they are recommended for impression materials.
- ❏ Disadvantages:
  - ○ They corrode and discolour metal when mixed
  - ○ They are toxic and produce irritation with physical contact.

Beta-propiolactone (BPL)

- ❏ It is the condensation of ketone and formaldehyde with a boiling point of 163°C
- ❏ It is effective against the microbes and viruses
- ❏ It is activated by alkylation
- ❏ Efficiency at the time of fumigation is more than formaldehyde
- ❏ Used in sterilisation of vaccines, graft tissues and biological material.
- ❏ Advantage:
  - ○ Can be used to sterilize vaccines and enzymes.
- ❏ Disadvantage:
  - ○ It has cariogenic potential.

Question 3

Write a short note on rubber dam kit?

Answer

Rubber dam kit consists of the following:
- ❏ Rubber dam sheet
- ❏ Rubber dam punch
- ❏ Rubber dam clamps
- ❏ Rubber dam clamp forceps
- ❏ Rubber dam frame/holder
- ❏ Rubber dam stamp
- ❏ Rubber dam lubricant
- ❏ Waxed dental floss
- ❏ Plastic tray for holding the clamp
- ❏ Scissors.

Rubber Dam Sheet

- ❏ Made of latex
- ❏ Available sizes: 5 × 5 inches (12.5 × 12.5 cm)
- ❏ 6 × 6 inches (15 × 15 cm)
- ❏ Colours: blue, green, black, dark brown
- ❏ Sheet surface: dull and shiny side.

Rubber Dam Holder

- ❏ It is a U-shaped metal/plastic frame which maintains the borders of the rubber dam in position (**Fig. 2.1**)
- ❏ It has small projections for borders of rubber dam.

Rubber Dam Frames

- ❏ Young frame
- ❏ Nygaard–Ostby frame
- ❏ Safe T-frame.

Rubber Dam Clamp (Retainers)

- ❏ It consists of 4 prongs and 2 jaws connected to a bow
- ❏ It is used to anchor the dam to the most posterior tooth which has to be isolated
- ❏ It should be positioned so that it contacts four areas: 2 facial and 2 lingual
- ❏ It is used to retract gingival tissue.

Types

- ❏ Metallic: Carbon/stainless steel
- ❏ Non-metallic plastic.

Uses

- ❏ Upper central incisors and all cuspids: w7
- ❏ Upper laterals and all lower incisors: w212
- ❏ Premolars: w4
- ❏ Most molars: w56
- ❏ Mandibular molar anchor tooth: w7
- ❏ Maxillary molar anchor teeth: w8
- ❏ Terminal mandibular molar: w27.

Rubber Dam Clamp (Retainer) Forceps

- ❏ This is used in both the placement and the removal of the retainer from the tooth

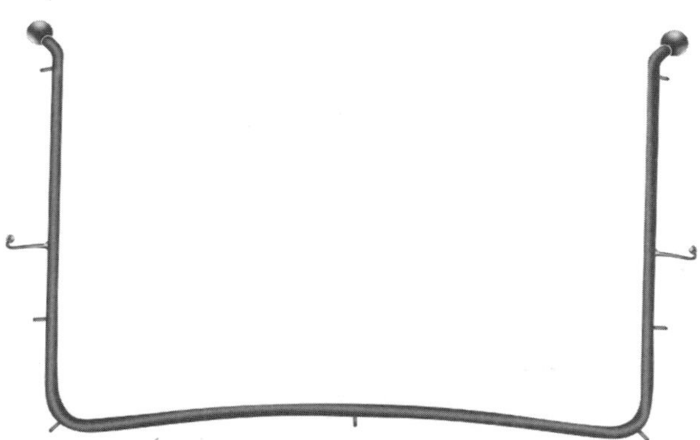

Fig. 2.1: Rubber dam holder.

- The rubber dam clasp holes are fitted into the projections of the retainer forceps which are of the size of the holes at working and are then taken to the desired tooth.

Rubber Dam Punch

- It is an instrument which has a rotating metal table with six holes of different sizes and a pointed puncher which is used to punch holes in the rubber dam
- The plunger should be centred in the cutting hole so the edges do not get chipped off at the point of closing.

Types of Holes Required

- Molars: larger holes
- Premolars, canines and upper incisors: medium holes
- Lower incisors: smaller holes.

Rubber Dam Templates

They are of the same size and shape, like the unstitched rubber dam.

- Holes on the templates are just like the tooth positioning
- The dam must be marked and punched with the template before putting it in patient's mouth.

Rubber Dam Napkin

- It should be placed between rubber dam and patient skin
- They are soft, absorbent and disposable.

Rubber Dam Lubricant

- They are applied in the area of the punctured holes
- Water soluble lubricants are preferred, e.g., soap
- It should not have unpleasant taste
- Cocoa butter and petroleum jelly are used as a lubricant which is applied on the corner of the mouth.

Waxed Dental Floss

- Used for listing interdental contacts
- For flossing of the rubber dam through tight contact area
- Bow is attached to dental floss so as to avoid aspiration in case of accidently swallowing of the retainers
- 12 inch of dental floss is recommended to be attached to the retainer.

Modelling Compound

It helps in the movement of the retainer.

SHORT NOTE

Question 1

Write a short note on OSHA?

Answer

Occupational safety and health administration (OSHA) is an agency in United States Department of Labour.

- It was established in 1971
- It is an agency which assures safe and healthful working conditions for working men and women by setting and enforcing standards and by providing training, outreach education and assistance.

Regulations

- Provide facilities related to hand wash after removing gloves. Washing off other skin immediately after contact with blood or any infectious material
- Safe handling of used needles and sharp objects
- Disposal of single use needles, wires, carpules and sharps
- Blood and contaminated specimen to be transported or stored into suitable closed container to prevent leakage
- Providing employees with safety training and equipment is at no cost to workers
- Providing a written schedule for cleaning of floor, work surface and equipment
- Inform about chemical hazards through training, labels, documents, colour coded systems, alarms
- Performing test at the work place by OSHA standards, such as sampling
- To be cautious about the instruments that can be reused so that no physical touch and contamination can occur before they are ready to be used
- Receiving copies of records of work-related illness and injuries in the work place.

CHAPTER 3

Dental Caries, Risk Assessment and Management

Question 1

Define and classify dental caries. Discuss various diagnostic methods of detection of dental caries. Discuss the sequelae of caries progress in dentin?

Answer

Definition

According to Sturdevant, Dental caries is defined as a multifactorial, transmissible, infection oral disease caused primarily by the complex interaction of cariogenic oral flora (biofilm) with fermentable dietary carbohydrate on the tooth surface over time.

Classification of Dental Caries

- According to location:
  - Primary caries
    - Pit and fissure caries
    - Smooth surface caries
    - Root caries.
  - Secondary caries.
- According to direction:
  - Forward caries
  - Backward caries.
- According to extent:
  - Incipient caries (reversible)
  - Cavitated caries (irreversible).
- According to rate:
  - Acute (rampant) caries
  - Chronic (slow) or arrested caries.
- According to histological depth of penetration:
  - Enamel caries
  - Dentinal caries.
- According to treatment and restorative design (**Fig. 3.1 to 3.6**):
  - Class I: Pit and fissure caries on the occlusion surface of posterior teeth
  - Class II: Proximal caries in the posterior teeth
  - Class III: Proximal caries in the anterior teeth not involving the incisal edge
  - Class IV: Proximal caries in the anterior teeth involving the incisal edge
  - Class V: Caries on the gingival third of the facial and lingual surfaces of all the teeth
  - Class VI: Caries on the incisal edges of the anterior and cusp tips of the posterior teeth without involving any other surface.
- According to number of tooth surfaces involved:
  - Simple caries: one surface involved
  - Compound caries: two surfaces involved
  - Complex caries: more than two surfaces involved.
- WHO classification:
  - D1: Clinically detectable enamel lesion with intact surfaces
  - D2: Clinically detectable caries in the enamel
  - D3: Clinically detectable caries in the dentine
  - D4: Lesion extending to the pulp.
- According to the appearance on the radiographs:
  - ED: no radiographic evidence of caries
  - E1: Lesion in outer one-half of enamel
  - E2: Lesion in inner one-half of enamel
  - D1: Lesion in outer one-third of dentine
  - D2: Lesion in middle one-third of dentine
  - D3: Lesion in the inner one-third of dentine.

Various assessment tools for diagnosis of dental caries:

- Patient history
- Clinical examination
- Nutritional analysis
- Salivary analysis
- Radiographic assessment.

Sequelae of caries progress in dentine. As caries spread in dentine three changes are observed:

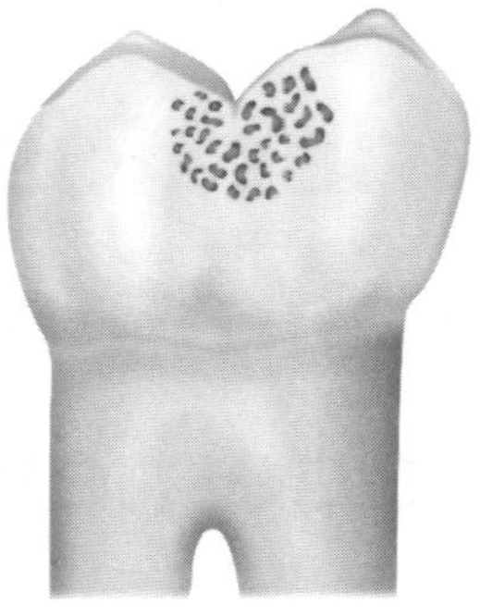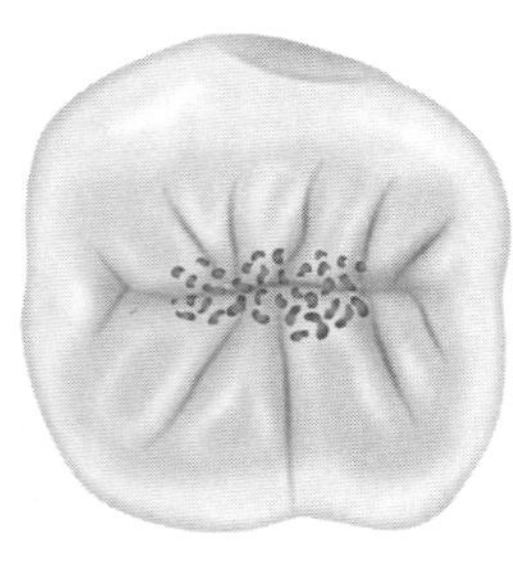

Fig. 3.1: Class I Caries

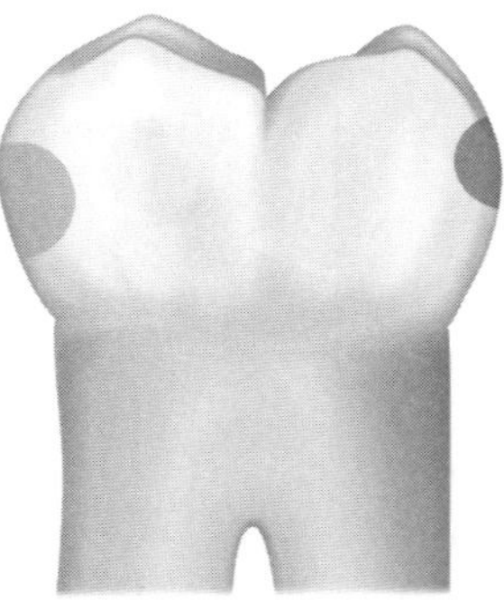

Fig. 3.2: Class II Caries

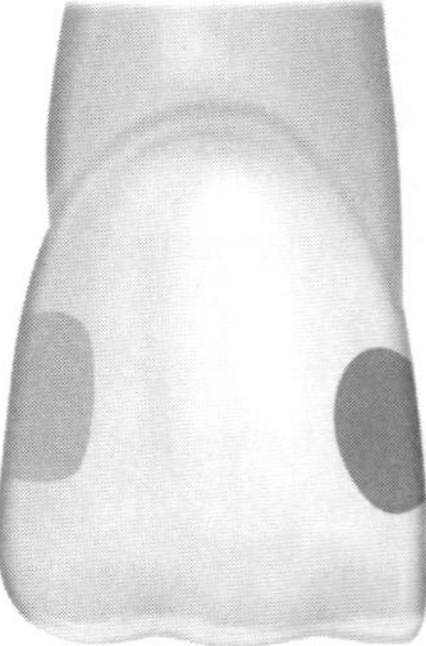

Fig. 3.3: Class III Caries

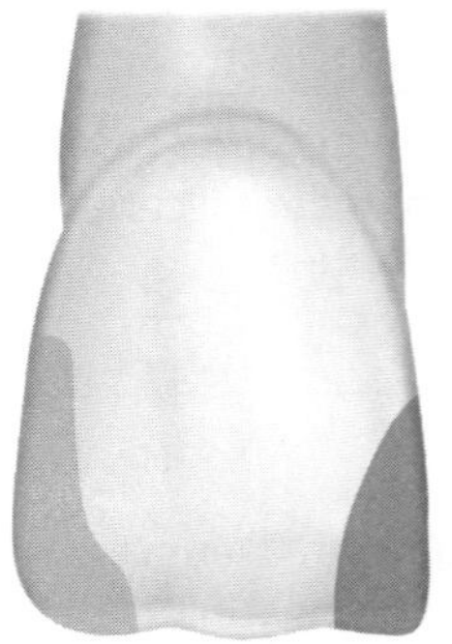

Fig. 3.4: Class IV Caries

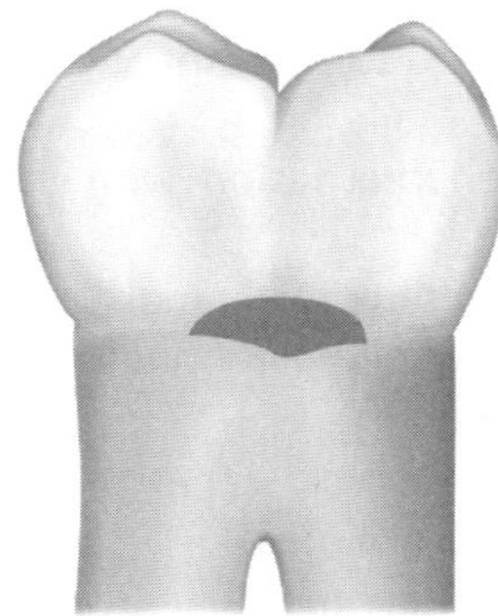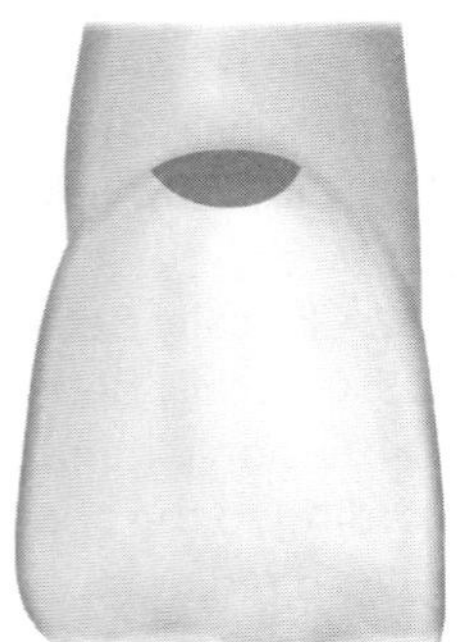

Fig. 3.5: Class V Caries

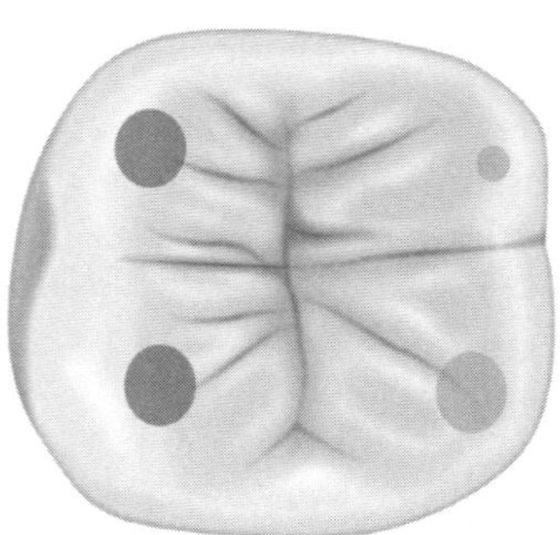

Fig. 3.6: Class VI Caries.

1. Demineralisation of dentine by weak organic acids
2. The organic content of dentine, i.e., collagen undergo dissolution and degeneration
3. Breakdown of structural integrity followed by bacterial invasion.

Zones of Carious Dentine

Zone 1: Normal dentine

Deepest zone of carious dentine have normal collagen, intertubular dentine and odontoblast processes.

Zone 2: Sub-transparent dentine

❑ Demineralisation of intertubular dentine happens
❑ Damaged odontoblast process and fine crystals are seen in the lumen of dental tubules
❑ No bacteria.

Zone 3: Transparent dentine

❑ Superficial to sub-transparent dentine softer than normal dentine, at intertubular dentine it exhibits mineral loss
❑ No bacteria
❑ This layer is capable of remineralisation.

Zone 4: Turbid dentine

- Dentinal tubules are widened and distorted because of penetration of bacteria
- Collagens are considerably demineralised and are irreversible
- This zone should be removed at the time of restoration because it is incapable of remineralisation.

Zone 5: Infected dentine

- Outermost zone
- Dentinal tubules and collagens are decomposed
- High bacterial concentration zone
- Should be removed to prevent the spread of infection.

Question 2

Write about the theories of dental caries?

Answer

Theories of Caries Formation

The Legend of the Worm

In the past it was believed that dental caries was caused by the living worms inside the tooth structure.

Endogenous Theories

Humoral Theory

According to this theory, the four elemental humours of the body, i.e., blood, phlegmy, black bile and yellow bile caused the imbalance leading to tooth decay.

Vital Theory

This theory suggested tooth decay originated from within the tooth itself, like bone gangrene.

Exogenous Theories

Chemical (Acid Theory)

According to Robertson (1835), tooth decay was caused by the acid formed by fermentation of food particles around the teeth.

Parasitic (Septic) Theory

- This was the first theory that released microorganisms with caries on a causative basis
- It was proposed in the theory that even though the caries starts with chemical process but the microorganisms continue to disintegrated in both enamel and dentine.

Miller's Chemico-parasitic Theory or Acidogenic Theory

According to WD Miller (1889), this theory combines both chemical and parasitic theory. It consists of two stages:

1. Preliminary stage: Decalcification of enamel and dentine
2. Large stage: Dissolution of the softened residue and the acid causing primary decalcification by fermentation of starches and sugar from the corners of the tooth.

Limitations

- Predilection of specific sites on a tooth
- Initiation of smooth surface caries
- Why some population is caries free?
- The phenomenon of arrested caries.

Proteolysis Theory

Proposed by Gottlieb and Gottlieb (1944). States that the proteolytic enzymes which are produced by the oral bacteria destroy organic matrix of the enamel causing dental caries.

Proteolysis Chelation Theory

- Schatz and martin (1955) stated in the theory that chelation process is responsible for the simultaneous microbial degradation of the organic components, i.e., proteolysis and the reason for dissolution of the minerals in tooth
- This theory suggests that even without acid formation demineralization of enamel can occur.

Sucrose Chelation Theory

- Eggers-lura (1967) proposed sucrose alone and not the acids that are derived from it
- It is capable of dissolution of enamel with the unionized calcium saccharates formation. The calcium saccharides and calcium complexing inter-mediaries require inorganic phosphate which is removed from the enamel by phosphorylating enzymes.

Levine's Theory

Levine (1977) stated that demineralisation and remineralisation of enamel is a continuous process and there is a constant exchange of ions between enamel and plaque.

Autoimmune Theory

Burch and Jackson (1966), stated that the partly inherited and partly mutated genes determine whether a site on tooth surface is at risk of caries attack.

Sulphatase Theory

Pincus (1950), stated that the bacterial sulphatase hydrolysed the mucotin sulphate of the enamel and chondroitin sulphate of the dentine which produced sulphuric acid causing the decalcification of the dental caries.

Question 3

Define caries activity test and mention it in detail?

Answer

It is defined as the total of new caries lesions and enlargement of existing carious cavities during a particular time period. It helps in the clinical management of patients.
- To determine, if there is need of preventive measures
- To evaluate and motivate the effectiveness of health education programs
- To manage restorative procedures
- Identifying high risk individuals.

Caries Susceptibility

It refers to the new lesions that may develop in a particular individual over a period of time.

Caries Activity Test

- Caries activity is the increments of active lesions over a state of time. It is the measure of speed of progression of a carious lesion
- Caries susceptibility is the inherent tendency of the host, the target tissue and the tooth to be affected by carious process.

Requirements

- Test should be reproducible as well as valid
- Should serve as an index and have correlation between the caries activity scores and the actual caries development
- Should be simple to perform and results should be obtained rapidly
- Should be expensive and applicable to all clinical settings.

Lactobacillus Colony Count Test

Hadley 1933

Estimation of acidogenic and aciduric bacteria is determined. Patients' saliva is the source of the test procedure.
- Saliva is collected by chewing paraffin
- The sample is vigorously shaken and the sample is taken
- Undiluted and diluted samples are spread evenly over liquefied agar (Rogosa's SL agar plate)

- Plate is incubated for 4 days at 37°C and the number of lactobacillus colonies that developed over that period of time as then counted (**Table 3.1**).

No. of organisms	Symbolic designation	Degree of caries activity
Table 3.1: Showing calculation of degree of caries activity		
1–1,000	+ve	Little or none
1,000–5,000	+ve	Slight
5,000–10,000	++ve	Moderate
10,000 and above	+++ve	Marked

Snyder Test

- Snyder test measures the ability of salivary micro-organisms to form organic acid from the carbohydrate medium
- Bromocresol green which is an indicator dye is the medium for the test
- The dye changes colour from green to yellow with pH
- Range at time intervals and estimation is done in 24, 48 and 72 hours.

Procedure

- Paraffin is chewed and saliva sample is collected in a test tube is cooled to 50°C which contains melted agar medium
- After solidification it is incubated at 37°C
- The acid produced is than monitored at the time interval of 24, 48 and 72 hours.

Alben's Test

- It is the modification of Snyder test
- The semisolid agar is removed from refrigerator but it is not heated
- Saliva sample which is unstimulated is again spitted into the test tube which is than incubated for 4 days and the acid formation is determined.

Swab Test

- Mostly used in young children because there is no collection of saliva required
- Swab test works on the same principle of Snyder test
- The sampling is done by swabbing the buccal surface of tooth with cotton
- The pH change is monitored after 48 hours to determine the acid produced.

Reductase Test

- ❑ This test measures the activity of the enzyme reductase which is present in salivary bacteria
- ❑ The saliva sample is mixed with diazoresorcinol, and after 15 minutes of mixing the colour change indicates caries activity **(Table 3.2)**.

Table 3.2: Reductase test measures caries activity			
Colour	**Time**	**Score**	**Caries activity**
Blue	15 minutes	1	Non-conductive
Orchid	15 minutes	2	Slightly conductive
Red	15 minutes	3	Moderately conductive
Red	Immediately	4	Highly conductive
Pink	Immediately	5	Extremely conductive

Saliva Flow Test

- ❑ It is a simple test which works on the principle that severely decreased salivary flow is related to caries susceptibility
- ❑ As the salivary flow is decreased, the viscosity is increased
- ❑ Salivary flow is determined by collecting paraffin stimulated saliva in a test tube over 5 minutes.

Home Method

- ❑ This method requires minimal equipments and not particular setup
- ❑ It can easily be performed by an individual at any place
- ❑ It also helps in educating the child patient to the problem of dental caries.

Procedure

- ❑ Aqueous solution of methyl red is used
- ❑ Aqueous methyl red is applied to the surface of the tooth with dropper
- ❑ Indication changes colour in the pH 6.3–4.2
- ❑ Red colour is developed in the area of plaque accumulation.

Question 4

Write a short note on caries diagnosis?

Answer

Caries diagnosis is defined as the process which involves risk assessment and the application of diagnostic criteria to determine the disease state.

Methods in detection of dental caries are:

Traditional Methods

- ❑ Clinical methods:
  - ○ Patients complaint
  - ○ Visual examination.
- ❑ Mechanical methods:
  - ○ Tactile examination
  - ○ Tooth separation
  - ○ Dental floss or tape.

Radiograph Methods

- ❑ Conventional radiographic methods:
  - ○ Intraoral periapical radiographs
  - ○ Bitewing radiographs.
- ❑ Advanced radiographic methods:
  - ○ Xeroradiography
  - ○ Digital radiographic methods
  - ○ Computer-aided radiographic methods
  - ○ Digital subtractions radiography.

Optic Methods

- ❑ Fibre optic transillumination
- ❑ Digital fibre-optic transillumination
- ❑ Optical coherence tomography (OCT).

Fluorescence Method

- ❑ Quantitative laser fluorescence
- ❑ Endoscopic filtered fluorescence method.

Lasers

- ❑ DIAGNOdent
- ❑ Dye enhanced laser fluorescence.

Other Recent Methods

- ❑ Caries detector dye
- ❑ Ultrasonic probe imaging
- ❑ Visible luminescent caries detector
- ❑ Vanguard electronic caries detector
- ❑ Electrical conductance measurement
- ❑ Alternating current impedance spectroscopy technique.

Patient's Complaint

Patient will always provide the clue regarding the presence of caries. Patients may have sensitivity to thermal changes with mild to moderate toothache.

Visual Examination

- ❑ Presence of grey hue at the marginal ridge can be a hint about the presence of proximal caries under the ridge
- ❑ Examination of tooth with good isolation reveals visual signs, signs like cavitation, brown discolouration and also pit and fissures helps in diagnosis of caries.

Tactile Examination

Use of Explorer

- Carved explorers are used in occlusal surface pit and fissures
- Detection of proximal caries are diagnosed with interproximal explorers.

Bitewing Radiographs

- It is the most important diagnostic method for the diagnosis of proximal caries in enamel and dentine
- Small radiolucent notch is seen below the contact area in enamel
- A dark triangular area in proximal area indicates proximal caries. The base of which is towards the external tooth surface.

Fibre-optic Transillumination

The teeth when examined with a fibre-optic light source the caries appear as darkened shadow because of lowered index of carious lesion with light transmission.

Lasers

- The use of diode-laser and DIAGNOdent detectors can be used for sound tooth structure on the occlusal surface

- The changes in caries induced teeth have increased fluorescence at specific wavelengths.

Caries Bacterial Dye

- Various dyes change colour when applied on a carious lesion, i.e., silver nitrate, alizarin stain and methyl red
- Originally, 0.5% basic fuchsin in propylene glycol was used
- But studies showed that basic fuchsin was carcinogenic, hence it was replaced.

Enamel Dyes

- Calcpin
- Procion
- Brilliant blue.

Dentine Dyes

- Acid red
- Basic fuchsine.

Ultrasonic Probe Imaging

- It works on sound wave theory, ultrasonic probe sends and receives sound waves from tooth surface
- Normal enamel: No echoes
- Initial lesion: Weak surface echoes
- Caries lesion: High amplitude echoes.

SHORT ESSAYS

Question 1

Describe the factors influencing caries incidence?

Answer

Four principal factors which interact with each causing dental caries (**Fig. 3.7**):

Primary Factors

- Host factor
  - Tooth factor
    - Location and morphology of the tooth
    - Chemical nature of tooth.
  - Saliva.
    - Composition, pH and antibacterial activity
    - Quality and quantity.
- Bacterial microflora
- Diet or substrate
  - Physical nature
  - Local factors.
    - Carbohydrate content
    - Fluoride content
    - Vitamin content
    - Protein and fatty content.
- Time.
  - Physical nature
  - Local factors.

Modifying Factors

- Saliva
- Sex
- Health
- Heredity
- Occupation
- Habitat
- Host factors
- Tooth factors.

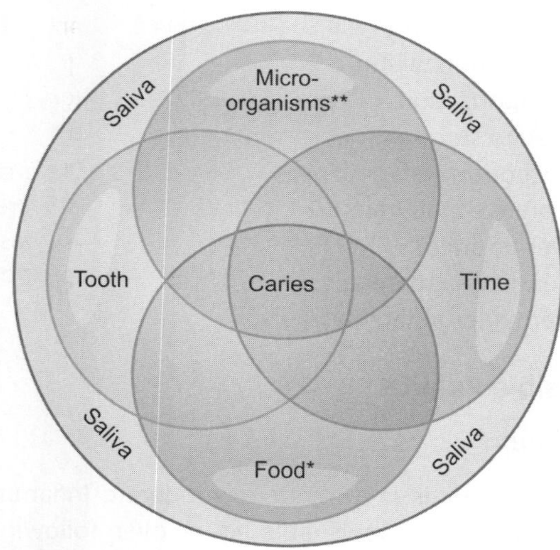

Fig. 3.7: Factors affecting occurence of dental caries

Morphology and Location of the Tooth

- Due to deep pit and fissures on the occlusal surfaces of the posterior teeth they are more susceptible to caries
- Mandibular first molar followed by maxillary first molar among permanent dentition are most susceptible to caries
- Impacted and malpositioned teeth are more prone to caries because the chances of food lodgement and plaque accumulation are much higher in them.

Chemical Nature of the Tooth Surface

Surface enamel is more resistant than subsurface enamel because of more mineral content and less water.

Saliva

- Due to the presence of fluoride, calcium and phosphorus in saliva, it helps in the remineralisation of the tooth
- Normal pH of saliva is 6–7, pH which helps in the maintenance of buffering capacity. Fall of which will lead to caries incidence
- Saliva contains secretory IgA, IgG, lysozyme, salivary peroxidase which have antibacterial properties
- Lesser salivary flow leads to xerostomia which in return act as a catalyst for caries
- Salivary flow is affected by:
  - Radiotherapy
  - Sjogren's syndrome
  - Certain drugs, like antidepressant, antihistamines, etc.

Bacterial Microflora

Dental caries occur in the presence of bacteria. The commonly associated bacteria in dental caries are *streptococcus mutans*, *lactobacillus* and *actinomyces*.

Substrate/Diet

Modern diet which consists of sticky food aids in plaque accumulation and host for the bacterial activity leads to increased incidence of caries.

Local Factors

Carbohydrate Content

- Refined carbohydrate is the primary factor in caries formation
- Polysaccharides, disaccharides or monosaccharides are carbohydrates which catalyse caries formation
- High intake of fermentable carbohydrate alongwith decreased oral hygiene leads to higher incidence of caries
- Dietary sucrose derived from sugarcane and sugar beet are called "arch criminal" in caries formation
- Sucrose is a primary source of energy to most of the cariogenic bacteria.

Fluoride Content

- Fluoride on enamel surface produces fluorapatite crystals which are more resistant to caries
- Fluoride plays a role in the prevention of caries
- Fluoride sources most accepted are water fluoridation, fluoride rinses, fluoride varnishes, fluoride dentifrices, etc.

Protein and Fatty Content

Some fatty products with antimicrobial properties have inhibited carbohydrate metabolism in plaque, e.g., aged cheddar cheese shows anti-acidogenic in plaque.

Vitamin Content

- Vitamin B6 has arginine rich peptides and pyridoxine has protective effect against caries
- Vitamin D helps in development of teeth. Deficiency of which leads to hypoplasia of teeth which in turn inhibits caries
- Food containing vitamin C, citric fruits, and beverages reduce tooth structure

Time

There is a time period in which the micro-organism produces acidic pH from the fermentation of carbohydrates.

Question 2

Classify pulpal lesions. Differentiate between reversible and irreversible pulpitis?

Answer

According to Ingle

- Bacterial
  - Coronal ingress
  - Radicular ingress.
- Traumatic
  - Acute
  - Chronic.
- Iatrogenic
  - Cavity preparation
  - Restoration
  - Intentional extirpation
  - Orthodontic movement
  - Periodontal and periapical curettage
  - Rhinoplasty
  - Intubation.
- Chemical
  - Restorative materials
  - Disinfectants
  - Desiccants.
- Idiopathic
  - Ageing
  - Internal resorption
  - External resorption
  - Hypophosphatemia.

Other Factors

- Preoperative factors
  - Cervical exposed dentine
  - Caries
  - Tooth surface loss-erosion: Attrition, abrasion, abfraction caries
  - Trauma
  - Tooth fracture: Enamel, dentine, pulp exposure
  - Periodontal disease
  - Tooth subluxation or avulsion.
- Intraoperative factors
  - Tooth preparation
  - Intracoronal
  - Extracoronal
  - Iatrogenic pulp exposure.
- Other restorative procedures
  - Local anaesthesia (LA)
  - Pin placement
  - Cavity cleaning
  - Impression taking
  - Temporization
  - Electro surgery
  - Orthodontics.
- Restorative materials
  - Dentie liners
  - Temporary materials
  - Permanent materials.

Reversible Pulpitis

Definition

Reversible pulpitis is a minor to moderate inflammation from which the pulp is able to recover following the removal of stimuli, which mostly is thermal and cold stimulus.

Features

- Cavities have not reached nerve yet
- Erosion only at the dentine
- Enamel fracture which has exposed dentine.

Clinical Features

- Pain range from no pain to mild to serve pain when they are stimulated
- Pain disappears when the stimulus is not acting upon
- Cold food triggers pain more than hot food.

Aetiology

- Trauma
- Thermal shock from cavity preparation
- Excessive dehydration of cavity from chloroform and alcohol
- Fresh amalgam restoration in contact with gold restoration
- Bacteria.

Histopathology

- Dilated blood vessels
- Odontoblast layer is disrupted
- Reparative dentine
- Presence of chronic inflammatory cells along with acute inflammatory cells.

Treatment Plan

- Prevention is the best treatment
- Proper base/varnish should be placed to prevent damage to the pulp

Irreversible Pulpitis

Irreversible pulpitis is a serious inflammation from where there is minimal chance of spontaneous recovery which is accompanied by an exudate and often pain, caused by a noxious stimulus.

Aetiology

- Bacterial
- Chemical
- Mechanical
- Thermal.

Clinical Features

- Pain with sudden temperature change mostly cold and sweet stimuli
- Pain is sharp piercing and shooting
- Pain can be intermittent or continuous
- Pain during change in posture like mostly bending over or lying down (changes in intrapulpal pressure)
- Pain in the adjacent tooth, to temple or sinus when upper posterior involvement of tooth is seen.

Diagnosis

- Deep caries exposing the pulp
- Greyish, scum like layer over exposed pulp and the surrounding dentine
- Eroded pulp surface
- Odour of decomposition in the area
- Thermal and electric test elicits pain and the pain is continued even after the removal of stimulus.

Histopathology

- Areas of abscess, necrotic tissues with microorganisms are seen
- Polymorphonuclear leukocytes infiltration, zone of fibroblastic proliferation and calcific masses may be present.

Treatment

- Pulpectomy
- Shaping, cleaning and obturation of pulp canal
- Post endodontic restoration.

Phoenix Abscess

- A phoenix abscess is a dental abscess that can occur immediately following root canal treatment
- Another cause is due to untreated necrotic pulp (chronic apical periodontitis)
- It is also caused by inadequate debridement during the endodontic procedure.

Bacteriology

- Staphylococci are frequently associated with pus formation
- It produces enzyme called coagulase which causes fibrin formation, which helps in walking of the lesion
- Coagulase promotes virulence by inhibiting phagocytosis.

Clinical Features

- When palpated clinically superficial abscess is fluctuant. There is tenderness on percussion
- There may not be swelling
- Patient may present with lymphadenopathy, malaise and fever
- Offending tooth is carious and mobile
- Formation of sinus tract that opens into labial mucosa
- The healing occurs by formation of granulation tissue post endodontic treatment.

Diagnosis

- No response to electric or thermal test
- Well defined periradicular radiolucencies seen on radiographs.

Histopathology

Presence of disintegrating polymorphonuclear cells (PMNLs) and cellular debris at the area of liquefaction surrounded by lymphocytes and plasma cells.

Treatment

- Drainage and RCT
- Repeating endodontic treatment with improved debridement
- Tooth extraction
- Antibiotics indicated to control the spread of systemic infection.

Question 3

Discuss secondary dentine. Differentiate between infected and affected dentine?

Answer

Secondary dentine is dentine that is formed and deposited in response to a normal or slightly abnormal stimulus after the complete formation of the tooth.

Types of Secondary Dentine

Physiological Secondary Dentine

- Regular uniform layer of dentine around the pulp chamber
- Due to physiological factors it is laid down throughout the life of the tooth
- This type of secondary dentine is produced more slowly than primary dentine

Reparative Secondary Dentine

- It forms around the pulp chamber as a result of irritation or attrition which is a form of tooth wear
- Loss of tooth structure can occur from tooth to tooth contact resulting in bruxism, which stimulates the development of natural protective measures, such as secondary dentine
- Differences between Infected and affected Dentine are enlisted in **Table 3.3**.

Table 3.3: Differences between infected and affected dentine

Infected dentine	Affected dentine
Superficial layer	Deeper layer
Soft and leathery in consistency	Dark in consistency
Light brown	Dark brown
High concentration of bacteria and collagen	Does not contain bacteria
Non-remineralisable	Remineralisable
Sensitive to touch	Non-sensitive to touch
Caries detecting dyes can stain	Not stained by caries detecting dyes
Should be removed	Should be pressured

Question 4

What are the principles and concepts of cavity preparation?

Answer

Various classifications for cavity preparations have been advocated. The more relevant classification pertaining to primary teeth and young permanent teeth are discussed below.

Black's Classification

Class I Lesion

Lesions that begin in the structural defects of teeth such as pits, fissures and defective grooves (**Fig. 3.8**).

Locations include:

- Occlusal surface of molars and premolars
- Occlusal two thirds of buccal and lingual surfaces of molars
- Lingual surfaces of anterior tooth.

Class II Lesions

They are found on the proximal surfaces of the bicuspids and molars (**Fig. 3.8**).

Class III Lesions

Lesions found on the proximal surfaces of anterior teeth that do not involve or necessitate the removal of the incisal angle (**Fig. 3.8**).

Class IV Lesions

Lesions found on the proximal surfaces of anterior teeth that involve the incisal angle (**Fig. 3.8**).

Class V Lesions

Lesions that are found at the gingival third of the facial and lingual surfaces of the anterior and posterior teeth (**Fig. 3.8**).

Class VI (Simon's Modification)

Lesions involving cuspal tips and incisal edges of teeth (**Fig. 3.8**).

Other Modifications

Charbeneu's Modification

- Class II: Cavities on single proximal surface of bicuspids and molars
- Class VI: Cavities on both mesial and distal proximal surfaces of posterior teeth that will share a common occlusal isthmus
- Lingual surfaces of upper anterior teeth
- Any other unusually located pit or fissure involved with decay.

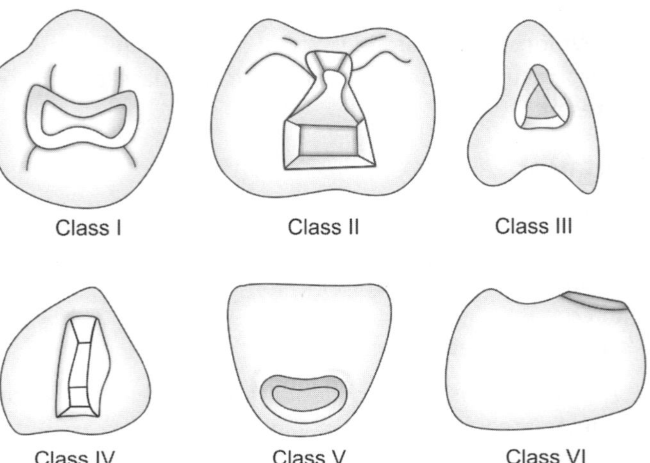

Fig. 3.8 Cavity preparations according to G V Black lesions

Sturdevant's Classification (Table 3.4)

Table 3.4: Sturdevant's Classification	
Cavity	**Feature**
Simple cavity	A cavity involving only one tooth surface
Compound cavity	A cavity involving two surfaces of a tooth
Complex cavity	A cavity that involves more than two surfaces of a tooth

Finn's Modification of Blacks' Cavity Preparation for Primary Teeth

- Class I: Cavities involving the pits and fissures of the molar teeth and the buccal and lingual pits of all teeth
- Class II: Cavities involving proximal surface of molar teeth with access established from the occlusal surface
- Class III: Cavities involving proximal surfaces of anterior teeth which may or may not involve a labial or a lingual extension
- Class IV: A restoration of the proximal surface of an anterior tooth which involves the restoration of an incisal angle
- Class V: Cavities present on the cervical third of all teeth. Including proximal surface where the marginal ridge is not included in the cavity preparation.

Baurne's Classification

- Pit and fissure cavities
- Smooth surface cavities.

Classification by Mount and Burne (1998)

This new system defines the extent and complexity of a cavity and at the same time encourages a conservative approach to the preservation of natural tooth structure. This system is designed to utilize the healing capacity of enamel and dentin (**Table 3.5**).

- The Three Sites of Carious Lesions
  - Site 1: Pits, fissures and enamel defects on occlusal surfaces of posterior teeth or other smooth surfaces
  - Site 2: Proximal enamel immediately below areas in contact with adjacent teeth
  - Site 3: The cervical one-third of the crown or, following gingival recession, the exposed root
- The Four Sizes of Carious Lesions
  - Size 1: Minimal involvement of dentine just beyond treatment by remmeralisation alone

- Size 2: Moderate involvement of dentine. Following cavity preparation, remaining enamel is sound, well supported by dentine and not likely to fail under normal occlusal load. The remaining tooth structure is sufficiently strong to support the restoration
- Size 3: The cavity is enlarged beyond moderate. The remaining tooth structure is weakened to the extent that cusps or incisal edges are split, or are likely to fail or left exposed to occlusal or incisal load. The cavity needs to be further enlarged so that the restoration can be designed to provide support and protection to the remaining tooth structure
- Size 4: Extensive caries with bulk loss of tooth structure has already occurred.

Table 3.5: Mount and Burne's Classification				
	Size			
Site	**Minimal 1**	**Moderate 2**	**Enlarged 3**	**Extensive 4**
Pit/fissure 1	1.1	1.2	1.3	1.4
Contact area 2	2.1	2.2	2.3	2.4
Cervical 3	3.1	3.2	3.3	3.4

Principles of Cavity Preparation

Conventional Concept (Black's Concept):

Dr. G. V. Black has described the concept of "extension for prevention" for cavity preparation. His basic idea was to prevent the recurrence of caries by placing the margins of restorations along selfcleansing areas.

- Incisors and canines: In these teeth the margins of the proximal cavities are placed beyond the contact area
- Molars and premolars: The contact between the adjacent tooth is broken. Occlusal step occupies the entire middle third of the tooth buccolingually. Buccal groove and other sharp grooves are included in the preparation
- Gingival third cavities: Cervical margin placed subgingivally and the mesiodistal extension placed in self cleansing areas.

Outline Form

The locations that the peripheries of the completed tooth preparation will occupy on tooth surfaces. It can be:
- Internal outline form
- External outline form.

Features

- Extend cavity margins to sound tooth structure
- Include all the fissures

- Extend outline form to provide sufficient access
- Cavity margins should be placed in self cleansable areas
- The pulpal floor and axial wall should have an average depth of 0.5 mm into the dentin
- Margins should be extended to include all defective enamel
- 0.2–0.3 mm clearance from the adjacent tooth while preparing the proximal box in class II cavities
- Margins of the cavity preparation should not be in contact with the opposing tooth
- If less than 0.5 mm of the tooth structure exists between two carious surfaces, then they should be joined.

Factors influencing outline form

- Embrasure area
- Contact with opposing tooth
- Caries index of the individual: High caries index—more tooth structure is included in the outline
- Position of the tooth in the arch
- Masticatory forces influencing mesiodistal extension
- Convexity of the tooth
- Extent of the carious lesion
- Proximity of the lesion to other defects in enamel
- Aesthetic consideration
- Partial edentulism
- Restorative material to be used
- Existing restorations.

Resistance Form

It is the shape given to the cavity to enable the tooth as well as the restoration to withstand the stresses of mastication to which it is subjected.

Features

- Flat pulpal and gingival walls, the formation of these walls perpendicular to occlusal forces
- Utilizing box form of cavity preparation
- Cavity prepared in such a way that strong cusp and ridge areas remain with adequate dentin support
- Rounded internal line angles to avoid stress concentrations
- Butt joint between the tooth and restoration
- Removal of unsupported enamel
- 90 degree cavosurface angle
- Adequate bulk of the restorative material
- Adequate depth and width of tile cavity
- Reverse curve in the case of class II cavities, when the proximal outline becomes offset buccolingually
- Gingival cavosuface bevel given in the case of permanent teeth

- The width of the cavity should not be more than $1/4^{th} – 1/5^{th}$ the intercuspal distance
- The pulpal floor should be 0.5 mm below the dentinoenamel junction
- The cavity wall should be divergent occlusally towards the marginal ridge areas.

Retention Form

It is comprised of those factors of cavity design that prevent the restoration from being displaced.

Features

- Parallel or an inverse taper of 5 degree under the triangular ridges of cuspal areas in the case of class I and class II cavities
- Retention cores and grooves as used in class III and Class V cavities. Occlusal dovetail in the case of proximal occlusal cavities where only one proximal surface is involved
- Pins placed into the dentine
- Acid etching of the enamel
- The proximal box of class II design is divergent gingivally to contribute to the retention form.

Convenience Form

It includes shaping the cavity to facilitate access for instrumentation, for condensation, adaptation and finishing.

Features

- Modifications of cavosurface margins for case of placement of restorative material
- Extension of buccal and lingual walls for visibility and access to deeper portions of the cavity
- The proximal lesion can be instrumented from the facial, or lingual embrasures in a tooth with wide, accessible embrasures and intact marginal ridges.

Removal of Any Remaining Infected Dentin

In case of a small carious lesion, the infected dentin would be completely removed as the above mentioned principles are achieved. However, when a large carious lesion exists, some amount of infected dentin still remains inspite of following the above procedures. In such cases the infected dentin has to be removed.

Finishing the Enamel Walls

It is the further development of specific cavosurface design and degree of smoothness that will bring about the maximum effectiveness of the restorative material being used.

Purpose

- To place the margins on sound tooth structure
- To have smooth walls and rounded angles
- To facilitate placement and finishing of the restorative material
- Placement of taper or bevel for the appropriate restorative material.

Cleansing of the Cavity

- The operating field should be kept clean and adequately isolated by the use of rubber dam, cotton rolls and high vacuum evacuation equipment
- Conditioning of the Cavity may be done in certain cases like bonding systems for amalgam and composite restorations.

Recent Concept

Cavity preparation for operative procedures now no longer adhere to Black's concept of Extension for prevention. Increased knowledge of preventive methods, advanced techniques, and improved restorative materials render the clinician to follow both conservative and preventive criteria which can be met by the present day dentistry based on the principle of construction with conservation.

The following principles should be considered while preparing a cavity according to the recent concept:

- Cavity designs should be dictated under the site and extent of the lesion and not by any preconceived notion of mechanical interlocking patterns
- Should not be in expectation of extending the cavity out to a caries free area
- The first choice of a restorative material should be one that displays some degree of biological activity and will therefore assist in the process of remineralization and healing of remaining tooth structure
- Only that part of the tooth crown that is irretrievably degenerated and broken down should be removed and the remainder even though demineralized and softened, should be retained and remineralized
- The first function of the restoration will be to eliminate any surface cavitation that has resulted from caries because in the continuing presence of defects on the surface it will not be possible to completely control plaque accumulation.
- Minimal intervention is therefore based on biological or therapeutic approach with following principles:
  - Repair rather than replacement of defective restorations
  - Disease control

- Remineralization of early lesions
- Reduction in cariogenic bacteria.

What are the modifications in cavity preprations in primary teeth. Write about class I, II, III cavity prepration?

Modifications of Cavity Preparation in Primary Teeth

All the principles of cavity preparation of permanent teeth also hold good for the primary teeth. However, few factors have to be taken into consideration while restoring the primary teeth. These include:

- The smaller tooth dimension of the deciduous dentition
- The thin enamel covering the teeth
- Broad contact areas
- Proximity of the pulp chamber to outer tooth surface
- Narrow occlusal table.

Class I Cavities

- Width of isthmus: Should not be more than 1/3rd the intercuspal distance due to narrow occlusal table
- Depth: Should not be more than 0.5 mm into dentine
- Pulpal floor: Should be saucer shaped. Any remaining carious lesion removed using round bur in slow speed
- Use of preventive resin restoration advocated rather than conventional cavity preparation including all pits and fissures.

Class II Cavities

- Due to presence of broad contact areas, gingival floor of proximal box should be wide so as to place margins in self cleansing areas
- Proximal box: should coverage occlusally. Its walls:
  - Should be parallel to external tooth surface
  - Should not be flared
  - Occlusal walls should be in straight line to avoid any stress points.
- Axial wall: should follow contour of tooth.
- Axiopulpal line angle: should be rounded. Angle of walls and floors should be gently rounded
- Gingival seat: should not be beveled rather than follow enamel rods inclination
- Amalgam strength at isthmus: can be increased by adequate depth of preparation
- Retention: Improved by U shaped retention groove along enamelodentinal junction of proximal box

- When cavity margins exceed that of an ideal preparation mainly in mandibular first primary molar an overlay of distobuccal cusp is prepared
- Weakend cusp is reduced to level of pulpal floor of occlusal preparation
- Mesiodistally cusp should not be reduced more than 1/3ʳᵈ the crown's mesiodistal length
- Avoid mesiobuccal pulp horn from exposure in case of small first molars
- Since contact with canine is a point contact, proximal box extension and gingival flare can be minimized
- Proximal box should allow passage of explorer tip between its margins and adjacent tooth.

Class III Cavity

- When the contact is open, the outline is triangular with base towards the gingival aspect of the cavity
- Gingival cavity wall is inclined occlusally to parallel the enamel rod direction
- Retention pits can be placed at the axiobuccogingival and axiolinguogingival point angles
- A dovetail may be placed in the middle one third of the lingual surface of the tooth
- This helps in gaining access to the carious lesion and in facilitating retention of the restoration.

Question 6

Write about matrices used for restoring the tooth?

Answer

Matrice is a temporary wall created opposite to axial walls and Surrounding areas of tooth structure that were lost during preparation.

Objectives

The matrix should achieve the following functions:
- Displace the gingiva and rubber dam away from the cavity margins
- This improves the accessibility during the restorative procedures
- Assure dryness and non-contamination of the operating field
- Provide shape to the restoration during setting of the restorative material
- Maintain shape during hardening of the restoration.

Matrices for Class I Cavity (Compound Cavity)

Double banded Tofflemire.

Matrices for Class II

- Single banded Tofflemire
- Ivory matrix No. 1
- Ivory' matrix No. 8
- Black's matrices
- Soldered hand or seamless copper band matrix
- Anatomical matrix
- Auto-matrix
- S-shaped matrix band
- T-shaped matrix band.

Matrices for a Cavity Preparation for Amalgam Distal of Cuspid

- S-shaped matrix
- Tofflemire
- Transparent celluloid strips.

Matrices for Class III for Tooth Coloured Restorations

Transparent celluloid strips

Matrices for Class IV for Tooth Coloured Restorations

- Celluloid strips
- Aluminum roil (non-light cure)
- Transparent crown form matrices
- Anatomic matrix
- Modified S-shaped band or copper, tin, aluminum foil (non-light cure).

Matrices for Class V Amalgam Restorations

- Window matrix
- S-shaped matrix.

Matrices for Class V Tooth Coloured Restorations

- Anatomic matrix (non-light cure)
- Aluminum or copper collars (non-light cure)
- Celluloid strips (light cure).

Sectional Matrix with G-rings (Retainers) for Posterior Composites

CHAPTER 4

Fundamentals of Tooth Preparation

LONG ESSAYS

Question 1

Define cavity preparation. Write the various concepts of cavity design for amalgam restorations?

Answer

- Cavity: It refers to a defect in the tooth enamel or in both enamel and dentine due to carious process
- Cavity preparation: It is the mechanical alteration of a defective, injured or diseased tooth to best receive a restorative material, which will re-establish the normal form, function and aesthetics of the tooth.

Outline Form

This forms the occlusal portion just like pit and fissure lesions but the difference being the external outline is extended proximally towards proximal surface that is defective.

Establishing the Occlusal Slip

A punch cut is made in the pit close to the involved proximal surface using a high speed bur.

- A number 245 bur is used
- The long axis of bur is kept parallel to the long axis of tooth
- Initial depth should be 1.5–2.0 mm (**Fig. 4.1**).

Central fissures are included while the outline is extended to maintain uniformity in depth of pulpal floor.

- Isthmus width should be narrow as null as possible. It should not be wider than one-fourths of the intercuspal distance
- Slight occlusal convergence to facial, lingual and proximal walls are given that provides retention for amalgam restoration
- On distal pit area a dovetail is given which prevents mesial displacement of the restoration.

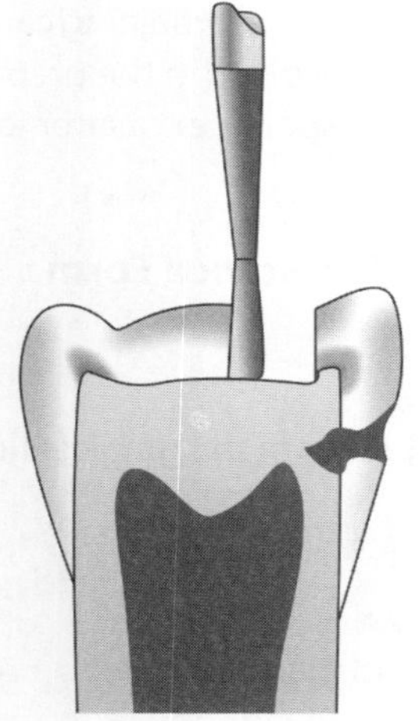

Fig. 4.1: Extend the bur keeping it parallel to the long axis of tooth

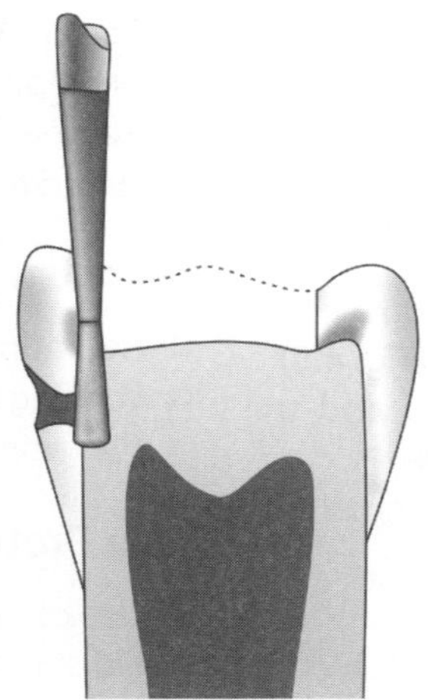

Fig. 4.2: Extend the preparation ending short by 0.8 mm of cutting through marginal ridge

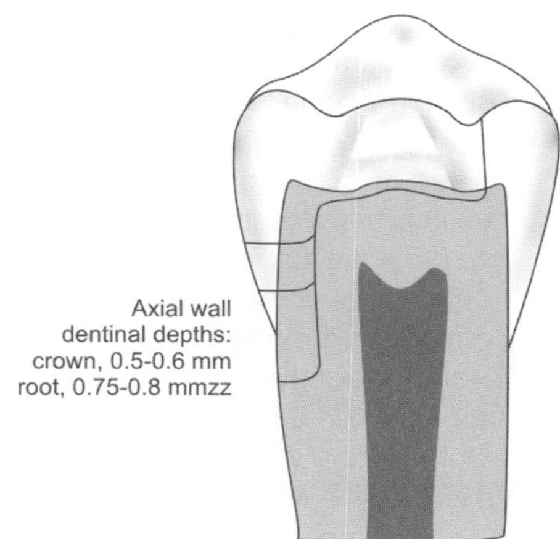

Fig. 4.3: Proximal cutting should be sufficiently deep into dentin

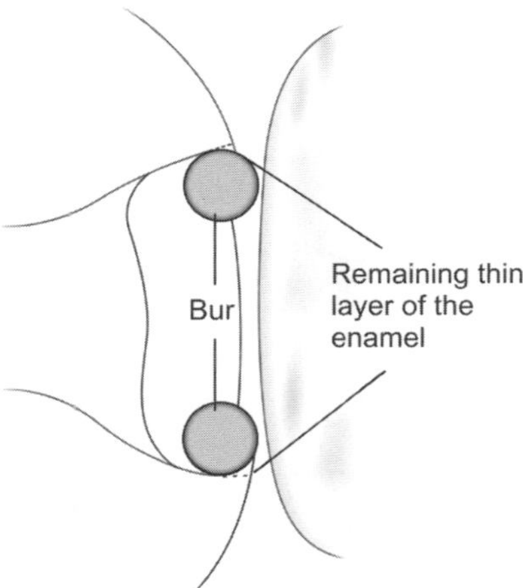

Fig. 4.4: A small slice of enamel is kept at contact area so as to prevent accident damage to adjacent tooth

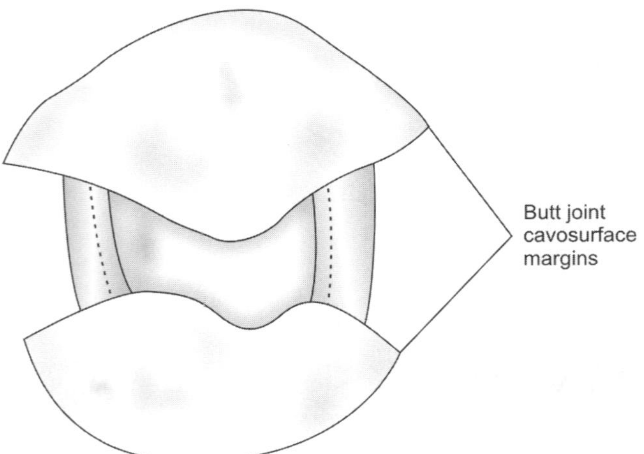

Fig. 4.5: The cavosurface margins should be 90° with occlusal convergence

Extending Occlusal Step Proximally

- Outline form is determined by the faciolingual position of the contact and the extent of carious lesion
- Preparation is extended towards the proximal surface while establishing the pulpal depth
- It should be 0.8 mm short of cutting through mesial marginal ridge (**Fig. 4.2**)
- The retentive locks are prepared into the axiolingual and axiofacial line angles (**Fig. 4.3**) proximal cutting into dentine should be 0.5–0.6 mm.

Preparation of Proximal Box

- To clear the contact area faciolingual preparation is widen
- Proximal cut is diverged gingivally
- This is done to gain good retention and to conserve the marginal ridge
- Small amount of enamel is left at the contact area to prevent damage to the adjacent tooth (**Fig. 4.4**)
- Use matrix bond to avoid contact
- Using a chisel or enamel hatchet fracture the enamel in the region of the contact
- Proximal margins should have a cavosurface angle of 90° and proximal box should converge occlusally (**Fig. 4.5**)
- It should be done to keep the tooth strong and the occlusal forces on the amalgam should be lesser
- Clearance of facial and lingual margins of proximal box should be 0.2–0.5 mm.

Primary Resistance Form

- There should be flat pulpal and gingival floor
- It should have cavosurface angle of 90°
- It should include the weakened tooth structure

- It should pressure tooth structure by maintaining minimal width of the preparation
- All the internal unit and point angles are rounded
- Cusp capping is done to pressure the cuspal strength.

Primary Retention Form

- It prevents the restoration from being displaced
- Retention form is increased by:
  - Two to five percent occlusal convergence of the buccal and lingual walls
  - By giving an occlusal dovetail.

Final Tooth Preparation

- Remove all the debris and correct all cavosurface angles and margins
- Removal of old restorative materials, remaining caries and deep pit and fissures that are involved in the preparation
- Removal of soft caries with spoon excavator or slow speed round bur.

Secondary Retention and Resistance Form

- Retention grooves are placed
- Locking the proximal box
- Placement of slots and pot holes in the gingival floor.

Pulp Protection

- Use of pulp protecting material
- Finishing of enamel walls and margins
- All unsupported enamel is removed
- Beveling of enamel portion of the gingival wall with gingival margin trimmer (GMT)

- ❑ Cavosurface angle should be 90°
- ❑ Finally clean the preparation with wally and air spray
- ❑ Dry it with moist air.

Question 2

Define fissure sealant, pit, fissure and occlusal sealants and classify pit and fissure sealant?

Answer

Fissure Sealant

A fissure sealant is a material that is placed in the pits and fissures of teeth in order to prevent or arrest the development of dental caries.

Fissure sealants are defined whereby pits and fissures that occur principally on the occlusal surfaces of the molar and premolar, teeth are occluded by application of fluid materials, which are then polymerized.

Pit

It is defined as a small pinpoint depression located at the junction of developmental grooves or at terminals of those grooves. The central pit describes a landmark in the central fossae of the molars where developmental grooves join (Ash, 1993).

Fissure

It is defined as deep clefts between adjoining cusps. They provide area for retention of caries producing agents. These defects occur on occlusal surfaces of the molars and premolars, with tortuous configuration that are difficult to assess from the surfaces. These areas are impossible to keep clean and highly susceptible to advancement of the carious lesion, (Orbans, 1990).

Occlusal Sealants

Occlusal sealants are defined as the application and mechanical bonding of a resin material to an acid etched enamel surface thereby sealing existing pits and fissures from the oral environment.

Classifications

Pits and fissures are broadly classified into four varieties:
- ❑ A shallow groove
- ❑ Complete penetration of the enamel
- ❑ The fissure may end blindly
- ❑ The end of fissure may open into an irregular chamber.

Nagano (1960) described four principal types of fissures, based on the alphabetical description of shape.

- ❑ V type
- ❑ U type
- ❑ I type
- ❑ IK type.

The shallow, wide V and U shaped fissures tend to be self-cleansing and somewhat caries resistant. Deep, narrow I shaped fissures are quite constricted and resemble a battle neck. They have a narrow slit-like opening with a larger base as it extends toward the dentino-enamel junction. These caries susceptible, I shaped fissures may also have a number of branches. Similarly, IK shaped fissures are also very susceptible to caries. Usually, non-invasive technique is recommended for U and V shaped fissures and invasive technique for I and IK type fissures.

Pit and fissure sealants can be classified in different ways.
- ❑ According to the chemistry of materials it may be of three types with different resin systems:
  - ○ Alkyl cyanoacrylates
  - ○ Polyurethane
  - ○ BIS-GMA.
- ❑ According to the method of polymerization
  - ○ Ultraviolet-activated sealants
  - ○ Self-cured or chemically cured sealants
  - ○ Light-activated sealants.
- ❑ According to the filler particles incorporated in the sealants
  - ○ Filled
  - ○ Unfilled.
- ❑ According to the coloring pigments incorporated into the sealants.
  - ○ Clear
  - ○ Tinted/endowed sealants.

Mitchell and Gordon (1990) stated that the sealants can be differentiated in the following ways:
- ❑ Polymerization methods
  - ○ Self-activation (mixing two components)
  - ○ Light activation
    - ➤ First-generation: Ultraviolet light
    - ➤ Second-generation: Self-cure
    - ➤ Third-generation: Visible light.
  - ○ Fourth generation: Fluoride releasing.
- ❑ Resin systems
  - ○ BIS–GMA
  - ○ Urethane acrylate.
- ❑ Filled and unfilled

❑ Clear or tinted: Clear sealants have been shown to have better flow characteristics than tinted or opaque, but this can be an advantages or disadvantage depending on the position of the tooth to be sealed. Although the retention rates of the two types are similar, colored sealants are more easily appreciated by the patients and monitored by the dentist at subsequent recalls.

RJ Simonsen (1981) listed the advantages of coloring the sealants.

❑ Ease in detection which makes recall examinations much easier and faster
❑ Ease in application, for example, one can more easily detects the materials, where the material is placed and that if it is present in the amount desired
❑ Provision of a visible primary preventive service that increases patient and parents acceptance.

RIPA (1993) classified fissure sealant into four generations:

1. Ultraviolet activated
2. Auto polymerizing
3. Visible light cured
4. Fluoride containing sealants.

Question 3

Write a short note on classification of the tooth preparation?

Answer

Classification of Tooth Preparation

GV Black (1947) classified tooth preparation based on anatomic areas involved and the associated type of treatment. He classified tooth preparation into five original classes. Later class VI was added to the original classification by Simon.

Class I

All pit and fissure restorations are included in this class. Class I restorations can be divided into three groups:
1. Restoration on occlusal surface of premolars and molars
2. Restoration on occlusal two-thirds of the facial and lingual surfaces of molars
3. Restoration on lingual surface of maxillary incisors **(Figs. 4.6 - 4.8)**.

*Class I cavity preparation has eight (8) line angles and four (4) point angles.

Class II

All restorations on proximal surface of posterior teeth:
1. MO: Mesio-occlusal preparation
2. DO: Disto-occlusal preparation
3. MOD: Mesio-occlusal distal preparation **(Figs. 4.9 - 4.11)**.

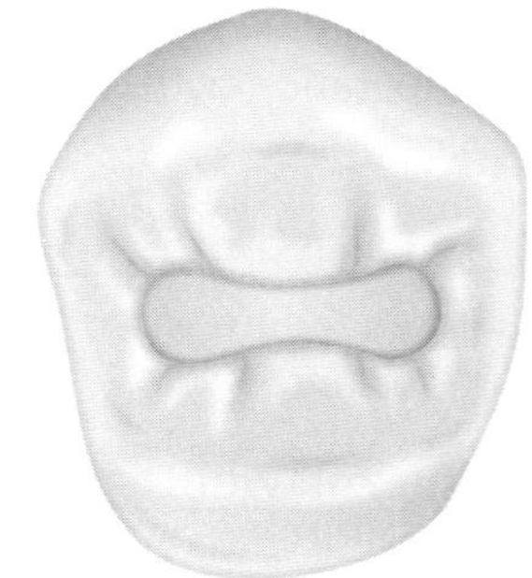

Fig. 4.6: Typical class I cavity preparation on maxillary premolar

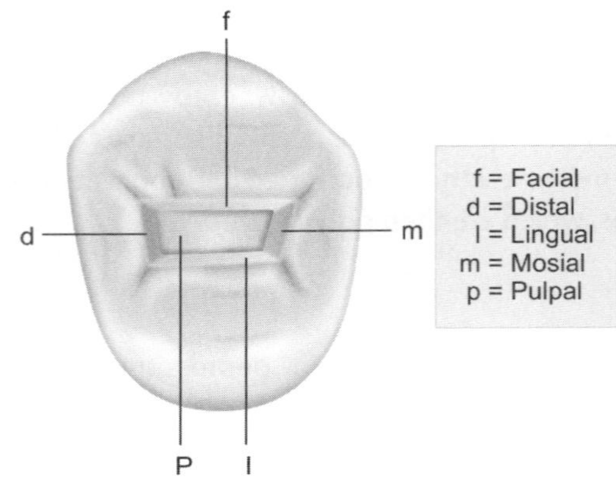

Fig. 4.7: Schematic representation of class I cavity preparation walls

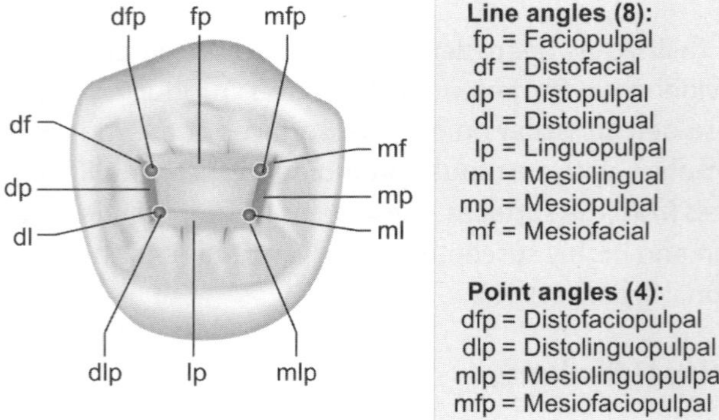

Fig. 4.8: Schematic representation of class I cavity preparation line angles and point angles

*Class II cavity preparation has eleven (11) line angles and six (6) point angles.

Class III

Restoration on the proximal surfaces of anterior teeth and do not involve the incisal edge **(Figs. 4.12 - 4.14)**.

*Class III cavity preparation has six (6) line angles and three (3) point angles.

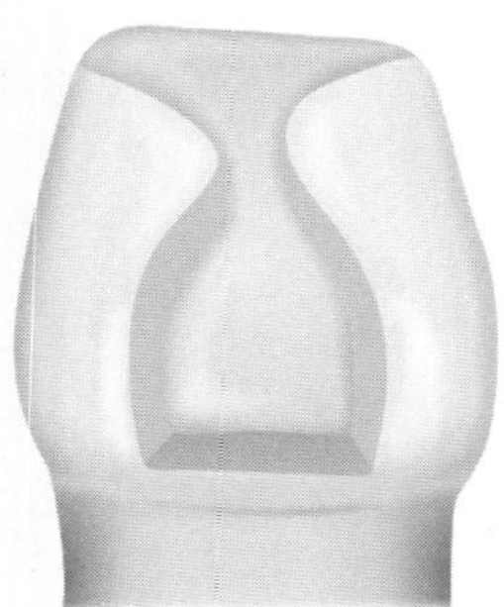

Fig. 4.9: Typical class II mesio-occlusal cavity preparation on maxillary premolar

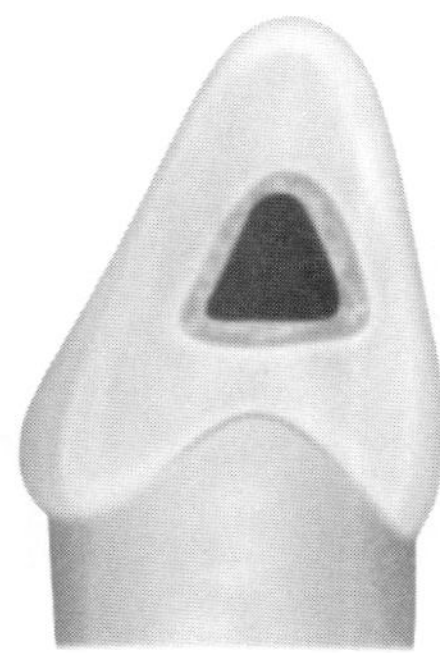

Fig. 4.12: Class III cavity preparation on maxillary central incisor

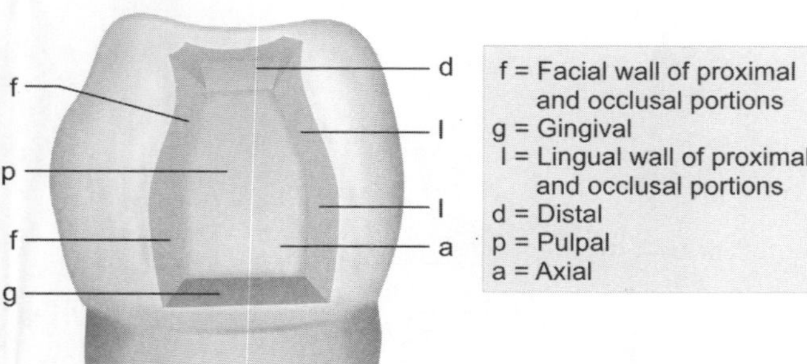

Fig. 4.10: Schematic representation of class II cavity preparation walls

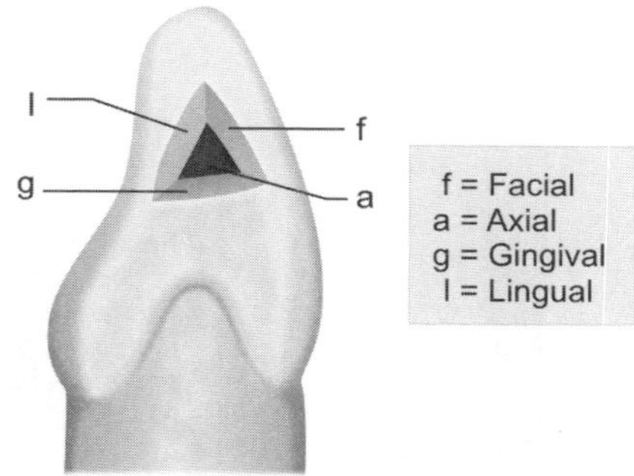

Fig. 4.13: Schematic representation of class III cavity preparation walls

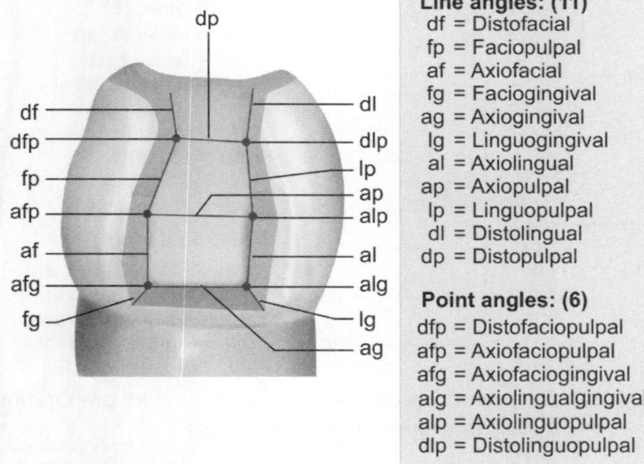

Fig. 4.11: Schematic representation of class II cavity preparation line angles and point angles

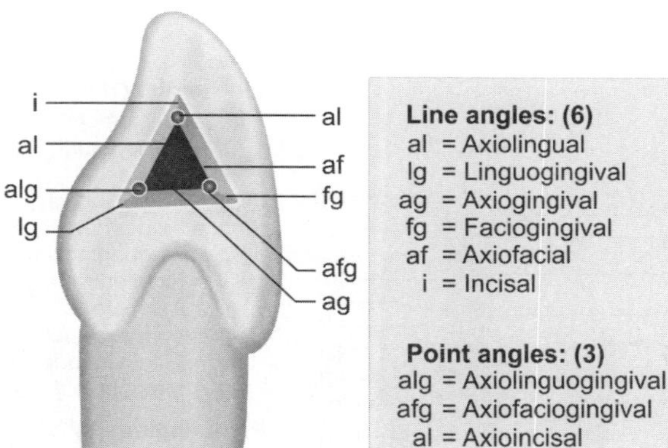

Fig. 4.14: Schematic representation of class III cavity preparation line angles and point angles

Class IV

Restoration on the proximal surfaces of anterior teeth that do involve the incisal edge **(Figs. 4.15 - 4.17)**.

*Class IV cavity preparation has eleven (11) line angles and six (6) point angles.

Class V

Restoration on the gingival third of the facial third of the facial or lingual surface of all teeth (except pit and fissure lesion) **(Figs. 4.18 - 4.20)**.

*Class V cavity preparation has eight (8) line angles and four (4) point angles.

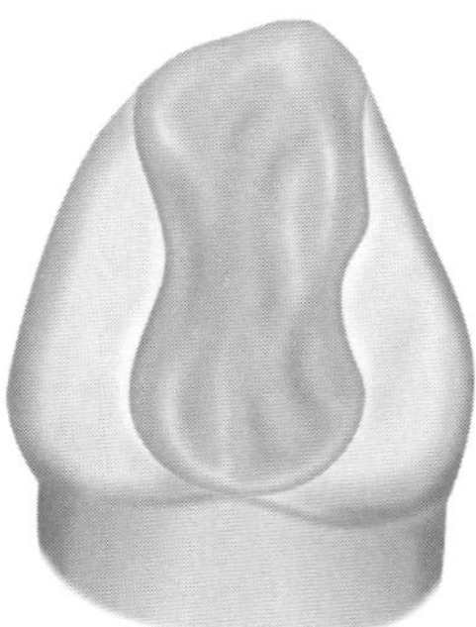

Fig. 4.15: Class IV cavity preparation for inlay on maxillary canine

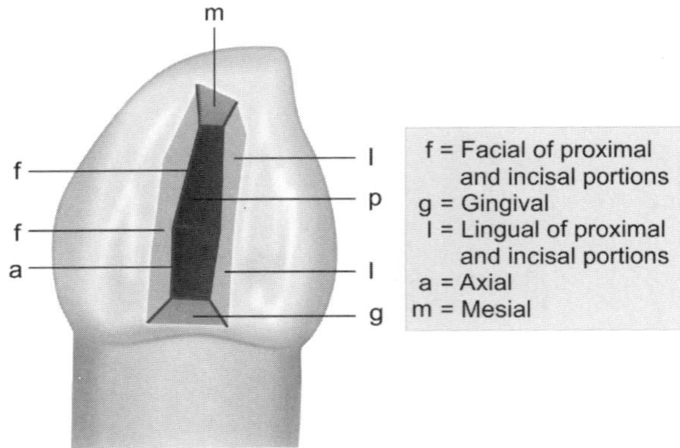

Fig. 4.16: Schematic representation of class IV cavity preparation walls

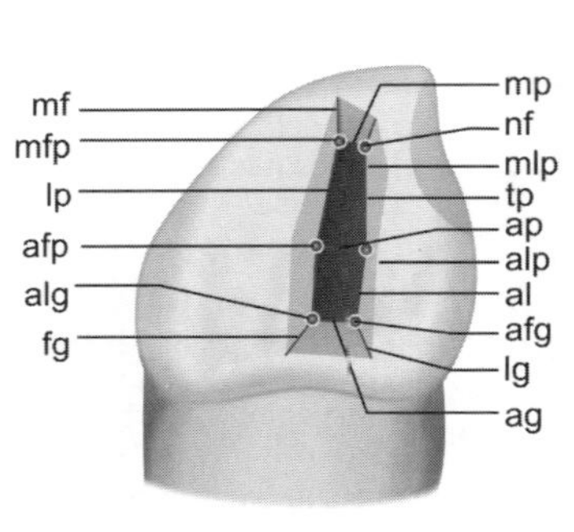
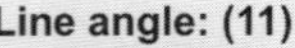

Line angle: (11)

mf = Mesiofacial
tp = Faciopulpal
nf = Axiofacial
fg = Faciogingival
ag = Axiogingival
lg = Linguogingival
al = Axiolingual
ap = Axiopulpal
lp = Linguopulpal
ml = Mesiolingual
mp = Mesiopulpal

Point angles: (6)

mfp = Mesiofaciopulpal
afp = Axiafaciopulpal
afg = Axiofaciogingival
alg = Axiofinguogingival
alp = Axiolinguopulpal
mlp = Mesiolinguopulpal

Fig. 4.17: Schematic representation of class IV cavity preparation line angles and point angles

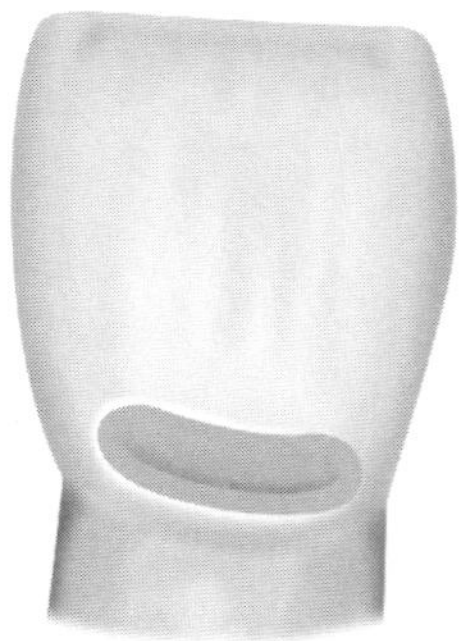

Fig. 4.18: Class V cavity preparation

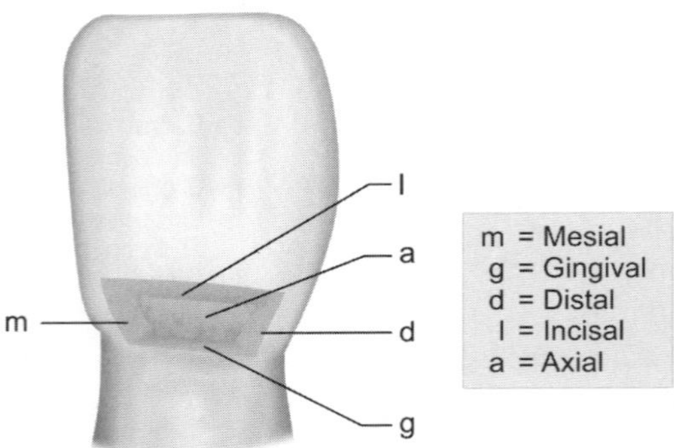

Fig. 4.19: Schematic representation of class V cavity wall

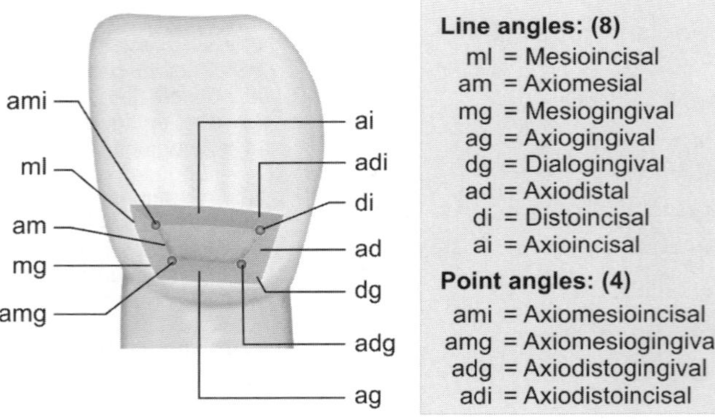

Line angles: (8)

ml = Mesioincisal
am = Axiomesial
mg = Mesiogingival
ag = Axiogingival
dg = Dialogingival
ad = Axiodistal
di = Distoincisal
ai = Axioincisal

Point angles: (4)

ami = Axiomesioincisal
amg = Axiomesiogingival
adg = Axiodistogingival
adi = Axiodistoincisal

Fig. 4.20: Schematic representation of class V cavity preparation line angles and point angles

Class VI

Restoration on the incisal edge of anterior teeth or the occlusal cup height of posterior teeth.

*Class VI cavity preparation has eight (8) line angles and four (4) point angles.

SHORT ESSAYS

Question 1

Cavity preparation for class III composites?

Answer

Conventional Class III

Steps

Outline of tooth preparation is determined by the extent of lesion.

- The bur entry is preferred from the lingual side to conserve estethesis, color match is not required, unsupported facial enamel can be saved for bonding, discoloration in future is less visible
- Labial approach is given when the labial enamel is involved
- Malignated teeth
- When there is damage only in the root surface
- When carious lesion is not deep
- It is kept at 0.75 mm.

Beveled Conventional Class III Tooth Preparation

It is indicated in:
- For replacing existing restoration that is defective at the crown portion of anterior tooth
- For larger preparation.

Steps

Caries is approached lingually with small round bur.

- Bur is moved incisogingival direction
- Tooth preparation should be same as that of existing carious lesion
- Initial depth of axial wall should be 0.7 mm deep gingivally
- 1.25 mm deep incisally
- Axial wall should follow the tooth contour
- It should be convex outwardly
- Removal of all infected dentive or restoration is done in final preparation with a spoon excavator
- Calcium hydroxide is placed to protect the pulp
- External walls should be perpendicular to enamel surface **(Fig. 4.21)**
- Prepare retentive grooves and cover along gingiva axial line angle and inciso axial line angle.

Modified (Conventional) Class III Tooth Preparation

It is indicated in: Small to moderate class III.

Steps

- Bur entry is done from palatal surface
- Extent and design depends on the extent of the carious lesion **(Fig. 4.22)**
- It does not have definite axial wall depth
- The walls diverge from axial depth show scoop shape
- Finally, the preparation is cleaned and pulp protection is provided.

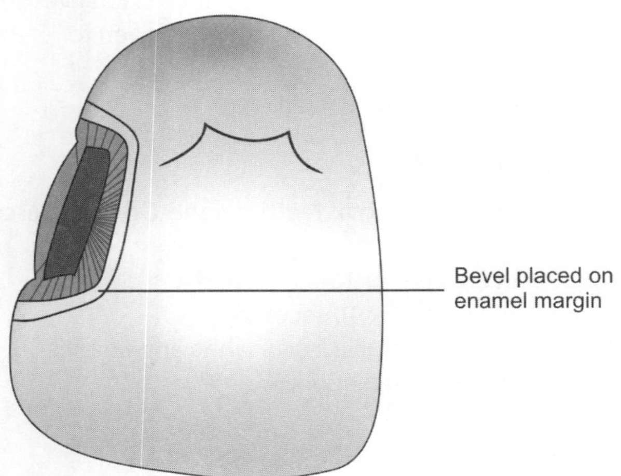

Fig. 4.21: Beveled class III tooth preparation for composites

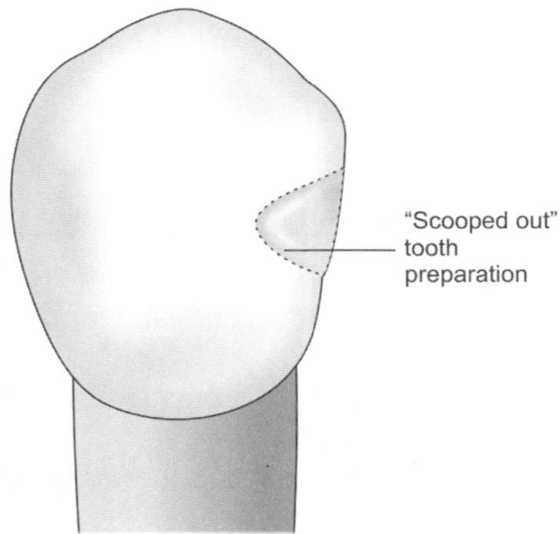

Fig. 4.22: Extent of preparation is determined by extent of caries

SHORT NOTES

Question 1

Explain extension for prevention?

Answer

Extension for prevention is placing the margins of preparations at areas that would be cleaned by the excursions of food during chewing.

- In this the margins of the restoration are placed on line angles of the tooth
- The occlusal surface is extended through pits and fissures
- Buccal and lingual extending of proximal unit angles through embrasures and cervically below the gingival margin
- It prevents recurrence of decay in the tooth surface of adjoin restoration
- It results in self-cleaning embrasure areas.

Question 2

What is air abrasion?

Answer

- It is also known as advanced particle beam technology or microabrasion
- It is done by involving high energy sand blasting of tooth surface
- This works on the method that abrasion particles are emitted in a particular, well defined shape that is focused on the target
- Particle: Size 25–30μ
- Pressure: 60–120 pound per square inch pressure
- Most common in the AL_2O_3 dust.

Question 3

Discuss reverse class II amalgam restoration?

Answer

- In class II cavity preparation extension of proximal area is important for eliminating caries and for breaking the proximal contacts
- In cases where the teeth have broader contacts reverse S-shape curve is given
- It is done to widen the box and it removes less tooth structure **(Fig. 4.23)**
- Excessive flare should be avoided as this will make proximal walls pass the axial angle through the cusp
- This then results in weakening of tooth and more prone to fracture.

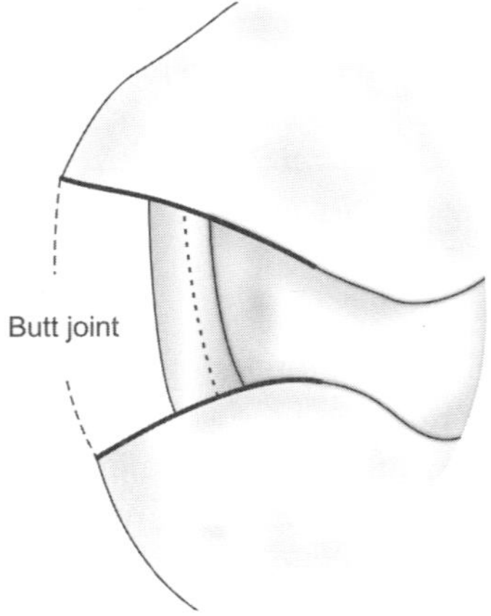

Fig. 4.23: Reverse curve is given to the proximal walls by curving them toward the contact area

Advantages

- Triangular ridge is prevented in the cusp
- Conserves the tooth structure
- Increases the resistance form.

Question 4

What is acid etching?

Answer

- It is a process of increasing the surface reactivity by demineralization the superficial calcium layer and thus cleating the enamel tags. These tags are responsible for micro-mechanical bonding between tooth and restorative resin
- Acid used is 37% phosphoric acid time given for etching is 15–20 seconds
- It is supplied in liquid and get form

Steps for Bonding

- Cleaning and washing of teeth is done. Dry it to descent any contaminants
- Apply acid etchant for 15–20 seconds
- Wash it with water for 10 seconds
- After wash it should give frosty white appearance
- Bonding agent is than applied.

Properties

- It cleans debris from enamel surface increases the enamel surface for bonding agent
- Products micropores which have mechanical interlocking appearance.

Question 5

What is enameloplasty?

Answer

It is defined as removal of sharp and irregular enamel margins of the enamel surface by rounding or saucering it and converting it into a smooth groove making itself clearing area.

Indications

- In case where caries thickness is one-third of that of enamel present
- When there are shallow fissures that cross lingual and facial ridge
- It does not extend the outline form so if a fissure cannot be converted into a groove it should not be implemented.

Question 6

Define attrition, abrasion and erosion?

Answer

- Attrition: Attrition is defined as mechanical wear of opposite teeth commonly seen on the contacting occlusal, incisal and proximal surfaces
- Abrasion: Abrasion is defined as loss of tooth material by mechanical wear other than contacting surfaces. It is common due to improper brushing and use of abrasive tooth powder
- Erosion: Erosion is defined as loss of dental hard tissue as a result of a chemical process which does not involve bacteria.

Question 7

What is smear layer?

Answer

Smear layer is an iatrogenically produced layer which decreases both sensitivity and permeability of dentinal tubules.

It has two compounds:

1. Superficial smear layer: This is the layer which is loosely attached to the underlying dentin till the depth of 1–1.5 mm
2. Smear plugs: This occludes the dentinal tubules. It extends till the depth of 1 mm.

Question 8

What is cavosurface angle?

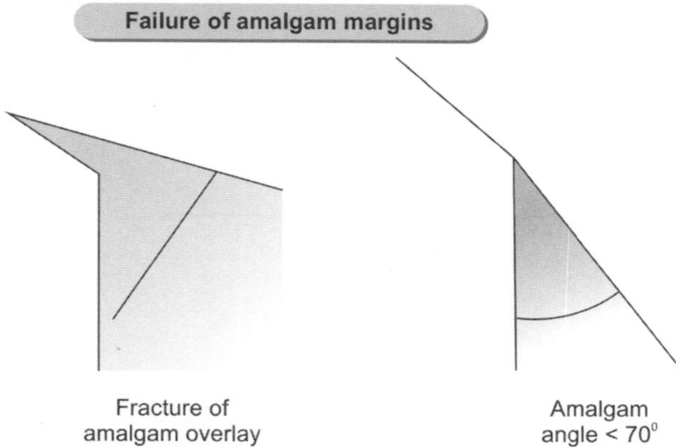

Fig. 4.24: Cavosurface margins should be 90° for amalgam fracture of restoration can occur if angle is acute or obtuse

Answer

- It is defined as the angle of the tooth structure which is formed by the junction of a prepared wall and the external tooth surface
- It should be a butt joint
- If the cavosurface angle is acute the enamel margin may fracture under load
- If it is obtuse it will fracture under masticatory stress **(Fig. 4.24)**.

Question 9

Explain tunnel preparation?

Answer

It is the preparation made for removal of proximal caries by making an access through occlusal surface while leaving the marginal ridge intact.

Indications

- It is indicated in tooth which won't last more than 5 years
- In posterior teeth, with incipient proximal lesions patients with low caries index.

Contraindications

- When the proximal decay undermines the marginal ridge
- When there is occlusal load on marginal ridge.

Question 10

What is prophylactic odontotomy?

Answer

- It is a technique where minimum cavity preparation is one and amalgam restoration is given
- This procedure is not used now.

CHAPTER 5

Dental Cements

Question 1

Define and classify dental cements. Discuss in detail glass ionomer cements (GIC)?

Answer

Definition

A dental cement is a substance that hardens to act as a base, liner, filling material or adhesive to bind devices or prosthesis to the tooth structure or to each other (**Table 5.1**).

Ideal Requisites

- Should be non-toxic, non-irritant to pulp and other tissues
- Should not be soluble in oral fluids
- Cements which are used under metallic restoration should protect the pulp from thermal changes
- Should be ideally adhesive to enamel and dental and gold alloy, porcelain, acrylic but not to dental instruments.
- Should be bacteriostatic.

Classification

- Type I: Luting
- Type II: Restorative applications
- Type III: Unit or base applications.

According to Anusavice, Based on the use of Cements

Table 5.1: Type of cements and their use

Cement	Principal use	Secondary use
Zinc phosphate	Luting agent for restorations and orthodontic bands	Intermediate restoration, base
$ZnPO_4$ with AG/Cu salts	Intermediate restorations	
Zinc oxide eugenol (ZOE)	Intermediate restoration, luting agent, base, pulp capping agent	Root canal sealer, periodontic bandage
$CuPO_4$ (red/black)	Intermediate restorations	
Polycarboxylate	Luting agent, base	Intermediate restoration
Silicophosphate	Anterior restorations	
Glass ionomer	Coating for eroded/ abraded areas, luting	Pit and fissure sealant, base, anterior restoration
Resin	Luting agent	Intermediate restoration
Calcium hydroxide	Pulp capping agent, base	

Glass Ionomer Cement (GIC)

According to Kenneth J. Anusavice, Glass ionomer is the generic name of a group of materials that use silicate glass provider and aqueous solution of polyacrylic acid.

Composition

Powder (Table 5.2)

Table 5.2: Powder composition

Compound	Age	Properties
Acid soluble calcium fluoroaluminosilicate glass		
Silica (SiO_2)	41.9%	Increases translucency, skeletal structure
Alumina (Al_2O_3)	28.6%	Increases opacity, skeletal structure
Aluminium fluoride (AlF_3)	1.6%	Decreases fusion temperature, anticariogenicity, increases translucency, increases working time and strength

Calcium fluoride (CaF$_2$)	15.7%	Acts as flux, increases opacity
Sodium fluoride (NaF)	9.3%	Anticariogenicity
Aluminium phosphate (AlPO$_4$)	3.8%	Decreases melting temperature
Fluoride components		Act as ceramic flux
Lanthanum, strontium barium, zinc oxide (ZnO)		Provide radiopacity

Liquid

- Polyacrylic acid: In the form of copolymer with itaconic acid, malic acid and tricarboxylic acid
- Increases reactivity of liquid
- Decreases viscosity
- Reduces tendency for gelation
- Tartaric acid
- Improves handling characteristics
- Increases working time
- Shortens setting time
- Water (most important)
- Reaction medium
- Hydraulic reacting product
- Amount of water in liquid critical as too much results in weak cement and too little impairs reaction and subsequent hydration.

Classification

Wilson and Mclean (1988)

Type-I : Luting Cement

- For cementation of crowns, bridges, inlays and orthodontic appliances
- Powder / liquid ratio - 1.5:1
- Fast Set with early resistance to water uptake
- Ultimate film thickness 25μm or less
- Radiopaque.

Type-II: Restorative Cements

- Restorative Aesthetics
- Restorative Reinforced.

- Restorative Aesthetics - Auto Cure and Dual Cure
  - For any application requiring an esthetics restoration, the only limitation is not under occlusal load
  - Powder / liquid ratio 2.8:1 to 6.8:1
  - Excellent shade range and translucency
  - Autocure cements have a prolonged setting reaction and remain subject to water loss and water uptake for atleast 24 hrs after placement they require immediate protection from the oral environment
  - Most auto cure cements are radiolucent
  - Dual cure cements are immediately resistant to water uptake or water loss, they do not require sealing
  - Dual cure cements are radiopaque
  - Particle size ranges from 20-50 μm.

- Restorative Reinforced
  - For use where esthetic considerations are not important but a rapid set and good physical properties are required
  - Powder / liquid ratio 3:1 to 4:1
  - Fast set with early resistance to water uptake, can be trimmed and polished immediately after initial set, remain susceptible to dehydration for 2 weeks after placement
  - Radiopaque.

Type-III: Lining or Base Cement

- Can be autocure or dual cure
- Can be used as either lining or a base depending on powder / liquid ratio used
- Powder / liquid ratio 1.5:1 for use as a lining material under other restorative materials
- Powder / liquid ratio 3:1 / greater for use as a base or dentin substitute in combination with other restorative material
- Physical properties improve as the powder content increases
- Radiopaque.

According to the Application

- Type I: Luting Cements
  - They flow readily to form a thin film.
- Type II: Restorative Materials
  - Aesthetic filling material : These are viscous pastes which have good colour and translucency
  - Reinforced filling material : These metal filled pastes are radiopaque and some what more wear-resistant than the unfilled cements.
- Type III: Fast-setting lining cements. These flow readily and are opaque to both light and x-rays
- Type IV: Fissure sealing cements. These have good flow
- Type V: Orthodontic cements. These are viscous and set rapidly
- Type VI: Core build-up cements. These are viscous, radiopaque pastes which set rapidly. Some contain finely divided metal powder.

Mclean et al 1994 - Classification

Glass Ionomer Cement

Consists of basic glass and an acidic polymer. It sets by an acid-base reaction between these components. This GIC embraces 2 subgroups.
1. Glass Polyalkenoates.
2. Glass polyphosphonates.

Resin Modified Glass Ionomer

Hybrid materials that retain a significant acid base reaction as part of their overall curing process. A feature of these materials is that they will set in the dark however the process is lower than conventional glass ionomers. It is used not only as base but also as filling materials.

Polyacid Modified Composite Resin

These materials may contain either or both of the essential components of GIC, but at levels insufficient to promote the acid base reaction in the dark. They have high aesthetic qualities of composite resin.

The Vitremer Tri-cure System

Modification of the glass ionomer formulation with a visible light curing resin component improves the physical properties of the cement, simplifies clinical handling of the material, and significantly reduces operating time.
In addition to the light curing mechanism vitremer hardens by acid/base, glass ionomer reaction and a chemical "dark cure" catalyzed by a reduction/oxidation reduction. The dark cure is perhaps important in deeper restorations in which light beam penetration may not be sufficient for completion of light hardening phase.

Composition

The glass of cement sets as a result of a reaction between an acid and a base; the product of the reaction, a hydrogel salt, acts as a binding matrix.

Glasses

The composition of the glass can be varied greatly, although these are based on ion leachable calcium aluminosilicates. The composition of the original ionomer glass,

SiO_2	-	30.1%
Al_2O_3	-	19.9%
$Al F_3$	-	2.6%
$Ca F_2$	-	34.5%
$Na F$	-	3.7%
$AlPO_4$	-	10.0%

The three essential constituents of dental ionomer glasses are Silica (SiO_2) alumina (Al_2O_3) and calcium fluoride or calcium fluorite (CaF_2). When fused together they form a glass suitable for cement formation. Other components, such as cryolite and aluminium phosphate are also added.

The different types of calcium fluroalumino-silicate glasses that may be employed in glass ionomer cement formulations are

$$SiO_2 \quad - \quad Al_2O_3 \quad - \quad CaF_2$$
$$SiO_2 \quad - \quad Al_2O_3 \quad - \quad CaF_2 \quad - \quad AlPO_4$$
$$SiO_2 \quad - \quad Al_2O_3 \quad - \quad CaF_2 \quad - \quad AlPO_4 \quad - \quad Na_3AlF_6$$

Conventional

Glass Ionomers is the generic name of the group of materials that use silicate glass powder and an aqueous solution of poly acrylic acid. This acquires its name from its formulation of glass powder and an ionomeric acid, which contains carboxyl groups.

The glass ionomer powder is an acid soluble calcium fluoro alumino silicate glass.

Three essential constituents of glass are: Silica (SiO_2), Alumina (Al_2O_3) and Calcium fluoride (CaF_2)

Glasses high in silica more than 40% are clear and transparent. Increase in CaF_2 and AlF_2 increases opacity. The glasses are prepared by mixing together finely ground constituents (20-50 μm) melted in a sillimanite crucible between 1,100°C to 1,300°C for 40-150 min in an electric furnace.

The melt is cooled by pouring on a steel tray when the mass appears dull red, it is plunged into water. The glass first so obtained is ball milled passing through a sieve mesh with openings of dimensions depending on the required particle size for luting or for restoration.

The Glass Ionomer powder has the following composition (**Table 5.3**):

Table 5.3: Glass Ionomer powder composition

Component		Weight %
Quartz	SiO_2	29.0%
Alumina	AlO_3	16.6
	AlF_3	5.3
Fluorite	CaF_2	34.2
Cryolite	Na_3AlF_6	5.3
	$AlPO_4$	9.9

Metal Modified Glass Ionomers

Two Systems Available

The first is that of mixing spherical silver amalgam alloy powder with the restorative type of glass ionomer powder. This cement is referred to as silver alloy admix.

The second involves fusing glass powder to silver particles through high temperature sintering of a mixture of the two powders. This is commonly referred to as to ceremet. Ceremet ionomers are manufactured by intimate mixing of glass and metal powders which are then compressed in a hydraulic press; Pelletising is carried out at high pressure (> 300 MPa). During the operation it was found favourable to evacuate the pelletising chamber at pressure around 800°C and the sintered metal glass cermet when ground to a fine powder retains its characteristics because the metal powder remains its firmly bonded in the glass cermet powders and are more rounded than conventional glass powder because of the lubricating effect of silver.

The silver-cermet cement has low fracture strengths and cannot be used to replace cusps and marginal ridges, but does have enhanced wear resistance. Class I Ketac Silver restorations surrounded by strong cusps and ridges do not need high fracture resistance because the protective surrounding tooth structure absorbs forces of impact and associated stresses of occlusion and mastication.

Resin Modified Systems (RMGI) or Resin Reinforced Glassionomer (RRGR)

The powder consists of fluoro aminosilicate glass and the liquid contains 15-25% resin component in the form of HEMA together with < 1% poly reversible groups and a photo initiator. Some manufactures incorporate further trace chemicals into the liquid to create an oxidation reduction reaction there by enhancing the set in any remaining unset resins and reducing the susceptibility to water uptake.

Poly Acid Modified Composite (Compomers)

Newest member of the family of restorative materials available for paediatric restorative dentistry.

Composition

The resin contains functional groups of poly carboxylic acid and methacrylate combined in one molecule.
- Fluoride containing glasses as fillers.
- Acid Monomer
- Catalyst.
- These are hydrophilic resins.

The Vitremer Tri-cure System (3M Dental Products Division)

It consists of four components:
1. Primer: Consisting of the Vitrebond copolymer, HEMA (2-hydroxyethlymethacrylate), ethanol and photo-curing agents. The purpose of the primer is to modify the smear layer and completely wet the tooth structure to accommodate the glass polyalkenoate acid/base bonding reaction.
2. Glass Powder: Consisting of fluoroaluminosilicate glass particles. The powder also contains a proprietary reduction/oxidation system using "microencapsulated", potassium persulfate and ascorbic acid that catalyzes a methacrylate "dark cure" of the cement.
3. Liquid: Consisting an "aqueous solution of polyacrylic acid modified with pendant methacrylate groups" (Internal communication, 3M Dental Products Division). Also in the liquid solution are the Vitrebond copolymer, HEMA, water and photoinitiators for the visible-light curing reaction.
4. Resin gloss: Consisting of a clear, BIS-GMA/TEGDMA visible-light polymerizing, dental-bonding-resin liquid.

Setting Reaction

The setting characteristics of the glass-ionomer cement are central to its science, and some understanding of the setting reaction, even if only in outline is needed to appreciate the scientific technology of glass-ionomer cements and the correct clinical usage of them in dental surgery.

Stages of Setting Reaction

Stage I : Dissolution

The surface layer of the glass particles attacked by polyacid to produce a diffusion-based adhesion between the glass particles and the matrix. Approximately 20-30% of the glass is decomposed and ions (including Ca, Al and fluoride ions) are released leading to the formation of a cement sol.

Stage 2 : Precipitation of Salts, Gelation and Hardening

During this stage Ca and Al ions bind to polyanions via carboxylate groups. The initial clinical set is achieved by cross linking of the more readily available Ca ions. This reaction is relatively rapid forming a clinically `hard' surface within 4-10 minutes from the start of mixing.

Maturation occurs over the next 24 hours as the less mobile aluminium ions become bound within the cement matrix, leading to more rigid cross-linking between the poly (alkenoic) chains. Fluoride and phosphate ions form insoluble salts and complexes.

Sodium ions contribute to the formation of an orthosilicic acid on the surface of the particles and, as the pH rises, this converts to a silica gel which assists in binding the powder to the matrix.

Stage 3 : Hydration of Salts

Associated with maturation phase is a progressive hydration of the matrix salts, leading to the sharp improvement in the physical properties.

Properties of GIC

Biocompatibility

GIC is biocompatible. Their ability to bond chemically to tooth structure ensures that they provide an excellent marginal seal, thus eliminating the secondary caries, while their slow release of fluoride acting as a reservoir confers resistance to caries. They are not only biotherapeutic, but they are also bioactive because there is an active exchange of ions between the tooth structure and restorative materials.

Resistance to Plaque

It has been shown that bacterial plaque fails to thrive on the surface of glass ionomer, this in turn means that there is a high level of tolerance in surrounding soft tissues.

Streptococcus mutans is the major pathogen found in dental plaque and it is thought that it is unable to thrive in the presence of fluoride. Thus the response of all soft tissues to glass ionomer restorations is favourable.

Pulp Response to Glass Ionomer

The pulpal response to glass ionomer materials is favourable. The freshly mixed material is very acidic with the pH ranging between 0.9 and 1.6. However dentine is an excellent buffer and even thin layers of dentine remaining between the restoration and the pulp are sufficient to prevent a reduction of pH within the pulp tissue. A mild inflammatory response has been noted by several authors but, as the pH rises again within the first hour, the inflammation will resolve within 10-20 days.

Recent work suggests that glass-ionomer can be used to cover and protect a mechanical or traumatic exposure of an otherwise healthy pulp because formation of a dentin bridge can occur in spite of the lowered pH.

Sensitivity to Luting Materials

It has been suggested that glass ionomers can be the cause of post insertion sensitivity when used as a luting agent under full crowns. In a tooth which requires a crown, it is likely that the pulp has already become inflamed as a result of its original condition and the following preparation procedures. It is therefore desirable to treat it

with considerable care. Do not remove the smear layer by conditioning or scrubbing the dentine in an attempt to develop adhesion. For preference, seal the dentine tubules by applying a mineralising solution or a resin dentine bond at the time of cavity preparation and before recording the impression. Then, at the time of cementation, mix the cement at the correct powder.

The reasons for selecting a glass-ionomer for cementation of indirect restorations include:

- ❑ Thixotropic flow properties
- ❑ Excellent ultimate film thickness
- ❑ Fluoride release
- ❑ Low solubility.

Solubility and Disintegration

In a clinically relevant organic acid solution, such as lactic acid the solubility of glass ionomer is low compared with zinc phosphate and zinc polycarboxylate cements. Solubility in water is less than that of silicate cements, but slightly greater than that several other cements, including resin materials. However, the surface of glass ionomer cements can be damaged in the presence of low pH, such as occurs during application of some topical fluoride solutions.

Acid phosphate fluoride solutions has a pH of 3.0, whereas neutral sodium fluoride is about pH 6.5. Therefore, it is possible for roughening of the cement surface to occur if a phosphate fluoride solution is applied regularly.

Fluoride Release

Glass-ionomer cement has a cariostatic effect. The spread of caries is arrested at the restoration/cavity wall margin. Protection is conferred on the enamel of the crown for some distance from the restoration. The influence of fluoride is found in a zone resistance to demineralization which is atleast 3mm thick around glassionomer restoration. This favourable result has been attributed to the release of fluoride from the cement and its movement into adjacent enamel.

Fluoride exert their anticarious effect by three different mechanisms:

1. Presence of fluoride ions greatly enhances the precipitation into tooth structure of fluorapatite from Ca and Po_4 ions present in saliva. This results in enamel becoming more acid resistant
2. Incipient, non-activated carious lesions are remineralized by the same process
3. Fluoride has antimicrobial activity.

Dimensional Change

A free standing specimen of a glass ionomer material will if correctly manipulated and protected from early exposure to moisture, show a volumetric setting contraction of approximately 3% which develops slowly through the setting process. In the presence of adhesion, through ion exchange with tooth structure, the shrinkage is controlled and, in view of the time taken for the setting reaction, there is a degree of stress relaxation leading to a reduced marginal discrepancy.

Resistance to Fracture

One of the major limitations of glass ionomer is their susceptibility to brittle fracture. Compared with hybrid composite resins and dental amalgams, glass-ionomer materials are weak and lack rigidity. Clinical use should avoid situations that subject the restoration to heavy occlusal load or bending. There is a difference in strength among various glass-ionomers, with a substantial difference between the original autocure glass-ionomers and composite resins or amalgams. The resin-modified glass ionomers are stronger, with the best of them showing more than double the fracture resistance; they are nearly as resistant as the microfill composite resins.

Abrasion Resistance

Immediately after placement, glass ionomers are less resistant to abrasion than composite resin, but their resistance improves considerably as they mature. So long as the material is well supported and protected with remaining tooth structure, abrasion resistance is satisfactory. Abrasion results in loss of matrix, there will be an increase in surface roughness over time with exposure of internal porosities.

Thermal Diffusivity

This property governs the insulating efficiency of a material under transient conditions. Thermal diffusivity increases with increased P/L ratio. Therefore Type III lining cement shows a higher value than type II restorative cements. Despite its silver content, the silver cermet behaves as a cement rather than as a metallic material and has a diffusivity lower than that of polycarboxylate cements.

Colour and Translucency

Restorative Esthetic materials both autocure and resin modified, provide adequate colour matching and translucency, although translucency will take several days to develop in the autocure cements. The greatest problem with the autocure type is that it may be seriously affected by early exposure to water; therefore, careful sealing immediately after placement is essential. If colour selection is correct, careful clinical placement, with final contouring undertaken at least 24 hours later, can lead to entirely satisfactory results. If the colour match or translucency is not satisfactory after maturation over 1 week, the restoration may be laminated with composite resin.

Radio Opacity

It is desirable that an interproximal restoration in a posterior tooth be able to be differentiated radiographically from dentine or recurrent caries so that changes can be reliably monitored. These cements can be made radiopaque through the selection of an appropriate glass or the inclusion of radiopacifiers such as barium sulphate or metals such as silver.

Microleakage

Analysis of microleakage over a period of time indicated that the gap size of the restorations restored with microfilled resin and bonding agents may increase with time and the glass ionomer restorations and microfilled resin restorations showed decrease in gap size with time. The glass ionomer restorations showed a faster rate of decrease in gap sizes.

Adhesion to Tooth Structure

Glass ionomer cements have the important property of permanently adhering to untreated enamel and dentine under the moist conditions of the mouth. They share this property with the zinc polycarboxylate cements. Whether the cement penetrates the acquired pellicle on enamel or bonds to it is uncertain, but it does react with the smear layer on cut dentine.

This is an important attribute for a filling material and, to a lesser degree for a luting. Glass ionomer cements also bond to other reactive polar substrates, such as the base metals. Acid etching or other surface roughening procedures are depreciated, for the bonding is of a chemical rather than a micromechanical nature. About 80% of maximum bond strength is developed in 15 minutes but strength is developed in 15 minutes.

Bond to Mineralised Tissue

One of the most important characteristics of glass-ionomer materials is their ability to adhere chemically to mineralised tissues. The probable mechanism of adhension is based upon both diffusion and absorption phenomena. Adhesion is initiated by the polyalkenoic acid when freshly mixed material contacts the tooth surface. Phosphate ions are displaced from apatite by carboxyl groups, each phosphate ion taking a calciums ion with it to retain electrical neutrality. The setting of the material and dissolution of the enamel or dentine surface result in buffering of the polyacid, a rise in local pH and reprecipitation of minerals at the cement-tooth interface.

Bond to Collagen

Adhesion to the organic component of the dentin may also occur through either hydrogen bonding or metallic ion bridging between the carboxyl groups on the polyacid and the collagen molecules of the dentin. The strength of the union has not yet been measured because failure, under normal circumstances, is cohesive in the cement.

Conditioning the Tooth Surface

Logically, adhesion will take place best in a clean environment. Various agents have been proposed to remove some or all of the smear layer and possibly preactivate the enamel or dentine. Low molecular weight acids such as citric acid or hydrogen peroxide were recommended initially, but the most desirable material has proved to be a low - concentration polyacrylic acid, applied for a brief period and then washed thoroughly from the tooth surface. Polyacrylic acid is a part of the glass ionomer system; therefore any remaining residue will not interfere with the setting reaction.

Both glass ionomer and the tooth structure have a high surface energy and application of the polyacrylic acid will lower the surface energy of the tooth and thus increase the wettability of the surface and encourage the adaptation of the material to the tooth.

Polyacrylic acid is a mild acid with a high molecular weight and will not demineralize the tooth surface, unduly or penetrate the dentin tubules. After an application time of 10 seconds, plugs will still be present in the dentine tubules, discouraging dentin fluid flow and helping to keep the cavity dry until the restoration is in place.

Clinical Consideration

GIC in Restorative Dentistry

Placement Routine

The following routine is recommended for the placement of any glass-ionomer material.
- Prepare the cavity surface as smooth as possible
- Clean the tooth surface, where access permits, using a slurry of plain pumice and water
- Apply a liberal coat of 10% polyacrylic acid for 10 seconds
- Wash vigorously with air-water spray for 10 seconds
- Dry lightly but do not dehydrate the surface

The glass ionomer is now immediately syringed into place the supported positively with a matrix to assist adaptation between the glass ionomer and the dentine and enamel

Dispensing and Mixing

Glass ionomers are available commercially in two forms.
- Encapsulated, for mechanical mixing.
- Powder and liquid supplied separately, for hand-mixing.

Capsules

There are several types of capsule available and use of such a system provides a consistent and satisfactory powder: liquid ratio. This results in standardised mixings and setting times, and ensures optimum physical properties.

A further advantage lies in the fact tat the capsule also acts as a syringe for placement of the mixed material into the cavity.

Hand Mixing

The principal objective in mixing these materials is to wet the surface of each glass particle, without dissolving the powder completely in the liquid. The strength of the set cement lies in the remaining glass particles rather than in the matrix.

Therefore, the mix should under taken quickly on a cool dry glass slab without spreading the mix around or spatulating heavily. The powder should be dispensed onto the slab, then divided in half and mixed in two parts. The first part should be incorporated by gently but rapidly rolling the powder into the liquid within 10 seconds.

Now, include the second part entirely, leaving no residue, and finish the mixing within a further 15 seconds. The finished mixed material should be 'glossy wet' on the surface and the working time should now be between 60-90 seconds.

Technical Considerations

Critical Procedures for G.I. Restorations

To achieve a long-lasting restoration several conditions must be satisfied. They include appropriate cavity surface preparation to achieve the bonding, proper mixing to obtain a workable mixture, and surface finishing and protection during the maturing of the cements.

Surface Preparation

Clean surfaces are essential to promote adhesion. A pumice wash can be used to remove the smear layer that is produced during cavity preparation. The purpose of the pumice debridement is to remove the fluoride rich surface layer that may compromise the surface conditioning process.

Low molecular weight acids such as citric acid or hydrogen peroxide were recommended initially but the most desirable material has proved to be a low concentration polyacrylic acid applied for a bried period of 10 seconds then washed thoroughly from the tooth surface. Polyacrylic acid is a part of the glass-ionomer system, therefore any remaining residue will not interface with the setting reaction.

Both glass-ionomer and the tooth structure have a high surface energy and application of the polyacrylic acid will lower the surface energy of the tooth and thus increase the wettabiling of the surface and encourage the adaptation of the material to the tooth.

Question 2

Write about dental amalgam. Classify and mention setting reactions and properties?

Answer

Dental amalgam is an alloy of mercury, silver, copper and tin which may also contain palladium, zinc and other elements to improve handling characteristics and clinical performance. The general term AMALGAM is also used as a synonym by the dental profession.

Advantages

- Ease of handling
- Wide range of applications
- Optimal dimentional changes
- Physical characteristics comparable to enamel and dentine
- Biologically stable
- Economical.

Disadvantages

- Poor esthetics
- Marginal degradation is prominent in low copper alloy
- Excessive cavity cutting
- Less tensile strength
- Base is required as it as a good thermal conductor of heat
- Galvanic current can be produced in association which gold fillings
- Oral lichen planus is reported with silver amalgam.

Composition

GV black and ADA No. 1

Silver	-	68-72%
Tin	-	25-27%
Copper	-	2.6%
Zinc	-	0.3%

Composition by percentage of elements by weight.

Low Copper

Lathe cut or spherical

Silver	-	65-77
Tin	-	26-28
Copper	-	2-5
Zinc	-	0-2
Palladium	-	0
Indium	-	0

High Copper

Admixed
Lathecut

Silver	-	40-70
Tin	-	26-30
Copper	-	13-30
Zinc	-	0-1
Palladium	-	0
Indium	-	0

Spherical

Silver	-	40-70
Tin	-	0-30
Copper	-	20-30
Zinc	-	0
Palladium	-	0
Indium	-	0

Unicompositional

Silver	-	40-60
Tin	-	22-30
Copper	-	15-30
Zinc	-	0-1
Palladium	-	0-4
Indium	-	0

Alloy mercury reaction:

AgSn (Y)	-	untreated particles
AgHg (Y1)	-	first phase
3xHg (Y2)	-	second phase

Setting Reactions

For Lathe-cut low copper alloys. When amalgam alloy is mixed with mercury the alloy particles gets dissolved in mercury.

$$Ag_3Sn + Hg \longrightarrow Ag_2Hg_3 + Sn_{7-8}Hg_3 + Ag_3Sn$$
$$(\gamma) \qquad\qquad (\gamma_1) \qquad (\gamma_2) \qquad (\gamma)$$

For admixed high copper alloys
This reaction occurs in two phases.

Initial Reaction

$$Ag_3Sn + Ag - Cu + Hg \longrightarrow Ag_2Hg_3 + Sn_{7-8}Hg_3 + Ag_3Sn + Ag - Cu$$
$$(\gamma) \qquad (eutectic) \qquad\qquad (\gamma_1) \qquad (\gamma_2) \qquad (\gamma) \qquad (unreacted)$$

Second Phase:

It involves silver copper phase (Ag-Cu)

$$Sn_{7-8}Hg + Ag - Cu \longrightarrow Cu_6Sn_5 + Ag_2Hg_3 + Ag - Cu$$
$$(\gamma_2) \qquad (eutectic) \qquad (\eta) \qquad (\gamma_1)$$

For Unicompositional Silver Alloy

Ag-Cu phase is absent and the reaction is directly with silver, copper and tin phases.

$$Ag - Sn - Cu + Hg \longrightarrow Ag_2Hg_3 + Cu_6Sn_5 + (unconsumed$$
$$(alloy\ particles) \qquad (\gamma_1) \qquad (\eta) \qquad alloy\ particles)$$

Silver

- ❑ Increased strength
- ❑ Decrease flow
- ❑ Increase setting expansion
- ❑ Resist tarnish and corrosion
- ❑ Reduce setting time increase setting process
- ❑ Whitens the alloys.

Tin

- ❑ Reduces strength
- ❑ Helps in amalgamation since it has great affinity for mercury
- ❑ Controls the reaction between silver of mercury
- ❑ Increase the setting time
- ❑ Decrease the setting expansion
- ❑ Reduces the resistance to tarnish and corrosion.

Copper

- ❑ Increased strength
- ❑ Reduce flow
- ❑ Increase setting expansion
- ❑ Copper makes the alloy less susceptible to imperfections
- ❑ During manipulation.

Zinc

- ❑ Prevents oxidation during manufacturing
- ❑ Contributes to cleanliness workability
- ❑ If mercury containing alloys get contaminated which water results in delayed expansion
- ❑ Makes the alloy less susceptible to imperfection.

Indications

Class I Preparation

It is used in Class I preparation which are moderate to large and specially in patients with heavy occlusion loads.

Class II Preparation

- ❑ It is used in large cavity preparation when there is heavy occlusion
- ❑ When there is extension of the root surface
- ❑ When proper isolation cannot be gained.

Class III Preparation

Amalgam is used in Class III preparation only if isolation is not possible.

Class V Preparation

- ❑ Used in Class V preparation when esthetic is not a problem
- ❑ It is used when preparation is entirely on root surface
- ❑ When proper isolation cannot be gained.

Class VI Preparation

It is used in Class VI preparation only to restore cusp tips.

Tooth with Poor Prognosis

It is used in the teeth with no definitive pulpal prognosis.

Teeth having Fractured Cusp

These teeth can be restored using pin and slot at the time of amalgam restoration.

In Post-endodontic Restoration

- ❑ In case of grossly decayed teeth amalgam is used as a primary foundation base
- ❑ It is used as restorative material after pulp therapy.

Contraindications

Esthetics

- ❑ Amalgam is not preferred when esthetic is of importance
- ❑ They are contraindicated Class IV and V and sometimes in Class III also.

Small Class I and Class II Preparations

Small to moderate Class I and Class II preparation should be avoided with amalgam restoration as they can be restored with composite to preserve the tooth structure.

In Grossly Decayed Teeth

As grossly decayed teeth and the remaining tooth structure cannot be reinforce by amalgam it should be contraindicated and these teeth should be restored by cast restorations.

SHORT ESSAYS

Question 1

Write a short note on cermet cement?

Answer

- Also called as cermet ionomer cements or metal modified glass ionomer cement. It is the fusing of glass powder to silver particles through sintering that can be made to react with polyacid to form the cermet
- Sintering is done at pressure of 300 MPa at 800°C
- 5% titanium dioxide is added for the aesthetic improvement.

Metal Modified GIC are of Two Types

1. Silver alloy admixed: Spherical amalgam alloy powder when mixed with Type II GIC powder is called miracle mix.
2. Cermet: Silver particles are bonded to glass particles.

Indications

- Used as core build up materials
- Served as root caps of teeth under the over dentures
- Lining for silver amalgam restoration
- Temporary restoration.

Contraindications

- Anterior restoration
- Areas with high occlusal load.

Properties

- Mechanical
  - Strength: 105 MPa
  - Fracture toughness low
  - More resistant to wear than Type I, II GIC.
- Anticariogenic
  - Due to release of fluoride ions
  - Fluoride release is less due to the metal casting in cermet.
- Aesthetics.
  - Poor due to metallic phase leads to greyish colour tint.

Question 2

Write a short note on resin-modified glass ionomer cement?

Answer

- Also known as hybrid ionomer
- It is defined as hybrid cement that sets via an acid base reaction and partly via a photochemical polymerisation reaction
- Developed by Antonucci, McKinney and SB Mitra.

Classification

Depending upon the predominant components:

- Resin-modified glass ionomer cement (RMG1), e.g., Fuji II LC, Vitremer
- Polyacid modified composite (PMC), e.g., Dyract, VariGlass VLC.

Composition

Powder

- Fluoroaluminosilicate: leachable glass
- Initiator for light curing
- Initiator for chemical curing
- Polymerizable resin.

Liquid

- Water
- Polyacrylic acid
- Methacrylate and hydroxyethylmethacrylate (HEMA) monomer.

Uses

- As bases and liners
- Restoration of Class I, III or IV cavities
- As pit and fissure sealant
- For repairing damaged amalgam cores
- As core build up
- Root surface caries
- As adhesive for orthodontic brackets.

Setting Reaction

- It is set partly by acid-base reaction and partly by photochemical polymerisation
- In some polymerisation there is chemical initiator mechanism involved.

Properties

- Strength
  - Compressive strength is slightly lower to conventional glass ionomer cement
  - Tensile strength is slightly higher because of plastic deformation, before fracture.
- Hardness: 40 KHN
- Adhesive to tooth: Reduced (reduced carboxylic acid in the liquid. Also by interruption of chemical bond by resin matrix)
- Adhesion to restorative materials:
  - Used as liner and bases
  - They have higher bond strength compared to composite.
- Marginal adaptation: due to polymerisation it shows greater shrinkage on setting
- Anticariogenicity: it is anticariogenic due to fluoride release
- Aesthetics: less translucent
- Pulp response: mild.

Question 3

Write a short note on compomers?

Answer

- It is defined as resin based composite material containing silicate glass filled particles and methacrylate and acidic monomers as matrices
- Compomers = Glass ionomers + composites
- They are also called as polyacid modified composites
- They are polymer-based composites that have been modified to permit fluoride release from glass or matrix phases
- They possess both the properties of glass ionomer and composites.

Composition

Powder

- Strontium aluminium fluorosilicate glass
- Metallic oxides
- Self and light cured initiators.

Liquid

- Polymerisable methacrylate/carboxylic acid monomer
- Multifunctional acrylate/phosphate monomer
- Diacrylate monomer
- Water.

Properties

- Compressive strength   –   100 MPa
- Elastic modulus   –   3.6 GPa
- Bond strength   –   18–24 MPa with dentine
- Setting time   –   3 minutes
- Solubility   –   Low
- Fluoride release   –   Yes.

Question 4

Write a short note on atraumatic restorative treatment?

Answer

- Also known as ART.
- It is a technique that permits the basic restorative procedures in places without the modern auxiliary equipment such as water, electricity and power driven tools
- Introduced by Jo Frenclean in 1996
- Only hand instruments are used to remove carious lesions.

Indications

- Only in cavities that are small and not deep
- Cavities that are accessible to hand instruments
- Restoration in deciduous teeth
- Small to moderate pit and fissure caries
- Mentally retarded, physically disabled of and special child
- Public health programs.

Advantages

- Less trauma and to conserve sound tooth structure
- Painless
- Cost effective
- Friendly procedure for children and fearful adults
- For special child.

Technique

- Isolate the carious lesion with cotton rolls
- Use hand instrument to remove the carious lesion

- Carious tissues which are soft should be removed with spoon excavator
- Removal of soft and over hanging tissue to be removed before restoration
- Restored with GIC
- Excess GIC should be removed after restoration.

Indications

- For fixed partial dentures
- Cementation of cast alloy, porcelain fused to metal (PFM)
- For bearing low stress area, e.g., Class III and V cavities.

Question 5

Write a short note on zinc oxide eugenol cement?

Answer

- They are cements that have low strength
- They are less irritating of all the dental cements and have an obtunding (soothing pain) effect on the dentine that is exposed
- It is been used since 1890.

Classification

- Type I: Temporary cementation
- Type II: Permanent cementation
- Type III: Temporary filling material and thermal insulating ball
- Type IV: Cavity liners.

Supplied As

- Powder and liquid
- Two paste system.

Composition

Table 5.4: Composition of zinc oxide eugenol cement

Powder		
• ZnO	Principle ingredient	69%
• White rosin	To reduce brittleness of set cement	29.3%
• Zn stearate	Accelerator and plasticizer	1%
• Zn acetate	Accelerator and improves strength	0.7%
• Mgo	Acts with eugenol	
Liquid		
• Eugenol	Reacts with zinc oxide (ZnO) and magnesium oxide (MgO)	–85%
• Olive oil	Plasticizer	15%

Setting Reaction

- It is a chelation reaction
- $ZnO + H_2O \rightarrow Zn\,(OH)_2$
- Hydrolysis of ZnO + 0 hydroxide
- $Zn\,(OH)_2 + 2HE \rightarrow ZnE_2 + 2H_2O$
  (base)   (acid)   (salt)
- Acid-base reaction to form chelate
- Setting time 4–10 minutes.

Properties

Mechanical Properties

- Compressive strength: 3–5.5 MPa
- Tensile strength: 0.32–5.3 MPa
- Modulus of elasticity: 0.22–5.4 GPa.

Thermal Properties

- Same as dentine
- Coefficient of thermal expansion: $35 \times 10{-}6/°C$.

Solubility and Disintegration

- Highest among cements
- They disintegrate in fluids
- (0.4%–wt).

Thickness of Film

- Higher than other cements
- 25 microns.

Adhesion

Does not adhere with enamel or dentine

Biological Properties

- Ph: 6.6–8.0
- Less irritating among all cements
- Pulpal response: minimum
- Bacteriostatic
- Obtundant.
- Optical properties : opaque.

Manipulation

- **Powder/liquid ratio:** 4 : 1 to 6 : 1 by weight.
- Measured quantity of powder and liquid are taken on a glass slab and mixed with a stainless steel spatula.
- Small increments are added until it is mixed properly.

Two Paste System

Equal amount of paste is squeezed onto the glass until a uniform colour is seen.

Modified Zinc Oxide Eugenol (ZOE) Cements

- ❑ Erythrocyte binding protein (EBA) alumina modified cements
- ❑ Increase in mechanical properties seen.

Composition

Powder

- ❑ ZnO — 70%
- ❑ Alumina — 30%

Liquid

- ❑ EBA — 62.5%
- ❑ Eugenol — 37.5%
- ❑ Polymer reinforced ZOE cement.

Composition

Powder

Finely divided natural resin.

Liquid

- ❑ Eugenol
- ❑ Acetic acid: accelerator
- ❑ Thymol: antibacterial agent
- ❑ Used as:
  - ○ Luting agent
  - ○ Temporary filling material
  - ○ Cavity lines.

CHAPTER 6

Dental Amalgam Restoration

LONG ESSAYS

Question 1

Define dental amalgam. Discuss composition, classification, indications, contraindications, advantages and disadvantages?

Answer

Dental amalgam is an alloy made by mixing mercury with a silver-tin dental amalgam.

Composition

Low Copper Alloy

- Ag   -   65%
- Sn   -   29%
- Cu   -   2–5% (6%)
- Zn   -   0–2%

High Copper Alloy

- Admixed:
  - Ag - 65–70%
  - Sn - 17%
  - Cu - 9–20%
  - Zn - 1–2%
- Single composition or unicomposition:
  - Ag - 60%
  - Sn - 27%
  - Cu - 13–30%
  - Zn - 0–2%

Functions of Individual Alloying Metals

Silver

- Major constituent in alloy
- Whitens alloy
- Decreases creep
- Increases strength

- Increases setting expansion
- Increases tarnish corrosion.

Tin

- Controls reaction between silver and mercury
- Decreases setting expansion
- Decreases strength and hardness
- Decreases tarnish and corrosion resistance.

Copper

- Decreases brittleness
- Increases strength and hardness
- Increases setting expansion.

Zinc

- Acts as scavenger
- Increases plasticity
- Decreases tarnish and corrosion
- Prevents oxidation of alloys during manufacture
- Causes delayed expansion, if amalgam alloy is contaminated with moisture during manipulation.

Palladium

- Increases hardness
- Whitens alloy.

Mercury

Sometimes present in alloy powders in range of 2–3%, they are called Pt amalgamated alloys which increase the rate of reaction.

Classification

- Based on amalgam particle geometry:
  - Lathe cut alloys
  - Spherical alloys
  - Admixed alloys.

- Based on amalgam alloy size:
  - Regular cut
  - Fine cut
  - Micro-fine cut.
- Based on copper content:
  - High copper amalgam. Copper content > 6 %
  - Low copper amalgam. Copper content < 6 %.
- Based on zinc content:
  - Zinc containing amalgam. Zinc content > 0.01%
  - Non-zinc Containing amalgam. Zinc content < 0.01%.
- Based on addition of noble metals:
  - Palladium
  - Gold
  - Platinum
  - Indium.
- Based on generation:
  - 1st generation: 3 parts Ag + 1 part Sn (peritectic)
  - 2nd generation: 3 parts Ag + 1 part Sn + Cu + 1 % Zn
  - 3rd generation: Blending spherical Ag-Cu (eutectic) to original powder
  - 4th generation: Alloy Cu to Ag and Sn up to 29% ternary alloy
  - 5th generation: Ag + Cu + Sn + In
  - 6th generation: Alloy Pd (10%), Ag (62%) and Cu (25%) to 1st, 2nd and 3rd generations.
- Based on composition:
  - Unicomposition (same chemical composition)
  - Admixed (spherical eutectic high Cu + lathe cut low Cu).
- Based on number of alloyed materials:
  - Binary: Ag–Sn
  - Ternary: Ag–Sn–Cu
  - Quaternary: Ag–Sn–Cu–In.

Indications

- Used in moderate to large Class I and II restorations
- Class V and VI restorations
- Badly broken teeth which require pulp evaluation before final restoration
- Those teeth that require increased resistance and retention form before the process of crown placement or metallic onlay
- Tooth with fractured cusp
- Post endodontic restorations.

Contraindications

- Aesthetic critical areas
- Class II and V restorations
- Small to moderate restorations in posterior teeth.

Advantages

- Easy to use
- High compressive strength
- Excellent wear resistance
- Long term clinical result
- Low cost
- Less technique sensitive
- Self-sealing
- Maintains good anatomic form.

Disadvantages

- Poor aesthetic
- Non insulting
- Brittle
- It weakens tooth structure
- Mercury toxicity
- Can be corroded and also prone to galvanic action
- Less conservative.

Question 2

Describe the properties of dental amalgam. Write in brief the factors affecting quality of dental amalgam?

Answer

Properties of Dental Amalgam

Compressive strength:
- American National Standards Institute (ANSI)/American Dental Association (ADA) specification no ≠ 1
- Compressive strength is 80 MPa after 1 hour of setting
- It is stored in compression
- Work tension and shear strength
- So at the time of amalgam restoration it should be designed so that it receives maximum compressive forces and minimum tensile or shear forces
- Most common fractures of amalgam restoration occurs at the margins
- Leading to corrosion and secondary caries
- Amalgam strength – 31 MPa
- Amalgam and its strength is described in **(Table 6.1)**.

Table 6.1: Amalgam and its strength

Amalgam	1 hour (MPa)	7 Days (MPa)
Low copper	145	343
Admixed high copper	137	431
Single composition high copper	-	-

Factors Affecting Amalgam Strength

Trituration

Trituration is a process in which the alloy particles are brought in contact with the mercury.

- It is done to reduce the particle size and to increase the surface area, which in turn increases the rate of amalgamation
- Over and under trituration decreases the strength of any amalgam
- Over trituration leads to cracks in crystals
- Under trituration will lead to interfaces formation as the maximum strength is achieved with mixing till the coherent mass of matrix.

Mercury Content

- Mercury content is important so that each alloy particle is wetted thoroughly
- Under and over mercury content or mixing flaw will lead to dry granular mix resulting in rough, pitted surface. Also strength is compromised.

Condensation

- It is the process that is required to squeeze out mercury (Hg) (for Lathe-cut alloy)
- Increased condensation pressure leads to decreased porosity and greater strength
- Normal condensation pressure leads to adequate strength.

Porosity

- Reduces the strength of set amalgam
- Results in corrosion and ultimately fracture of the restoration.

Amalgam Hardening Rate

- Strength of amalgam improves with time
- According to ADA specification: Strength of amalgam after 1 hour should be 80 MPa
- 70% of strength is gained after 8 hours
- Patient should be instructed not to bite from the site of amalgam restoration for that amount of time, i.e., 8 hours.

Dimensional Changes

- Manipulation of amalgam leads to expansion or contraction
- Contraction leads to micro leakage, secondary caries and plaque accumulation
- Expansion leads to excessive pressure on pulp leading to post-operative sensitivity
- Ideal example is the initial contraction for approximately 20 minutes after the beginning of trituration and after that expansion happens.

Delayed Expansion

This expansion starts of the 3–5 days after restoration. It can continue for months. Reaching value equal to greater than 400 μm.

- The expansion happens, if the zinc containing amalgam is contaminated with water during condensation or at the time of trituration, expansion at large proportion is seen
- Due to electrolytic acid of zinc and water hydrogen is produced
- This hydrogen is then collected within the restoration. This internal pressure at high levels causing amalgam restoration to creep, followed by expansion
- This contamination can occur anytime during the procedure
- Expansion causes pressure on pulp and causes throbbing pain
- Pressure on pulp can be up to = 200 Lb/sq. in

Creep

It is defined as time dependent plastic deformation of a material under a static or dynamic load.

- Creep in amalgam is a slow process
- Higher creep = greater chances of marginal breakdown
- Low copper amalgam: 0.8–8%
  High copper amalgam: 0.4–1%
- According to ADA specification no ≠ 1 the creep value should be less than 3%.

Minimising Creep Rates

- By minimizing mercury alloy ratio
- Reducing condensation pressure
- Proper timing and handling in trituration.

Tarnish and Corrosion

- Amalgam restorations are prone to tarnish and corrode in the oral environment
- Tarnish depends mostly on individual oral cavity environment and the alloy used
- Corrosion occurs on the metal surface along the interface between tooth surface and the restoration
- This space between alloy and tooth permits micro leakage of electrolytes
- The build of corrosion products gradually seals this space. That is why dental amalgam is considered as self-sealing restoration
- Most common corrosion products in amalgam are oxides of:
  - Chloride
  - Tin

- Corrosion occurs when a gold restoration is placed in contact with amalgam restoration
- Corrosion is the result of difference in electromotive force of the two materials.

Factors Affecting Amalgam Quality

Factors administered by the operator
- Alloy selection
- Alloy mercury ratio
- Trituration
- Condensation
- Marginal integrity
- Anatomical features
- Final finishing.

Factors Administered by the Manufactures

- Alloy composition
- Heat treatment of alloy
- Method of alloy production, i.e., shape, size and method
- Alloy particle surface treatment
- Alloy form when it is supplied.

Question 3

Write in brief about manipulation of dental amalgam?

Answer

Manipulation of Dental Amalgam

This process is done in five ways:
1. Mercury alloy ratio.
2. Proportioning.
3. Trituration.
4. Mulling.
5. Consistency.

Mercury Alloy Ratio

- Mercury in excess was used to attain smooth and plastic mix for amalgam. The excess mercury caused toxicity and deleterious effect on both physical and mechanical properties of restoration
- So now excess mercury is reduced by two processes:
  - Squeezing out excess mercury using a squeeze cloth
  - By working each increment to the top after which removal of mercury rich amalgam from top of each increment.
- Although the best method is to reduce the original mercury ratio in the alloy (minimal mercury technique/earners technique)
- Recommended ratio mercury: Alloy is –1 : 1

- Recommended ratio of Lathe-cut alloy: 50%
- Recommended ratio for spherical alloy: 42%.

Proportioning

- Use of mercury and alloy dispensers most common: based on volumetric proportion
- Pre-weighted pellets are the most convenient methods The reason being that mercury in liquid form can be measured by volume using mercury dispensers
- Use of disposable capsules which contain pre-proportioned quantity of mercury and alloy are now widely used
- To prevent any amalgamation while storage both alloy and mercury are separated physically from each other
- New alloys are now available as self-activating capsules. They release mercury into the alloy chamber with oscillations of the amalgamator
- Mercury should never be added after trituration.

Trituration

Objectives

- It is used to wet all the surfaces of alloy particles with mercury
- It attains workable plastic mass
- Removes the oxide layer from the surface of alloy particles by rubbing
- Forming matrix crystals by dissolving alloy in mercury
- To keep matrix crystals small.

Types of Trituration

- It is done by hand, the use of mortar and pestle
- The drawbacks were not proper result and also it was technique sensitive
- The process was very time consuming.

Mechanical Trituration

- Amalgamators are used for better procedure and it saves time. Amalgamators works on speed mixing:
  - Low : 3200–3400 cycles/minute
  - Medium : 3700–3800 cycles/minute
  - High : 4000–4000 cycles/minute.
- The amalgamator speed is used as per the manufacturer's instruction.

Mulling

- Mulling is a process which improves the homogeneity of the mix and achieves a single consistent mix.

❑ The mix is placed on a dry rubber dam and is vigorously rubbed between thumb of one hand and the palm of second hand for approximate time ranging between 2.5 seconds

❑ After the mechanical trituration is done, mix is then triturated in a pestle free capsule for approximately 2–3 seconds.

Consistency of Mix

After trituration consistency should be:

❑ Smooth
❑ Shiny appearance
❑ Should be coherent
❑ Warm when removed from capsule
❑ It should not be granular.

Normal Mix

❑ Should be wet and plastic
❑ Should be smooth and soft in consistency and also shiny surface
❑ Should possess good compressive and tensile strength

Under-triturated Mix

❑ Dull appearance
❑ Grainy in consistency
❑ After carving gives a rough surface
❑ Rapid hardening at the time of mixing
❑ Low strength
❑ Prone to tarnish and corrosion.

Over Triturated Mix

❑ Plastic appearance and property
❑ Hard to remove from the capsule
❑ Working time is reduced
❑ Increased creep and contraction
❑ Low strength.

Question 4

Write in brief about setting reaction of low copper and high copper amalgams?

Answer

Low Copper Amalgam

❑ Silver-mercury compound: γ_1 (Gamma one phase which is Ag_2H_3) **(Fig. 6.1)**
❑ Tin-mercury compound: γ_2 (Gamma two phase which is $Sn_{7-8}Hg$)

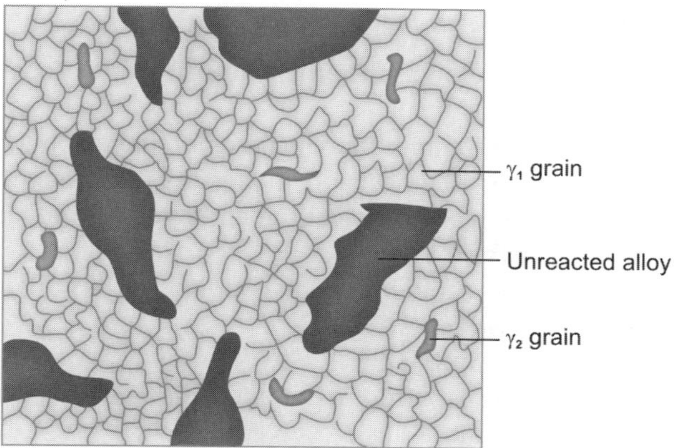

Fig. 6.1: Schematic diagram of final set low copper amalgam showing gamma one phase

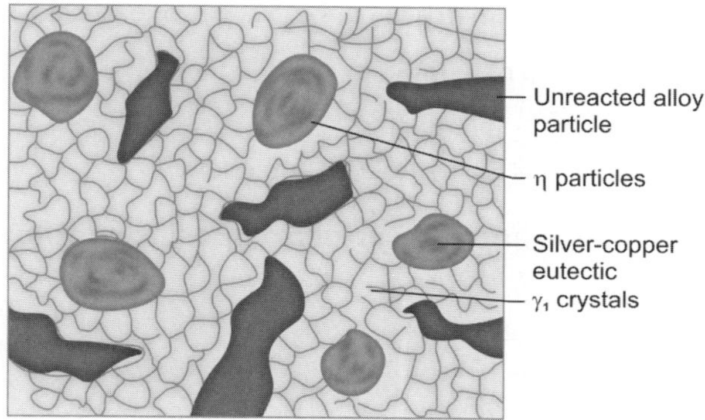

Fig. 6.2: Schematic diagram of final set low copper amalgam showing gamma two phase

❑ Solubility of silver in mercury is less than that of tin. So γ_1 phase precipitates first γ_2 and after that γ_1 and γ_2 crystals grow while the remaining mercury dissolves in alloy particle. That is the principle behind amalgam hardening when mercury disappears
❑ Alloy particles are surrounded and bound by solid γ_1 and γ_2 crystals
❑ The physical properties of hardened amalgam depend on the percentage of each microstructural phase **(Fig. 6.2)**
❑ The more unconsumed Ag–Sn particles that are retained, the stronger will be the amalgam in the final structure
❑ γ_2 phase – weakest and most prone to corrosion
❑ The percentage of γ_1 phase: 54–56% by volume
❑ Unreached alloy: 27–35% by volume
❑ γ_2 phase: 11–13% by volume.
❑ Reaction $\gamma + Hg \; \gamma_1(Ag_2Hg_3) + g2\,(Sn_{7-8}\,Hg)$
(Alloy particle) + unconsumed alloy particles (γ)

High Copper Amalgam

Two types of high copper alloy are as follows:

Admixed Alloys

At the time of trituration the amalgam particles dissolve in mercury.
- Tin dissolves 170 times more in mercury than copper
- Silver dissolves 10 times more in mercury than copper
- Silver and tin hence dissolves the entire mercury to form γ_1 and γ_2 phases
- Later γ_2 phase reacts with silver copper particles to form h (eta) phase which is CU_6Sn_5
- γ_2 phase is replaced by h
- Finally γ_1 particles surround the unreached silver–copper particles (**Fig. 6.3**).

Initial Reaction

$\gamma(Ag_3Sn) + Ag–Cu$ (eutectic) $+ Hg$
g1 + g2 + unconsumed alloy of both types of particles

Secondary Slow Reaction

$\gamma_2(Sn_{7-8}Hg) + Ag–Cu$ (eutectic)
$\gamma_1(Ag_2Hg_3) + h(CU_6Sn_5) + Ag–Cu$ (eutectic)

Single Composition Alloys/unicompositional Alloys

- Composition:
  - Silver : 60 wt%
  - Tin : 27wt%
  - Copper : 13 wt%.
- Formation of g1 and g2 phases forms when tin dissolves faster with mercury
- γ_2 phase then reacts with silver-copper phase forming h phase
- γ_1 phase grows and the matrix formed binds together the partially dissolved alloy particles
- η crystals look like-meshes of rod like crystals
- η crystals strengthen bonding between the alloy particles and g1 grains. There is an interlocking that is seen between h crystals and γ_1 grains.

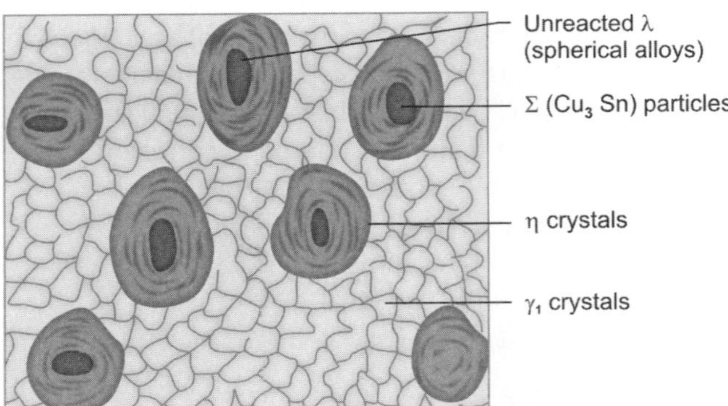

Fig. 6.3: Schematic diagram of final set high copper alloys

- This interlocking improves amalgams resistance to deformation
- Mostly no γ_2 phase or very little is found in single composition amalgam.

Reaction

$\gamma(Ag_3Sn) + e(CU_3Sn)\ Hg\ \ \gamma_1(Ag_2H_3) + \eta(Cu_6Sn_5).$

Question 5

Discuss in detail class I cavity for amalgam restorations?

Answer

Definition

All the pit and fissure restorations are called Class 1. They are divided into three groups:
1. Restorations on occlusal surface of premolars and molars.
2. Restorations on occlusal two-third of the facial and lingual surfaces of molars.
3. Restorations on lingual surface of maxillary incisors.

Procedure

Initial tooth preparation:
The outline form (**Fig. 6.4**):

Shape

- Maxillary premolar – Butterfly shaped (**Fig. 6.5**)
- Maxillary molar (not involving oblique ridge)
- Involving oblique ridge: H-shaped
- Maxillary 3rd molar
- G-shaped
- Mandibular 1st premolar
- Involving triangular ridge (**Fig. 6.6**)
  - Dumb-bell shape
- Does not involve triangular ridge
  - Snake eye (**Fig. 6.7**)
- Tricuspid premolar
- γ shape
- Mandibular 1st molar
- Elongated shape with two buccal and one lingual extension
- Mandibular 2nd molar
- Elongated shape with two buccal and one lingual extension (+ shaped).

Burs

- Number 245 inverted cone – amalgam cavity preparation
- Number 330 pear shaped-conservative amalgam preparation.

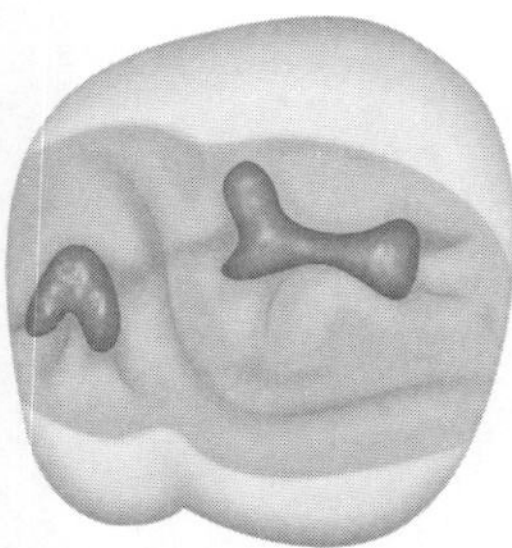

Fig. 6.4: Conservative class I cavity preparation of maxillary first molar leaving the oblique ridge intact

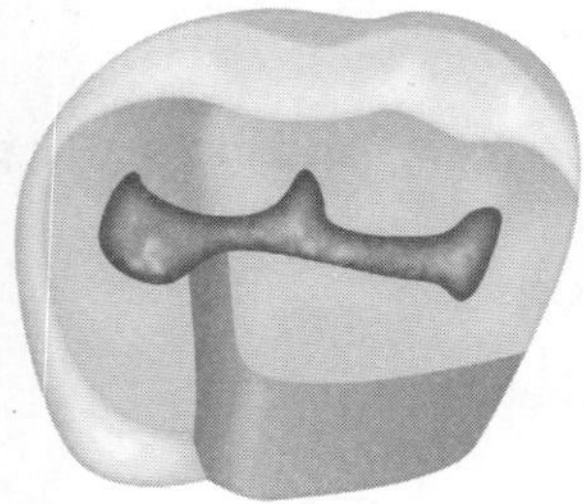

Fig. 6.5: Conventional class I cavity preparation on maxillary first molar including oblique ridge

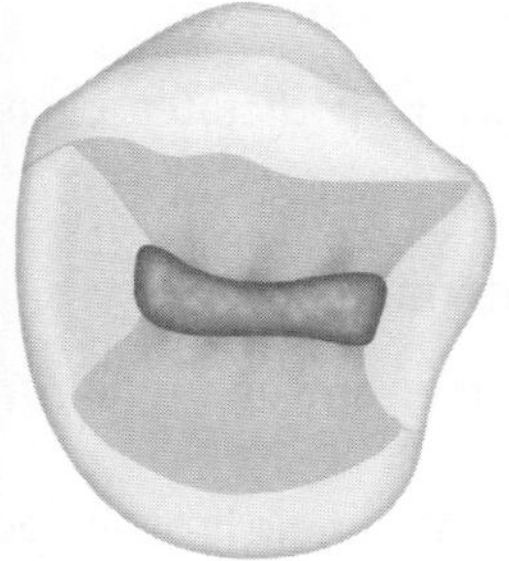

Fig. 6.6: Outline form of conventional class I occlusal cavity preparation

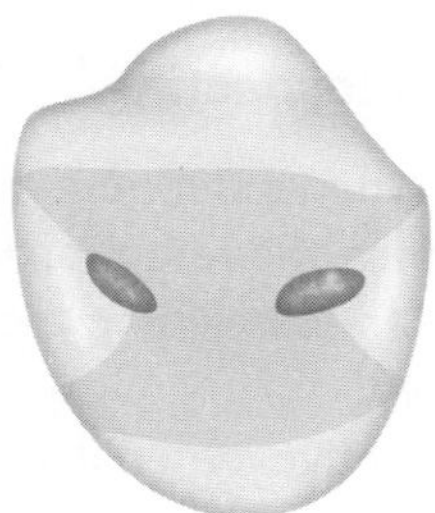

Fig. 6.7: Outline form of conservative class I cavity preparation of mandibular first premolar

Technique

- The tooth preparation is started by entering the most carious/deepest pit with a punch cut
- The bur is held parallel to the long axis of tooth

- In case both pits are equally carious, distal pit punch cut is given which provides increased visibility
- Pulpal depth at central fissure: 1.5 mm
- The outline form includes defective/faulty occlusal pits and fissure
- The distance between cavity margins to proximal surface should not be < 1.6 mm
- For premolar: 1.6 mm
- For molar: 2 mm
- At marginal ridge.
- Pulpal floor should be flat but at the same time should follow the contour of dentinoenamel junction
- Extension should follow from central fissure moving towards mesial pit
- Ideal faciolingual width: 1–1.5 mm
- Ideal faciolingual depth: 1.5–2 mm
- Enamel margins are made of full length enamel rods which rest on sound dentine
- Initial depth of pulpal floor is maintained so in case of restoration or caries present can be removed at the time of final tooth preparation.

Primary Resistance Form

- It is a box-shaped cavity with relatively flat floor
- There is minimum extension of external walls
- Sufficient depth required –1.5 mm
- To protect the tooth structure and prevention of encroaching of pulp horns is done by extending the preparation around the cusps
- Faults are included and margin placement should be done on smooth and sound tooth structure.
- Establishing ideal enamel margins
- In case two outlines are less than 0.5 mm apart, they are joined to make one outline by removal of weak enamel
- Preservation of strong marginal ridges
- Cavosurface angle should be 90%.

Primary Retention Form

- It is done by a parallel or slight occlusal convergence opposing the external walls
- Occlusal dovetail is given
- Marginal ridges should be conserved
- A slight undercut in the dentine is given near pulpal wall.

Convenience Forms

Convenience form gives adequate access and visibility for tooth preparation and also for instrumentation and condensation. A proper carving of amalgam is also included in this form.

Final Tooth Preparation

- Removal of remaining defective enamel and infecte dentine
- In case of deep pits and fissures:
  - Extend the pulpal floor **(Fig. 6.8)**
  - Depth of 2 mm is suitable
  - Bur no ≠ 245° is used.
- Removal of infected dentine is done by discoid type spoon excavator. Also carbide round bur is used
- Infected dentine should be removed till the time until there is hard and firm tooth structure
- Periphase dentinoenamel junction (DEJ) should be caries free
- It should be kept in mind that removal of carious dentine should not interfere in the resistance form.

Pulp Protection

- Varnish is used in ideal tooth preparation
- In deep carious excavation a thin layer of 0.5–0.75 mm base is applied
- Base should not be present on the cavity walls. It leads to dissolution in water and micro leakage through the gaps
- Base should be strong so it can withstand masticatory forces and amalgam manipulation
- Bases that can be used are:
  - Light cured resin modified glass ionomer (RMGI)
  - Desensitisers
  - Bonding systems.

Finishing the Wall

The cavosurface angle should be 90°. It should be made sure that all unsupported enamel is removed.

Cleaning

- Air spray and water is used to clean it thoroughly
- It should be dried with moisture
- Inspection for final approval.

Question 6

Describe the Class III cavity preparation for Class III amalgam preparation?

Answer

Definition

It is the restoration on the proximal surface of the anterior teeth that do not involve the incisal angle.

Indications

- On the distal surface of maxillary and mandibular canines
- For partial denture abutment teeth.

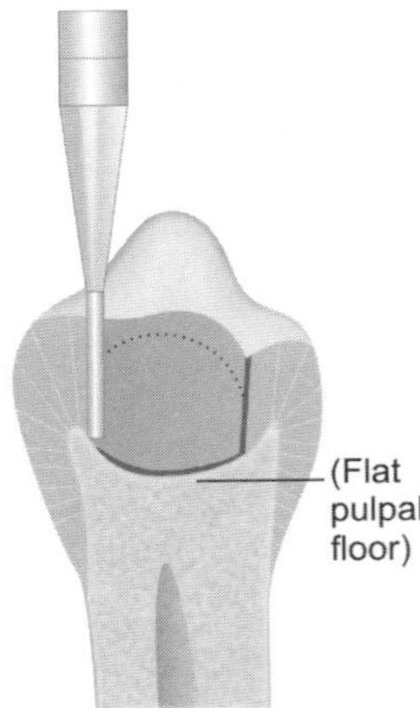

Fig. 6.8: Class I cavity preparation (Flat pulpal floor)

Contraindications

Areas where aesthetic is important.

Depth

Translation extent.

Occlusal Gingival Orientation

It is the bur tilt given. It dictates occlusal height of the "lock".

Finishing of External Walls

- Unsupplied enamel and marginal irregularities should be removed
- Only 90° cavosurface angle is given, occlusal cavosurface bevel is not indicated
- If bevelling the gingival margin is at distal surface, GMT (gingival marginal trimmer) is used.

Cleaning / Sealing / Inspecting

- Pulp is protected when it is required
- Secondary resistance and retention form.
- Both resistance of the remaining tooth structure against fracture from forces
- Resistance of restorative material against fracture.

Secondary Retention Locks

They prevent lateral displacement of restoration which in turn increases fracture strength of the restoration.

Four Determinants of Proximal Locks

- Position: Positioned 0.2 mm axial to the DEJ
- Translation: Direction of movement of axis of bur

- Round bur is used to remove hard caries slowly
- Spoon excavator (discoid type) is used in the removal of soft caries
- A partial extension of lingual and facial walls is done so:
  - The entire wall does not gets involved
  - For proper accessibility and visibility.
- 90° cavosurface angle
- The removal of defective enamel or infected dentine should not compromise resistance form
- Old restorative material should not be removed unless:
  - Its symptomatic
  - Shows evidence of recurrent caries.

Primary Retention Form

- An occlusal dovetail is given
- Also by the enhancement of occlusal convergence of lingual and facial walls.

Convenience Form

- An appropriate extension of the outline form during tooth preparation is done
- It is specific because of the following:
  - For the better access to lesion
  - To permit proper finishing
  - Access to condensing instrument
  - Periodic assessment
  - Self-care.

Final Tooth Preparations

Removal of any remaining defective enamel or infected carious dentine.

Primary Resistance Form

- Gingival and pulpal walls should be:
- Flat
- Perpendicular to forces directed along the long axis of the tooth
- Wall extension should be restricted so that strong cusps and ridges are preserved
- Occlusal outline form is restricted so that areas receive minimal occlusal contact
- To optimize the strength of amalgam and tooth structure a reverse curve is given at the junction of the occlusal cusp and at the proximal box
- Rounding of internal and external line and point angles so that to reduce stress concentration
- For resisting masticatory stress adequate thickness of restoration is given

- Length of axial wall from pulpal floor: 0.5–0.6 mm
- Apex occlusal and gingival seat base: triangular
- Extension of facial and lingual margins in proximal area into their respective embrasures.
- Proximal flare should be at right angles to the external tooth surface
- While preparation of proximal box a matrix band is used so that the bur does not come in contact with the adjacent tooth
- All the weakened enamel that is along the gingival wall is removed using enamel hatchet using a scraping motion
- A wooden wedge is placed in the gingival embrasure. It is done to depress the soft tissue and the rubber dam to protect them **(Fig. 6.9)**.

Gingival Seat

- Should be placed 1–2 mm supragingivally
- Subgingival margins placement are avoided
- Width of gingival seat:
  - Premolars: 0.6–0.8 mm
  - Molars: 0.8–1.0 mm.

Axial Wall

- It follows the faciolingual contour of the proximal surface of DEJ.
- It should be in dentine and parallel to the long tooth axis for:
  - Convenience form
  - Retention groove placement in axiolingual and axiofacial line angle without undermining the proximal enamel **(Fig. 6.10)**
  - Providing additional bulk of amalgam.

Advantages

- It is stronger
- Easier technique of placement
- Not expensive
- Easier finishing and polishing procedure.

Disadvantages

- Unaesthetic
- Metallic
- Can cause mercury contamination
- Requires 90° cavosurface margin, specific axial depth
- Requires secondary retentive features for a less conservative preparation.

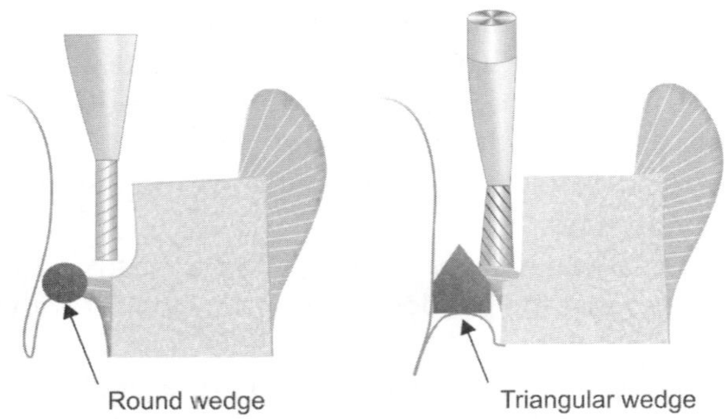

Fig. 6.9: Wedging required to protect gingiva during proximal box preparation

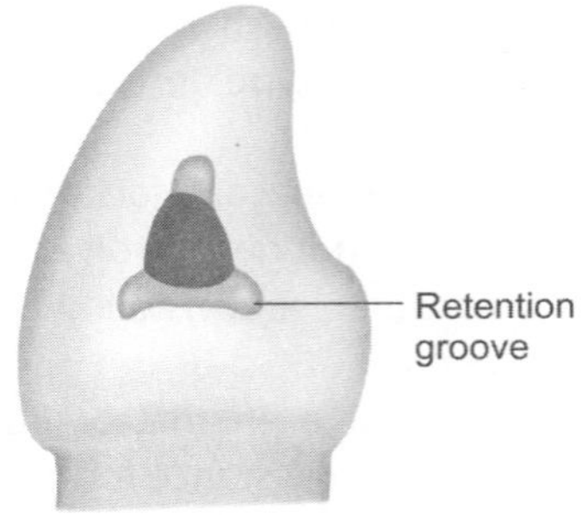

Fig. 6.10: Class III cavity preparation

Tooth Preparation

- Outline form is triangular with rounded corners
- Labial side conforms to the proximal surface anatomy more than the lingual surface
- Lingual side is the access point for the tooth preparation to conserve the enamel facial to the proximal contact
- Lingual dovetail indicated
- A Number 0.5 or Number 1 bur is used for small carious lesion
- The entry cut should be made gingival to the contact area
- Initial axial depth inside the DEJ = 0.50–0.6 mm on the root surface (cementum) = 0.75–0.8 mm
- The bur is positioned perpendicular to the long axis to the lingual surface and it is directed at a mesial angle. It should be as close as to the adjacent tooth

- The extension of facial margin is = 0.2, 0.3 mm into the facial embrasure
- At the axiogingival line angle. The cutting angle bisecting the angle between axial walls and gingival wall
- The direction of the gingival groove is slightly gingival/incisal than the axial groove
- At the axiogingivofacial and axiogingivolingual point angles two gingival grooves are placed instead of a continuous grooves for less retention
- After the proximal box preparation a lingual dovetail is placed but only if it is needed
- Axial depth of the dovetail = 1 mm
- Axial wall should be parallel to the lingual surface of the tooth
- GMT is used to bevel the axiopulpal line angle.

SHORT ESSAYS

Question 1

Discuss the cavity design for management of proximal carious lesions on posterior teeth with amalgam (Class II)?

Answer

Definition

It is defined as the restorations on the proximal surfaces of the posterior teeth.

Initial Tooth Preparation

Outline Form

Occlusal Outline Form

- The occlusal steps of Class II tooth preparation is similar to Class I

- The point of entry is a pit nearest to the involved proximal surface
- A punch cut is given
- Bur should be held parallel to the long axis of the tooth
- Initial depth at central fissure is 1.5 mm
- Depth on the prepared external walls is 2 mm
- Margins are extended to allow sufficient access.

Proximal Outline Form

- Objective of box preparation:
  - To include:
    - All caries
    - Existing restoration
    - Faults.
  - Forming a butt joint (90° cavosurface margin) **(Fig. 6.11)**.
    - Establishing 0.5 mm clearance with adjacent proximal surface lingually, gingivally and facially

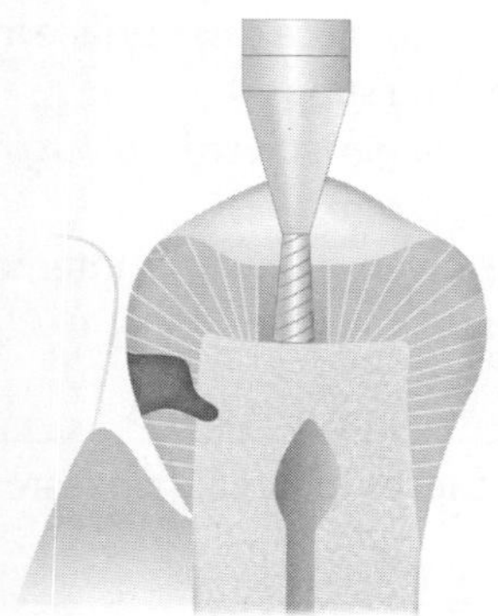

Fig. 6.11: Class II cavity preparation

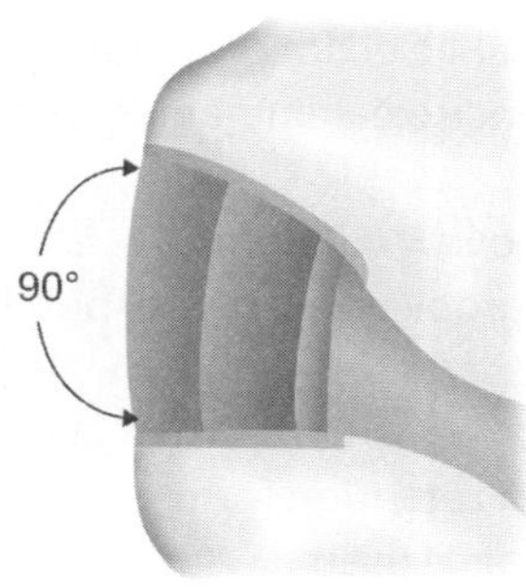

Fig. 6.12: Reverse curve is indicated when mesiofacial enamel wall is parallel enamel rod direction

- Initially the isolation of proximal enamel is done by proximal ditch-cut
- The final location of proximal box that is related to contact area is visualised for the prevention of overextension of margins of the prepared tooth
- The bur is directed gingivally and a little towards the mesial surface. So that it moves facially and lingually along the DEJ
- Extension of proximal ditch is done gingivally and beyond proximal contact area or it can be the area of caries, which ever is greater
- The occlusal step is slightly wide faciolingually to get additional width for proximal box
- A reverse curve is given, which results in occlusal outline form. The mesiofacial wall is perpendicular to the direction of enamel rods that conserves the facial cusp structure. The reverse curve lingually is minimum due to larger embrasure form (**Fig. 6.12**).

Advantages of Reverse Curve

- It conserves the tooth structure
- It preserves aesthetics
- The triangular of affected "cusp" ridge is prevented
- The gingival marginal clearance with the adjacent tooth should be 0.5 mm in case of small tooth preparation
- Tooth with even smaller lesions mesiofacial and mesiolingual margins is 0.2–0.3 mm.

Isthmus

- It is the junction between occlusal and proximal facial and lingual part in the preparation
- Width 1/4 of intercuspal distance
- This is done so as to remove the debris, to eliminate any moisture and to disinfect the cavity.

SHORT NOTES

Question 1

Write a short note on Class V cavity preparation for amalgam restorations?

Answer

Definition

Restorations on the gingival third of the facial or lingual surfaces of all teeth (except pit and fissure lesions).

Indications

- In premolars and molars where aesthetic is not important
- Class V defects caused by erosion, abrasion, hypoplasia, attrition, aplasia or hypocalcification.

Contraindications

Anterior teeth where aesthetics are of real importance.

Tooth Preparation

- A number ≠ 2 or 4 round carbide bur or a tapered fissure bur is used
- The axial wall is deeper at the incisal wall: 1–1.25 mm
- At roof surface = 0.75 mm
- Depth inside the DEJ = 0.5 mm

- It allows placement of retention grooves
- Number ≠ 1/4 bur is used for preparation of two retention grooves, i.e., at incisoxial line angle and at gingivoaxial line angle
- Depth of the groove = 0.25 mm
- Four retention grooves prepared but foul axial point angles of the preparation
- Angle forming chisel is used when access is not proper for preparation of retention form
- Number ≠ 33.5 bur is used
- Rubber dam or a retraction cord is required for isolation to protect gingiva at the time of Class V tooth preparation for gingival margins, which is apical to the gingival crest
- The apical restoration is extended around the line angle, if the distal surface is sound. It prevents the need for Class II cavity preparation
- If Class V outline reaches the old proximal restoration, extend it slightly into the bulk of proximal restoration
- If Class V and Class II need to be done on the same tooth:
  - Class II is done first
  - Class V is done prior to Class II so as to prevent damage to matrix band and the wedge that are needed for Class II restoration.

Question 2

Write a short note on class VI cavity preparation for amalgam restoration?

Answer

Class VI

Restorations on the incisal edge of anterior teeth or the occlusal cusp heights of the posterior teeth.

Indications

- Severe attrition with underlying dentine caries
- Sensitivity to cold and hot food
- Food impaction
- Sharp enamel edges that cause lip, tongue and check bite
- Hypoplastic cusp tip those are prone to caries.

Tooth Preparation

- Restoration procedure is quite similar to that of Class I tooth preparation for amalgam
- Isolation is done using cotton rolls
- Small tapered tissue bur is used for entry cut

- Extension is done to place cavosurface margin on enamel with sound dentine support
- 90° cavosurface margin is given by diverging walls occlusally
- Pulpal depth = 1.5 mm
- Undercuts are given along the internal line angles to obtain retention.

Question 3

Describe various causes for amalgam restoration failure?

Answer

The failure of amalgam restoration is classified as:
- Mechanical failures
- Biological failures
- Technique failures.

Mechanical Failures

- Marginal fracture
- Improper manipulation
- Incorrect alloy-mercury ratio
- Tooth fracture
- Discolouration of tooth
- Bulk fracture of restoration
- Faulty finishing and polishing
- Excess masticatory stress leading to fracture.

Biological Failures

- Pain after restoration
- Tarnish and corrosion
- Pulp involvement
- Marginal leakage leading to secondary caries
- Delayed expansion
- Proximal overhangs
- Periodontium injury.

Technique Failures

- Improper selection of material
- Under/over triturated mix
- Improper cavity preparation
- Presence of $\gamma 2$ phase
- Inappropriate condensation
- Presence of moisture
- Inadequate proximal extension
- Premature contact with opposite tooth
- Inadequate depth of the preparation.

Question 4

Write a short note on differences between high copper and low copper amalgam alloys?

Answer

Table 6.2: Differences between high copper and low copper amalgam alloys

Low copper	High copper
More mercury is required for its reaction	Less mercury is required for its reaction
G1 phase is dominant	H(phase) is dominant
Due to G2 phase, its more prone to tarnish and corrosion	Due to copper rich phase less corrosion is seen
Compressive strength 145–343 MPa	Compressive strength 262–510 MPa
Copper content ≤ 6%	Copper content 6–30%
Produced by milling	Produced by atomisation
Has lathe-cut shape	Has spherical smooth shape
It is subjected to greater dimensional changes	Subject to lesser dimensional changes
Creep rate 0.8–8%	Creep rate 0.4%
Need less energy for amalgamation	Requires high speed and great energy
Less plastic, requires greater condensation pressure	More plastic requires lesser condensation and pressure

CHAPTER 7

Composite Resins

Question 1

Define and classify composite. Write briefly about ideal requirements, indications, contraindications, advantages and disadvantages?

Answer

According to Anusavice, Composites are defined as highly cross linked polymeric material reinforced by a dispersion of amorphous silica, glass, crystalline or organic resin filler particles or short fibres bonded to the matrix by a coupling agent.

Classification

According to Sturdevant

- On the basis of matrix composition:
  - Bisphenol A-glycidyl methacrylate (Bis-GMA)
  - Urethane dimethacrylate (UDMA).
- On the basis of polymerisation method:
  - Self-cured or chemically cured, or two component systems: Amine accelerators were used to increase polymerisation rates
  - Ultraviolet light curing: Most popular today, but its success depends on the access of high intensity light to cure the matrix material
  - Visible light curing: Most popular today, but its success depends on the access of high intensity light to cure the matrix material
  - Dual curing: Combining self-curing and light curing. The self-curing rate is slow and is designed to cure only those portions that are not adequately light cured
  - Staged curing: By filtering the light from the curing unit during an initial cure, it is possible to produce a soft, partially cured material that can be easily finished.

According to Lutz and Phillips (1983)

- On the basis of filler particle size and distribution:
  - Type 1: Macro-filled composite resin—referred to as "conventional" or "traditional" composite
  - Type 2: Micro filled composite resin—fillers are amorphous silica particles of 0.04 µm average diameter
  - Type 3: Hybrid composite resin:
    - Often known as "small-particle composites"
    - Contain combination of macro-filler particles with a proportion of micro-filler particles
    - Probably the most commonly used composite resins.

According to Marzouk

- Based on their chronological development:
  - First generation composites: Consists of macro ceramic reinforcing phases in an appropriate resin matrix
  - Second generation composites: They consist of colloidal and micro ceramic phases in a continuous resin phase which has best surface texture of all composite resins
  - Third generation composite: Hybrid composites in which there is a combination of macro and micro-(colloidal) ceramics in a ratio of 75:25
  - Fourth generation composites: They are also hybrid types, but instead of macroceramic fillers, these contain heat-cured, irregularly shaped, highly reinforced composite macroparticles with a reinforcing phase of micro (colloidal)-ceramics
  - Fifth generation composites: Hybrid composites in which the continuous resin phase is reinforced with micro ceramics (colloidal) and macro, spherical, highly reinforced, heat-cured composite particles
  - Sixth generation composites: They are hybrid types in which the continuous phase is reinforced with a combination of micro (colloidal)-ceramics. This type

shows higher percentage of reinforcing particles of all composites. They have the best mechanical properties.

According to Phillips

Based on particle size **(Table 7.1)**:

Table 7.1: Average particle size according to Phillips

Category	Average particle size (Per 1 m)
Traditional composite	8–12
Small particle filled composite	1–5
Micro filled composite	0.04–0.5
Hybrid composite	0.6–1.0

Ideal Requirements of Composite Resin

- The co-efficient of thermal expansion should be closer to enamel
- It should not absorb water
- There should be less polymerisation
- Should be wear-resistant
- Should have smooth surface texture
- Should be radio-opaque
- Should have higher modules of elasticity
- Should be less soluble in all oral fluids.

Indications

- Used as restorative material for mild-to-moderate Class I and II tooth preparations
- When aesthetic is an important criteria, e.g., in Class III, IV and V restoration
- In restoring Class VI where high occlusal stress is absent
- As a core built-up material for grossly damaged teeth
- As a pit and fissure sealants
- To restore abrasion or erosion defects in cervical areas of premolar, canines and incisors
- To restore the hypoplastic defects on the facial or lingual areas
- It is used as aesthetic enhancement materials:
  - In partial and full veneers
  - Tooth discolouration
  - Diastema closure.
- For indirect restoration cementation like inlays, onlays and crown
- For repairing fractured ceramic crowns
- Used for bonding orthodontic appliances.

Contraindications

- In areas where isolation is difficult
- Areas with high occlusal forces

- Where indirect restoration is indicated
- Lesions extending to root surface
- Patients with poor oral hygiene and high caries susceptibility
- When tooth preparation extends subgingivally
- When small lesion is present on the distal surface of canine.

Advantages

- They are highly aesthetic
- They require minimal tooth preparation and conservation of tooth structure is maintained
- It requires easy tooth preparation
- It has low wear resistance
- In case of poor bonding these can be marginal percolation
- It has postoperative sensitivity due to polymerisation shrinkage
- Large composite restoration does not last long, like amalgam restorations which are durable for years
- It is difficult to establish proximal contact and contours and finishing as well as polishing
- They have low thermal conductivity
- They possess good retention as it shows bonding with enamel and dentine
- Finishing can be done as soon as the curing process is done
- Does not require replacement rather it can be repaired
- It has no galvanism because of no metal present in it.

Disadvantages

- There can be secondary caries if there is polymerisation shrinkage-gap formation on the margins
- The process is difficult and time consuming
- More expensive
- Needs lot of isolation and steps
- It is very technique sensitive.

Question 2

Describe tooth preparation for Class III composite restorations?

Answer

Class III Composite Restorations

Definition: *'Restoration on the proximal surfaces of anterior teeth that do not involve the incisal edges'.*　　　*–Sturdevant.*

Factors Influencing Composite Restorations

- Age of the patient: In young patients with rampant caries, composite is avoided
- Caries index: In high caries index, risk of early dental caries is present
- Abnormal contacts and contours: In heavy stress bearing areas, it is avoided

- Inadequate isolation
- Patients who are not psychologically healthy.

Prerequisites

- Isolation of the working area
- Teflon-coated composite filling instruments
- Use of yellow filter for light or keep it at low intensity to avoid premature polymerization
- Use safety spectacles to prevent eyes from glare.

Tooth Preparation

There are three designs for tooth preparation depending on the dental tissue involved:

1. Conventional
2. Bevelled conventional
3. Modified.

Conventional

- This is indicated for root surface lesions (**Fig. 7.1A**)
- The outline form is determined by the extent of the lesion
- The lingual approach is used for the direct entry into the lesion by no. 1/2, 1 or 2 round bur:
  - For aesthetics
  - Conserving labial enamel
  - Less thermal changes in lingual area
  - Colour matching is not ideal.
- The indications for the labial approach are:
  - Labial enamel is involved
  - In rotated teeth with difficult lingual approach
  - Maligned teeth
  - Old restoration from labial approach
  - In labial approach cases, a labial bevel is given.
- The cavosurface angle is 90° between the tooth and the composite material
- The retention is achieved by:
  - The adhesive bonding to the tooth structure
  - Roughened tooth structure
  - Parallel or converging external walls
  - Retentive grooves and coves: Retentive grooves (**Fig. 7.1B**) may be isolated or continuous. It is located at least 0.5 mm from the root surface and prepared to a depth of 0.25 mm. Continuous groove is placed in external walls parallel to the tooth surface by no. 1/4 round bur.
- The external walls are located on the sound tooth structure with butt angle
- The depth of the preparation is 0.75 mm. For deeper carious area, the depth is increased at required points.

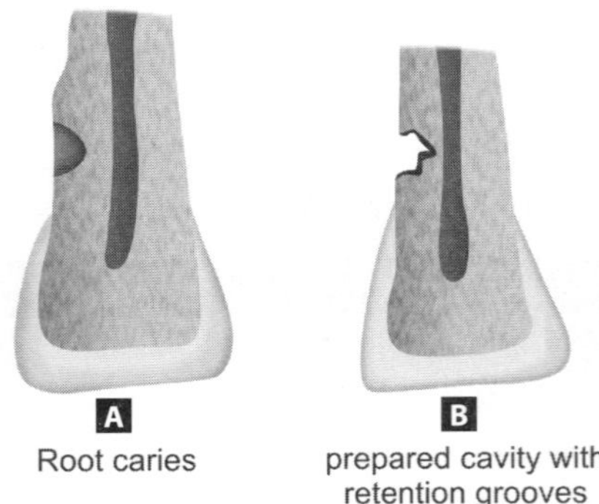

Fig. 7.1A & B: Class III conventional tooth preparation

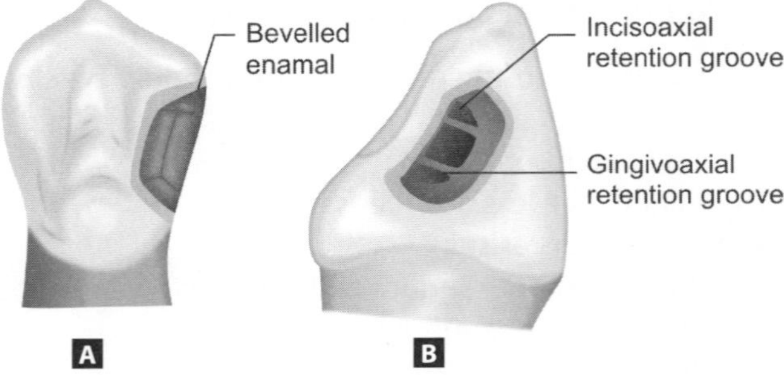

Fig. 7.2A & B: Bevelled conventional Class III tooth preparation

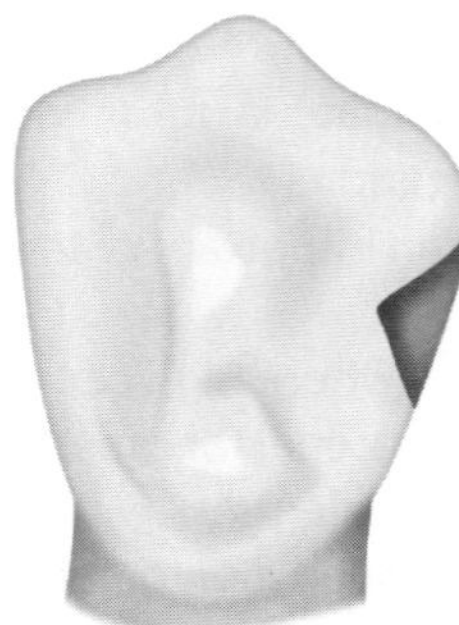

Fig. 7.3: Class III modified tooth preparation

Bevelled Conventional

- This is indicated for replacement of an old restoration or if large carious lesion is present which require increased retention
- The lingual approach is used by no. 1/2, 1 or 2 round bur for aesthetics
- The extent of the lesion determines the shape of outline form (**Fig. 7.2A**)
- Secondary caries and friable tooth structure is taken into consideration and removed by spoon excavator or slow speed round bur

- The depth of the cavity is 0.75 mm gingivally and 1.25 mm incisally or 0.2 mm into the dentine
- The axial wall should be convex or follow the contour of the tooth
- Calcium hydroxide liner is used for pulp protection, if required
- All the enamel margins are bevelled using flat and tapered fissure diamond bur at cavosurface margins. The bevel is 0.25–0.5 mm wide at an angle of 45° to the external tooth surface
- Bevels are not indicated on cementum covered root surfaces and in areas of heavy occlusal contacts
- Retentive grooves can be prepared in gingivoaxial and incisoaxial line angles with the help of 1/4 or 1/2 round burs. Depth of these grooves should be 0.2 mm into the dentine **(Fig. 7.2B)**

Modified (Conservative)

- Most commonly used preparation
- This is indicated for small to moderate class III lesions
- The carious tooth structure is scooped out conservatively resulting in concave areas **(Fig. 7.3)**
- The initial entry is done by lingual approach with a small round bur for aesthetics
- The bur should rotate "during entry and exit
- The outline form depends on the extent of the tooth structure
- There is no definite axial wall
- The external wall diverges outside from the axial wall
- The remaining caries is removed by spoon excavator or small round bur
- The internal line angles are rounded
- The pulp protection is done, if required.

SHORT ESSAYS

Question 1

Write a short note on class IV composite restoration?

Answer

Class IV Tooth Preparation

Definition: Restorations on the proximal surfaces of the anterior teeth that do involve the incisal edges.   -Sturdevant.

This is indicated in cases of incisal angle fracture due to trauma or caries.

Conventional

- This is indicated for lesions on the root surface or restorations in high stress bearing areas
- Preparation is box-like with facial and lingual walls parallel to the long axis of the tooth.
- Retention is achieved by dovetail, retentive grooves incisally and gingivally in the axial wall by 1/4 round bur 0.2 mm inside the dentinoenamel junction at a depth of 0.25 mm **(Fig. 7.4)**.

Bevelled Conventional

- This is indicated for large carious lesions
- The depth is 0.5 mm into the dentine
- The bevels are made at an angle of 45° with a width of 0.25–2 mm
- All the internal line angles are rounded **(Fig. 7.5)**
- Retention is gained by grooves, coves, undercuts, bevels and pins.

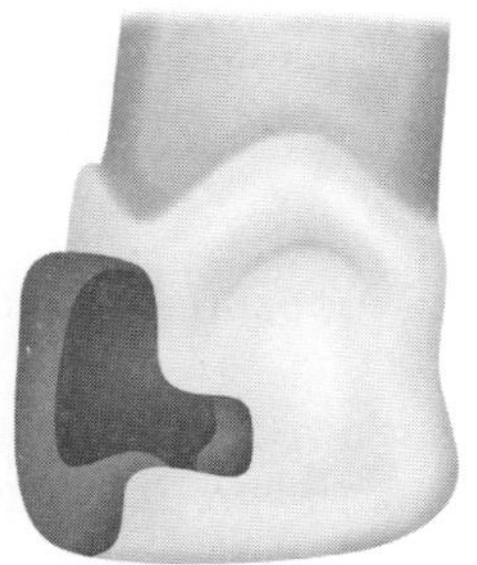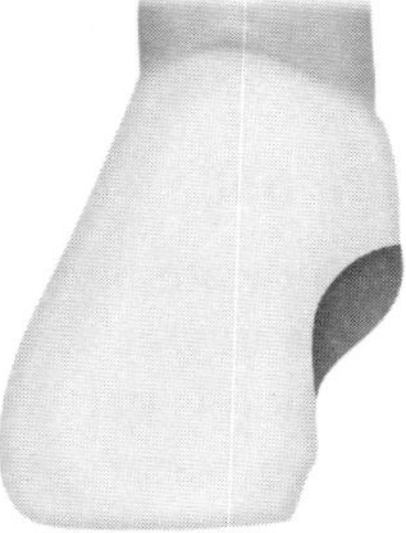

Fig. 7.4: Class IV conventional tooth preparation

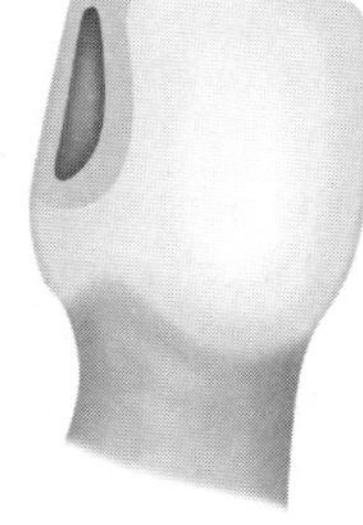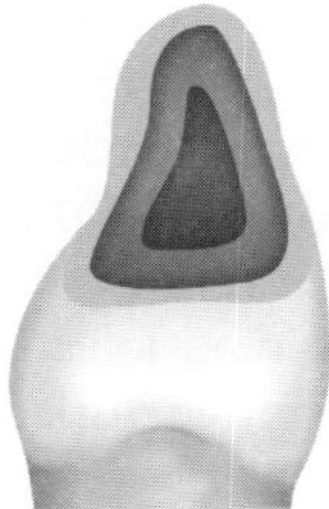

Fig. 7.5: Bevelled conventional class IV tooth preparation

Modified (conservative)

- This is indicated for small class IV lesions or traumatic defects
- The preparation is done in a conservative manner in a way similar to preparation for class III lesion

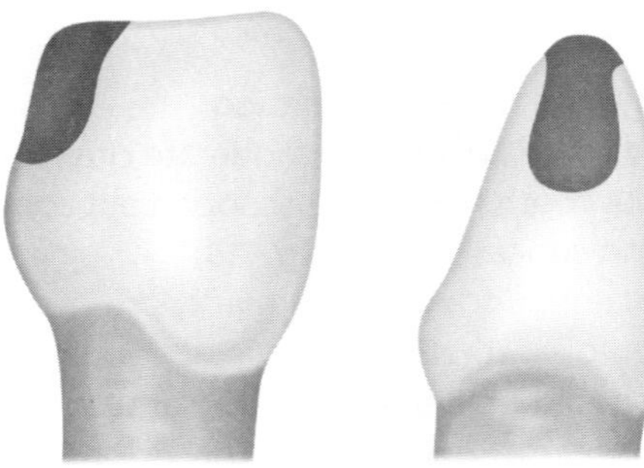

Fig. 7.6: Class IV modified tooth preparation

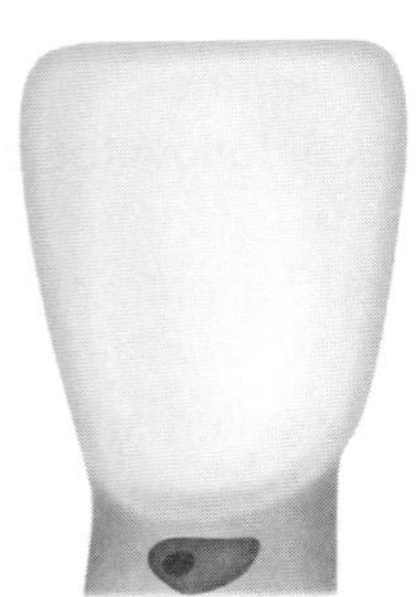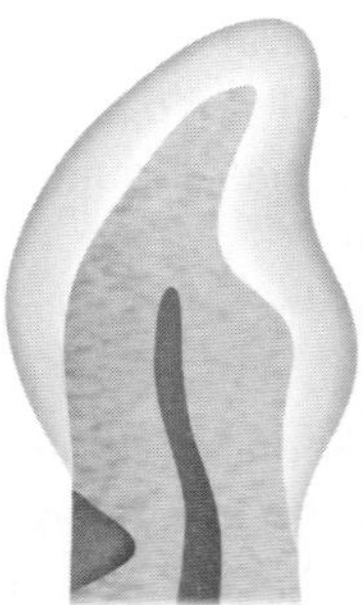

Fig. 7.7: Class V conventional tooth preparation or root surface

❑ Retention can be achieved by bevelling sharp cavosurface margins with a coarse flame-shaped diamond instrument **(Fig. 7.6)**.

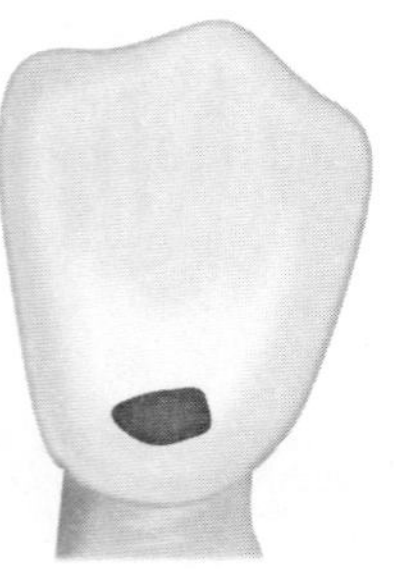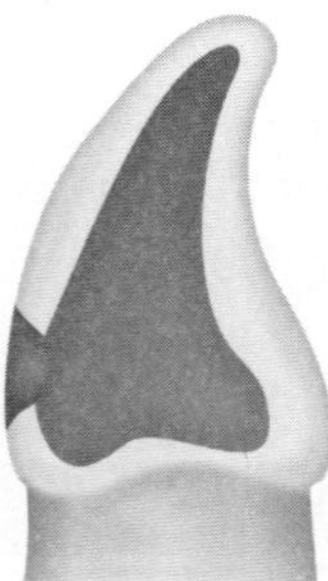

Fig. 7.8: Bevelled conventional class V tooth preparation

Question 2

Write a short note on class V tooth preparation for composite resins?

Answer

Class V Tooth Preparation

Definition: Restorations on the facial or lingual surface of the teeth (except pit and fissures).

Conventional

❑ This is indicated when present on root surface partially or completely
❑ If the lesion is partially on root surface and partially on the crown surface, then crown area is prepared using bevelled conventional or modified design and root surface is prepared by conventional design
❑ The preparation is box-like
❑ The initial entry is made at an angle of 45° to the tooth surface by a tapered fissure no. 700 or 701 bur
❑ Cavosurface angle is 90° **(Fig. 7.7)**
❑ The axial depth is 0.75 mm into the dentine
❑ The axial wall follows the external tooth contour
❑ The remaining infected material is removed by spoon excavator or slow-speed round bur
❑ Calcium hydroxide or glass ionomer liner is used, if required
❑ The retentive grooves are prepared in incisoaxial and gingivoaxial line angles using 1/4 or 1/2 round bur at a depth of 0.25 mm into the dentine
❑ The external walls should be occlusally divergent.

Bevelled Conventional

❑ This is indicated for replacing defective old restorations or large carious lesions

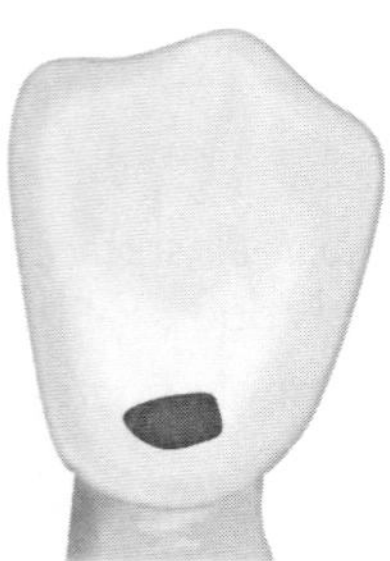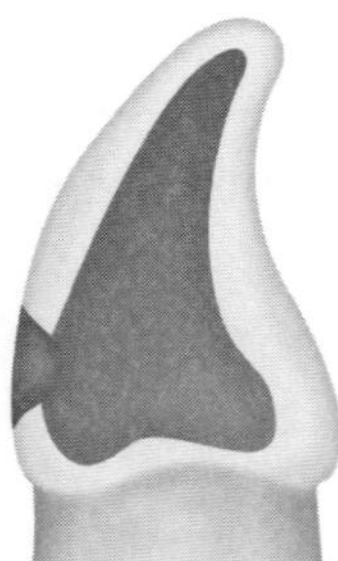

Fig. 7.9: Modified class V tooth preparation

❑ The axial depth is 0.2 mm in the dentine when retentive grooves are not placed and 0.5 mm when retentive grooves are placed
❑ The bevel is at an angle of 45° having a width of 0.25–0.5 mm **(Fig. 7.8)**
❑ Bevelling is done on enamel margins only.

Modified (Conservative)

❑ This is indicated for small and moderate carious lesions or decalcified and hypoplastic areas in cervical third of the tooth
❑ The preparation is having scooped-out appearance and divergent walls
❑ The axial wall can be in enamel or dentine **(Fig. 7.9)**.

Modifications in Class V Cavities

- When the carious lesion is on line-angles of buccal or lingual wall of teeth:
  - The outline form depends upon the size of the lesion
  - The shape is usually round or oblong
  - The depth of cavity is 0.5 mm inside the dentinoenamel junction
  - The short bevel is given wherever required for colour matching.
- When cervical lesion extends occlusally along the sides:
  - This can be unilateral or bilateral
  - The side of the occlusal wall is raised
  - The bevel can be placed all around.

Question 3

Define posterior composite. Write short notes on indications, contraindications, advantages and disadvantages of posterior composite?

Answer

It is a hybrid resin composite designed for use in posterior areas, where a stiffer consistency facilitates condensation in posterior teeth.

Indications

- Where aesthetics is a prime criterion it is a choice of material, e.g., premolars and 1st molar
- Used in small and moderate type of restorations
- It is used in patients with good oral hygiene and those with low caries index
- It is used when occlusal contact on the teeth that is restored is minimal
- Used in patients without parafunctional habits, e.g., clenching and bruxism
- It is used as core built-up material for full crown restorations
- In teeth where proper isolation can be done
- Used in large restorations in which the strengthening of weakened teeth structure is required.

Contraindications

- Where isolation is not possible
- Areas with heavy occlusal stresses
- Where all the occlusal contacts are on composites
- Areas where restorations are extended on to the root surfaces
- Patient with poor oral hygiene and high caries risk
- Patients with oral habits like clenching and bruxism.

Advantages of Resin Composite as a Posterior Restorative Material

- Aesthetic is the major positive
- Conservation of tooth structure
  - The preparation tends to be shallow
  - A narrow outline form allows less occlusal contact on restoration and reduces wear. It also improves integrity
  - It has rounded internal line angles
  - No extension for prevention.
- Adhesion to tooth structure
  - Reduced micro-leakage
  - Reduced recurrent caries.
- Improved retention
- Radiopacity
- Elimination of galvanic currents
- Low thermal conductivity
- Mercury free alternative
- Less post-operative sensitivity.

Disadvantages

- Polymerisation shrinkage: 2.6–7.1%
- Co-efficient of thermal expansion: 28–45 ppm/°C
- Requires more time for placement
- It is very technique sensitive
- Has decreased wear resistance
- Very low fracture toughness
- Water sorption
- Prior compatibility is unknown for some components
- Expensive.

Question 4

Write a short note about flowable and packed composites?

Answer

Flowable Composites

Flowable composites are modification of small particle filled and hybrid composites.

- They have low filler content
- Inferior physical properties:
  - Low wear resistance
  - Strength.
- Size of filler particles: 0.6–1.0 mm
- Inorganic filler content: 40–60% by weight.

Advantages

- Easy process and gives desired anatomy
- Good wettability
- Easy handling.

Essential Quick Review: Operative Dentistry and Endodontics

Disadvantages

- It has high polymerisation shrinkage
- Low wear resistance
- Low strength.

Packable Composites

Packable composites are hybrid composites which are more viscous so that they can be condensed like amalgam.

- Two major implications are seen in these composites:
  - Easy restoration of the proximal contact
  - Properties similar to amalgam.
- Higher polymerization shrinkage (should be placed in these layers)
- Flowable property allows it to adapt to the cavity giving it desired anatomy.

Indications

- Used in small size Class I restorations
- Used as pit and fissure sealants
- As marginal repair material

- As a cavity base or liner in Class II restorations
- Can be used in areas which have limited accessibility and minimal exposure to wear
- This majority consists of the basic material polymer rigid inorganic matrix material (PRIMM)
- Particles size: 100 mm
- Inorganic filler content: 65–81% by weight
- Tensile strength: 40–45 MPa
- Modules of elasticity: 3–13 GPa.

Advantage

- Used as restorative material in stress-bearing areas
- In Class II restorations, allowing easier proximal contact development.

Disadvantages

- Difficult handling
- Time consuming
- Poor aesthetics
- No studies in progress.

SHORT NOTES

Question 1

Write a short note on macro-filled composites?

Answer

They are also caused as conventional or traditional composites.

Composition

Inorganic filler particles are in the form of finely ground amorphous silica quartz.

- Size of particles: 8–12 mm
- Max. size can be: 50 mm
- Filler comprise: 70–80% wt of composite.

Properties

- Compressive strength: 250–300 MPa
- Tensile strength: 50–65 MPa
- Modules of elasticity: 5–15 GPa
- Co-efficient of thermal expansion: 25–35 ppm/°C
- Water sorption: 0.5–0.7 mg/cm^2
- Knoop hardness: 55 KHV
- Radiopacity: 2–3 mm
- Aesthetics: Polishing result in rough surface.

Clinical Considerations

- It has greater amount of initial wear than other composites
- Rough finish is seen at polishing
- They are more susceptible to discolouration and staining.

Question 2

Write a short note on micro-filled composites?

Answer

These composites were developed to overcome the problems of surface roughening and low translucency that were seen in macro-filled composites.

Composition

- Colloidal silica particles—0.01–0.04 mm. Filler loading is increased by grinding
- Pre-polymerised composite already loaded with silane treated colloidal silica
- Organic fillers:
  - Pre-polymerized particles
- Inorganic filler content:
  - 35–60% by weight.

Properties

- Compressive strength: 250–350 MPa
- Tensile strength: 30–50 MPa
- Modules of elasticity: 3–6 GPa
- Coefficient of thermal expansion: 50–60 ppm/°C
- Water sorption: 1.4–1.7 mg/cm^2
- Knoop hardness: 25–35 KHN
- Radiopacity: 2–3 mm
- Aesthetic: Polishing results in rough surface. It is due to faster wear of the resin matrix than the filler particles.

Clinical Considerations

- Greater amount of initial wear than other composites
- Polishing results in rough finish
- More susceptible to discolouration and extrinsic staining.

Question 3	

Write about differences between chemical cure and light cure resins?

Answer	

Following are the differences between chemical cure and light cure resins:

Table 7.2: Differences between chemical and light cure resins

Chemical cure resins	Light cure resins
They are activated by peroxide amine system	They are activated by light and accurate amount of wave length is required
Polymerisation occurs all through the bulk area of resin	Polymerisation is just towards the light-source in the centre
Working time in chemical cure is not controlled by the operator	Working inclined towards the light source

Single component system	Two component system
Shrinkage is more	Less polymerisation shrinkage
Less wear resistance	Greater wear resistance
Less aesthetic	Excellent aesthetics
More chances of air entrapment	Lesser chances of air entrapment
Less colour stability	Greater colour stability

Question 4	

Write a short note about advantages and disadvantages of light cure composites?

Answer	

Advantages

- No mixing and complicated technique is required
- It shows improved strength
- It shows less staining
- Porosity is less
- It has got better enhanced colour stability
- The operator can control the working time during the process
- Polymerisation happens only after light exposure.

Disadvantages

- It has a very limited curing depth. So, it requires built-up of 2 mm or less
- Poor accessibility in most posterior and interproximal locations
- Variable exposure time
- Sensitive to room illumination
- Very technique sensitive
- Expensive.

CHAPTER 8

Composite Resin Restoration

Question 1

Describe the restoration of Class III cavity using composite resin restoration?

Answer

Class III caries is smooth surface caries found on the proximal surfaces of the anterior teeth, usually slightly gingival to the proximal contact.

Consideration and Features of Class III Caries

- Does not involve the incisal angle of the tooth
- Facial and lingual approach is taken for preparation
- Lingual approach is preferred due to aesthetics
- The unsupported facial enamel is preserved for composite bonding
- Discolouration is less visible at the time of final restoration
- Caries are located more facially.

Conventional Class III Cavity Preparation

- These cavity preparations are indicated for root surface lesions
- The gingival portion is prepared using the conventional design, it is not usual to have the entire lesion on root surface.

Root Surface Lesions

- The outline form is prepared on the root surface
- Extension of external walls should be done perpendicular to the root surface
- The initial axial depth is maintained and should be protected with base, e.g., calcium hydroxide liner or glass ionomer base
- Grooves are placed on axiogingival and axioincisal line angles with a number $\neq$ 114 round bur giving a depth of 0.5 mm, so that these are better retentions of composite resin

- Round burs number 142 are used
- In the end, it is like a box pattern with defined external walls and also a 90° cavosurface angle design.

Large Class III Lesions

- The extensive Class III lesions that extend onto root surface, the coronal portion is then prepared using a bevelled conventional design
- The preparation of root portion is done in the conventional way using a butt joint margin and also making retention groove in the dentine.

Bevelled Conventional Class III Cavity Preparation

- This cavity preparation design is indicated to replace an existing old non-adhesive restoration, e.g., silicate or acrylic resin with composite
- Also can be implicated on large carious Class III lesions which require more resistance and retention
- Lingual approach is more preferred in this preparation
- Round burs are used in the beginning, close to the adjacent root at inciso-gingival level of caries
- Extend the preparation that is similar to the conventional design. The difference is instead of butt joint cavosurface margin a bevel is implicated by holding the bur perpendicular to enamel surface
- A flame shaped diamond bur point is used for preparation, which produces a cavosurface angle of 45°
- The bevel is 0.25–0.5 mm in width. Gingival margins and centric contact areas should be avoided.

Modified Class III Cavity Preparation

Indications

- Usually based on the extent of the caries. Mostly for small to moderate carious lesions
- The depth is limited to 0.2 mm into dentine

- It is done in most conservative way and lingual approach is most preferred
- The lingual approach is taken using a number 1 and 2 round diamond point bur perpendicular to the tooth surface
- Access is opened only to extent of caries
- A bevel is created by preparing a wall that diverges externally from the axial depth concavity
- Bevels may be placed on the enamel margin when required
- A flame shaped diamond is used.

Question 2

Describe the technique of restoring a fractured mesioincisal angle of 11 using composite resin?

Answer

Class IV Cavity Preparation for Composite

For Class IV cavity preparation following details should be considered:

Occlusion

The cavity design is determined by the amount of occlusal forces:
- Heavy occlusal forces: Increased resistance and retention form is necessary
- Minimal occlusal forces: Modified designs are adequate.

Shade Selection

This is one of the most important part in Class IV cavity preparation.
- Shade selection is important for the aesthetic point of view
- Dentinal portion: Opaque shades
- Enamel portion: Translucent shades
- Use of hybrid resin is recommended for dentine replacement. Micro-filled composites are used on the labial surface.

Conventional Class IV Cavity Preparation

- The cavity preparation is box-like facial and lingual walls should be parallel to the long axis of the tooth
- The gingival floor should be prepared such that it is perpendicular to the long axis. A round abrasive bur is used
- All weakened enamel should be removed. Initial axial depth should be maintained at 0.5 mm into dentine
- In case of deep caries, the remaining caries is excavated and pulp is protected by a sub-base, i.e., calcium hydroxide and glass ionomer base
- It is recommended that additional retention is gained by giving retention grooves that can be placed incisal and gingival at the axial wall. A round bur number ≠ 114 is used.

Conventional Class IV Cavity Preparation for Large Caries

- This design is applied for large Class IV cavities or when the old or defective restorations need to be replaced
- The outline form exhibits the preparation walls, which are perpendicular or parallel to the long axis of the tooth
- It is done by using a round diamond abrasive bur
- The weakened enamel is removed; excavation of infected dentine is done
- In the end enamel margin that are accessible are bevelled
- The bevel should be placed at 45° angle to the external tooth surface. A flame shaped diamond bur is used
- Bevel width range from 0.25–2 mm depending upon:
  - The tooth structure lost and amount of retention required.
- For extra retention a retention groove is placed at gingival wall.
  - Round bur number ≠ 14 is used.

Modified Class IV Cavity Preparation

- This design of cavity preparation is used in small carious lesions, defects or traumatic injuries. Mostly that fractures the incisal edge
- This preparation involves minimal tooth structure, is considered in case of carious defects. Retention is given by placement of bevel. A flame shaped diamond bur is used
- For traumatic injuries, fracture site is roughened and bevel is placed. A flame shaped diamond bur is used
- Bevel width: 1–2 mm
- It provides increased surface area of enamel for acid etching and bonding, helping in good retention
- Bevel also provides presentable aesthetic blending between enamel and resin.

Steps Involved in the Placement of Composite Resin

Acid Etching

It is defined as etching of dental surface with an acid to remove the smear layer and open enamel tubules, increase retention of resin sealant and promote mechanical retention.
- It is done using 37% phosphoric acid in the form of liquid or gel
- Gels are preferred because they can be confined to the specific area desired.
- They should be of contrasting colour
- Applied with a brush or syringe applicator
- The etching time ranges between 20–30 seconds for both enamel and dentine

- It should be thoroughly rinsed with a water spray for 5–15 seconds of the etching is done
- If the preparation is only restricted to enamel, the surface can be dried only with clean dry air
- The etched enamel gives a frosty white appearance because of removal of both prism cores and peripheries which creates microscopic irregularities
- In case preparation involves both enamel and dentine, a cotton pellets or blotting paper is used to dry the surface so that dentine is left visibly moist
- Acid etching of dentine removes the surface hydroxyapatite from the peri-tubular and inter-tubular dentine, thus opening the tubular which just leaves an interconnected layer of collagen fibrils
- If dentine is over dried, it results in poor bond because of the collapse of collagen network.

Bonding

- A micro-brush is used to apply bonding agent

- Bonding agent penetrates the enamel irregularities and bonds micro-mechanically by forming resin tags
- On dentine it penetrates the collagen and the dentinal tubules, which form a hybrid layer that consists of a resin-dentine inter-diffusion zone
- The bond to dentine is also by production of micro-chemical bonding.

Composite Resin Insertion

- The placement should be done in increments using a special composite carrier. The thickness of increment should be 1–2 mm
- Before light curing the material should be contoured
- The cavity should be filled and properly contoured using a matrix before final curing is done.

Finishing and Polishing

It is done by using burs, strips and stones.

SHORT ESSAYS

Question 1

Describe compomers?

Answer

Compomers are new variety of tooth coloured restorative material, that are developed by the combination of composites which provides durability with glass ionomer cements (GIC) which provide fluoride releasing ability.

Compomers = GIC cement + composite resin.

- There is high percentage of composite and very minimal proportion of GIC
- They are supplied as a single paste, light curable material inside a syringe or ampoule
- Composition:
  - Urethane dimethacrylate (UDMA)
  - Butane tetracarboxylic (TCB) acid with polymerisable hydroxyethyl methacrylate (HEMA) side chains
  - Strontium fluorosilicate glass: Reactive
  - Silicate glass filler containing fluoride
  - Photoinitiators
  - Stabilisers.

Setting Reaction

Light curing mechanism is implicated for hardening of components. Two stages of setting reactions are:

- Light curing causes polymerisation of UDMA and TCB resin
  - This in turn forms a three-dimensional (3D) network reinforced by filler particles.
- After the initial setting, the material absorbs water from the mouth
  - The carboxyl group present in TCB resin liberates metal from silicate glass particles in the presence of water
  - As a result, there formation of hydrogen similar to glass ionomer cements
  - This extra acid-base reaction crosslinks the entire matrix.

Properties

- They match hybrid composite resins when it comes to strength, fracture Toughness and wear resistance
- Optical properties are colour matching and are more superior to those of glass ionomer cements
- They release fluoride but to a lesser extent compared to the glass ionomer cements
- There is a rapid fall in fluoride release after the initial period. They do not possess any fluoride recharge capacity.

Clinical Applications

Indications

- Class III and V cavities
- They are better alternative to glass ionomer cements and composite resins.

SHORT NOTES

Question 1

Discuss micro-filled composites. What are its advantages and disadvantages?

Answer

Micro-filled composite resins are modified small particle composites which were developed to overcome the surface roughness and low translucency.

- The filler used colloidal silica
  - Particle size: 0.04–0.4 mm.
- Due to the very small particle size, they form a mass group leading to the formation of long chains
- This silica chain acts very similar to resin polymer chain which increases the viscosity of the micro-filled resins
- The filler content is kept low.
  - Low weight: 50%
  - By volume: 30–40%.

Advantage

It provides the smoothest surface finish among all composite resins.

Disadvantages

- They have inferior properties compared to the traditional composites due to increased matrix content
- They have much more water sorption
- High co-efficient of thermal expansion
- Decreased elastic modulus
- Low tensile strength
- Because of poor bond between clinically curved matrix and procured particles, there is increased wear.

Question 2

Discuss polymerisation shrinkage?

Answer

The process in which composite resins undergo shrinkage during polymerisation due to resin matrix presence is called as polymerisation shrinkage.

- It causes stress between the tooth structure and composite resin, which leads to marginal gaps and also enamel fractures
- Polymerisation shrinkage is negated by addition of fillers
- Hybrid composites shrink only 0.6–1.4%; micro, filled shrinkage 2–3%
- Also, polymerisation shrinkage can be reduced by incremental placement
- In this process, the shrinkage is allowed after placement of an increment before the next increment placement, leading to controlled polymerisation shrinkage.

CHAPTER 9

Direct Gold Restoration

LONG ESSAYS

Question 1

Discuss direct gold restorations. Write in brief classification, indications and contraindications?

Answer

Direct gold restorations are gold restorative materials that are manufactured for compaction directly into the prepared cavity.

Classification

According to Phillips

Direct filling gold (DFG) can be classified on the basis of its availability as below:

- Gold foil:
  - Sheath:
    - Cohesive
    - Non-cohesive.
  - Ropes
  - Cylinders
  - Laminated foil
  - Platinised foil.
- Electrolytic precipitate (crystalline gold)
  - Mat gold
  - Mat foils (mat gold plus gold foil)
  - Gold-calcium alloy.
- Granulated gold (encapsulated gold powder).

According to WJO'Brien

- Foil:
  - Platinised gold foil
  - Gold foil
  - Mat foil.
- Electrolytic:
  - Mat gold
  - Calcium alloy (e.g., electralloy).
- Powdered gold (e.g., golden): E-Z gold.

Indications

- Small Class I restorations pit and fissures of molar teeth, lingual surfaces of anterior teeth
- Class II restorations with minimum proximal caries
- Class III on the proximal surface of anterior teeth
- It is an ideal restorative material for Class V restoration in non-aesthetic zone
- Restoring small erosion on the tooth
- Class VI of incisal edges/cusp tip
- For repairing gold crowns
- For restoring hypoplastic defects on the lingual and facial surfaces.

Contraindications

- Expensive
- Teeth with poor prognosis
- Teeth with large pulp chamber
- Uncooperative patients
- Areas with high occlusal stress
- Root canal treated teeth
- Large lesions.

Question 2

Write in brief about Class I restoration with direct filling gold?

Answer

Tooth Preparation

Outline form for gold restoration is similar to amalgam. It is different than amalgam to a little extent:

- They have angular corners. In case of amalgam they are rounded
- Facial and lingual groove extensions have pointed terminations
- Sweeping curves in amalgam are more prominent than in gold restorations

- The outline form should extend to include lesion on the tooth surface
- The placement of the margins should be beyond the extent of pits and fissures
- Point angles and line angles are very definite and also very angular within the dentine
- The cavosurface margin is bevelled (partial enamel bevel 45°) to the direction of enamel rods. This helps in the easing of finishing and removal of rough enamel
- The preparation of external wall should be done in a way that they are parallel to each other
- Pulpal wall = 0.5 mm into the dentine. It should be of uniform depth
- Inverted cone should be used to give additional retention and small undercuts into the dentine
- Facial and lingual undercut are placed in the posterior tooth
- Incisal and gingival undercuts are placed on the anterior teeth.

Restoration

- Application of cavity varnish before the insertion of mat gold
- Before the gold is inserted into preparation it is degassed and cooled in air
- Condensation is followed with condenser that is 0.5 mm diameter
- Gold is compacted with the lines of force which are directed against the pulpal wall. Matching is done soon after the gold is stabilised. It should be done till the preparation is half filled
- It is followed by gold foil compacted into the preparation
- Using hand pressure pellets of suitable size are then degassed and inserted into the cavity
- Gold build-up is carried out till the cavosurface margin is covered with the foil
- Compacted surface should be saucer shape during the build-up
- To harden the surface flat beaver tail burnishes with heavy hand pressure is used to burnish gold
- Remove excess gold by cleoid discoid carver on the cavosurface margin and then again start the burnishing process
- To gain proper lustre of gold restoration flour of pumice, while rouge or tin oxide is applied on soft rubber cup in the low speed hand piece.

Question 3

Discuss gold foil in detail?

Answer

It is also known as fibrous gold.

- It is prepared by a cast ingot of 15 mm thickness which is beaten into 15–25 μm foils
- They are supplied in the form of sheets, cylinders, pellets, ropes and also partially pre-condensed laminates of various thicknesses
- Number of sheet of gold foils is placed over one another to form laminated gold foil
- Standard number ≠ 4 gold foil supplied as:
  - 4 × 4 inch sheet
  - 4 grains (0.259 g) weight
  - 0.15 μm thickness.
- Standard number ≠ 3 gold foil supplied as:
  - 3 × 3 inch sheet
  - 3 grains (0.194 g) weight
  - 0.38 μm thickness.
- Other foils:
  - Number 20—20 grains
  - Number 40—40 grains
  - Number 60—60 grains
  - Number 90—90 grains.

Types of Gold Foil

- Cohesive and non-cohesive gold foil
- Gold foil cylinders
- Gold foil pellets
- Preformed gold foils
- Platinised gold foil.

Cohesive Foil

- They are the types of gold foil which are free of surface contaminations
- To be cold welded at mouth temperature both the gold surfaces should be automatically cleaned
- During condensation cohesiveness of individual increment is prevented as gold attracts gases
- Gold foil supply by manufacturer is free of surface contaminations, but it can be contaminated during storage.

Non-cohesive Foil

- These gold foils are supplied by manufacturer with an absorbed protective gas film, e.g., ammonia gas
- Ammonia reduces adsorption which prevents premature cohesiveness of the sheets
- Non-cohesive gold could have adsorbed agents, like acidic gas and iron salts
- To restore the cohesive property of foil, the film is removed and heated
- They are used to build-up the bulk of a direct gold restoration.

Gold Foil Cylinders

- Gold foil cylinder foil is formed by rolling the cut segments of number ≠ 4 foils into the required width
- Foils that are rolled out to number ≠ 22 are:
  - Width 3.2 mm
  - Width 4.8 mm
  - Width 6.4 mm.
- Also number ≠ 60 and number ≠ 90 gold foils can be used as alternatives.

Gold Foil Pellets

Pellets of gold foil are rolled from 1/32, 1/64 or 1/28 sections cut from number ≠ 4 sheet foils.

- It is then marked and cut into square or rectangles
- The each piece is rolled into pellet form by placing them on finger-tip and corner tucked into centre.

Preformed Gold Foils

- Available in the form of ropes of cylinders
- These foils are carbonised or corrugated and are made of number ≠ 4 foils
- Corrugated gold foils are obtained by burning the foil between two sheets of paper in an air tight container
- Shrivelling of the paper in an air tight container removes carbon particles. After this process, gold exhibits superior welding properties
- The ropes and cylinders are rolled in various diameters and various lengths by cutting so that it fits the prepared cavity
- No preformed gold foils are provided by the manufacturer, but they can be manually prepared by placing desired number of sheets over another and then cutting them into the required shape.

Platinised Gold Foil

It is in a laminated structure. It is produced by:

- Pure platinum foil is sandwiched between two number 4 pure gold foils
- By cladding process in which the bonding layers of platinum and gold are bonded together during rolling
- The advantage of platinum is to increase hardness and wear resistance of the gold restorations.

Question 4

Define cold welding, wedging. Write in brief about condensation or compaction of direct filling gold?

Answer

- Cold welding: It is a process of forming atomic bonds between pellets, segments or layers as a result of condensation

- Wedging: It refers to the pressurised adaptation of the gold form within the space between the tooth structure walls or corners that have been slightly deformed elastically.

Condensation/Compaction

It is the process of increasing the density of the metal foil, pellets or powder through compressive pressure.

Objectives of Condensation of Direct Filling Gold

- Wedging of initial gold pieces between dentinal walls more at the starting points
- Wedging of gold pieces together by complete cohesion of space lattices in it
- It minimises the voids or eliminates them from critical areas, e.g., margins and surfaces
- Improving retention by adapting gold material to cavity walls and floor. This reduces micro leakage and reduces secondary caries.

Methods of Condensation

Hand Instrument

- Hand instrument is not sufficient to satisfy the objectives of condensation
- Used as only first step in a two-step process initially
- Mostly used as initial confinement of the material within the cavity.

Pneumatic Condensation

- Air compressed condensers are used
- Controlled air pressure allows condensation strokes to be adjustable in amplitude and frequency
- It is difficult to control condensation strokes
- It consists of knurled knob at the rear of the handpiece that regulates force
- Rheostat in electric motor regulates number of blows per minute
- More hardened and denser specimen than mallet.

Electronic Condensation

- It is the most efficient and controlled condensation method
- Amplitude of vibration in condenser is between 2 and 1502
- Frequency varies between 360–3600 cycles/minute
- Blow force is adjustable
- Lighter blow are preferred for greater patient comfort
- Produces good restoration.

Mallet/hand Condensation

- This is the oldest method
- It requires high skill for condensation
- It cannot be done alone, need of an assistant is required

- Mostly used for adaptation of denser cohesive gold into retention area
  - It is done after hand pressure is applied.
- Two types:
  - Long handled condensers
  - Small leather-faced mallet
  - It is flat and serrated at the face end
  - Condensation force is checked by tapping the thumb nail to its end
  - Force is decreased if tapping causes discomfort.

Procedure

- Piece of gold is placed in the prepared tooth
- Hand pressure is used first to place the gold
- A suitable condenser is then used for malleting at the centre of mass
- Also by lateral movement of the gold is compressed against surrounding prepared walls—which removes most void spaces, compact gold into line and point angles and against the wall.

SHORT ESSAYS

Question 1

Describe powdered gold?

Answer

- Powdered gold is supplied as:
  - Irregularly shaped particles
  - Pre-condensed pellets particles
  - Clumps of particles.
- They are prepared when gold is in molten state by comminution, chemical precipitation or atomisation
- Average size of gold powder gold powder 15 μm, maximum size = 74 μm
- Pellets are formed with atomised and chemically precipitated powders which are mixed with soft wax
- They are then wrapped with foil
- These pellets are cylindrical in shape so that they can be cut into several different diameters and lengths.

Advantages

- For the early stages of condensation it spreads laterally from the point of impact
- Overlaying with gold foil is highly recommended.

Goldent

- They are lightly pre-condensed to improve their handling
- An average 15 mm individual granule is gathered into the masses of irregular shapes of 1–3 mm
- They are enclosed in envelop of foil so that they possess better handling during condensation
- Composition:
  - Powder: 95%
  - Foil: 5%.
- Veneering is not required
- To improve its compacting properties the atomised spherical particles are thoroughly mixed with granules.

Stopfgold

- The gold powder is chemically precipitated which is subject to milling process, after the precipitation
- The individual particles are cut into strips after they are loosely sintered together
- Thickness: 0.7 mm and 1–1.5 mm
- It possesses high lustre due to the flat particles that produce reflection
- It gives cold welding ability because it has less porosity
- It has much better shear strength.

E-Z Gold

- They are new type of gold
- They are similar to powdered gold but are more user friendly
- They are provided as mixer of pull gold powder with wax wrapped in a gold foil
- More stickier than gold foil
- Softness is improved and working efficiency is better.

Question 2

Discuss degassing?

Answer

Degassing

The process of heating the foil or pellet immediately before carrying into the prepared cavity in order to remove volatile protective coating is called degassing.

Objectives

- To eliminate impurities from the surface and making the foil or pellet ready for cohesion
- To protect the surface from depositing any other impurities until cohesion takes place.

Methods

Piece Method

A single piece is annealed. It is done by using a simple alcohol and a gold foil carrier.

Advantages

- Selection of gold of desired shape is possible
- It eliminates the contamination that can happen between annealing and use.

Bulk Method

It is done by degassing of several gold pellets at same time.

Advantages

It is very convenient and takes less time.

Disadvantages

- Lot of gold is wasted
- There is unequal heating due to air currents so it possesses poor welding properties
- Sticking of pellets to each other is seen with the accidental movement during heating.

Degassing Done in Different Ways

- Open alcohol flame:
  - High energy reducing zone of the flame is used (middle zone)
  - Gold piece is held over the flame for 3–5 seconds individually before insertion with a gold foil carrier
  - Acetone free alcohol is preferred to alcohol or gas
  - If alcohol is used it should be pure methanol/ethanol.
  - Precautions:
    - Lamp should be free of contaminations and waxes on the surface
    - Wick is trimmed so that it produces clear blue light and flame 3/4 inch of height
    - It should be kept in mind that sulphur remnant from match stick should not adhere to the wick.
  - Advantages:
    - Pieces can be selected according to size required
    - Only the pieces which are needed to be desorbed can be picked
    - There is minimal contamination
    - It is more flexible, uniform and readily available.
- Mica:
  - Use of mica sheet is it can be used over any flame
  - Mica sheet is divided into several areas which indicate the timer as for how long gold is held over the mica sheet
  - Maximum time for gold to be heated on mica sheet is 5 minutes
  - The pieces should not be handed with stainless steel wire points to prevent contamination
  - Disadvantage: It is only convenient for gold foil.
- Electrical degassing:
  - Electrical degassing is the most standardised and controlled way
  - It has aluminium made heating compartments and an electric heater which controls time and temperature
  - Heater surface is divided. It is divided into small compartments to accommodate gold pieces
  - This in turn eliminate any chance of cohesion to occur before placement into prepared cavity
  - At temperature of 800°F, 5 minutes of heating is required
  - Advantages:
    - Time and temperature is in the hand of operator
    - Does not need manpower to perform.
  - Disadvantage: Powdered gold requires a temperature of 900–1200°F, which is not possible in electric degassing.

SHORT NOTES

Question 1

Write a short note on hazards of overheating and underheating of direct filling gold materials?

Answer

Overheating

- Overheating causes recrystallisation.
- It attracts impurities from the surrounded atmosphere when overheated
- Overheating of sintered gold causes over sintered situation causing adherence of the entire mass of the particles
- Causes complete melting of gold surface
- Overheating causes mass contamination and this leads to pieces of gold to adhere before inserting in the prepared cavity
- Makes gold stiffer, less ductile which is hard to compact.

Underheating

- Underheating causes pitting
- Porosity
- Failure to remove protective gases
- Makes it partially cohesive.

Question 1

Discuss dentinal hypersensitivity, various theories, diagnosis and management?

Answer

Dentinal hypersensitivity is characterised by short, stimuli typically thermal, tactile, osmotic or chemical and which cannot be ascribed to any other form of dental defect or pathology.

Aetiology

- Enamel loss due to:
  - Occlusal wear
  - Abfraction
  - Erosion
  - Tooth brushing
  - Parafunctional habits
  - Dietary erosion.
- Cemental loss due to:
  - Gingival recession
  - Periodontal disease
  - Periodontal surgery
  - Root planning.

Clinical Features

- Pain in response to heat, cold stimuli and to sweet and sour food
- This pain is similar to acute reversible pulpitis
- Difference in dentinal hypersensitive pain is that patient is able to locate the pain
- It is mild to moderate
- Pain intenses by stimuli like hot, cold sweet and sour
- Pain does not outlast the stimulus
- Normal radiographic appearance in the periapical region.

Theories of Dentine Hypersensitivity

- Direct innervation theory: This was the first theory put forward and it stated that nerve fibres which are present within the dentinal tubules initiate impulses when injured, causing dentinal hypersensitivity
- Odontoblast deformation theory/transducer mechanism: This theory states that the external stimuli when applied to exposed dentine the odontoblast and its processes are damaged. This leads impulse the nerve in pre-dentine and underlying pulp which in turn are proceeded to the central nervous system
- Hydrodynamic Theory:
  - This is most widely accepted of all the theories
  - It was proposed by Gysi in 1900
  - Validated by Brannstrom in 1996.
- This theory states that nerves within the tooth are triggered by hot and cold due to worn enamel and receding gums. Whenever exposed dentine is stimulated, there is a rapid movement of the dentinal fluid either outwards or towards the pulp.

Diagnosis

History

- Signs and symptoms
- Duration, type, frequency
- Dietary changes.

Clinical Examination

- Visual
- Physical
- Pocket depth
- Percussion
- Response to cold air.

Radiographic Examination

Periapical lesions should not be considered.

Management

- ❑ Desensitisation by occluding dentinal tubules. Two mechanisms are involved:
  - ○ Formation of smear layer over exposed dentin: It is done by blocking dentinal fluid movement by occluding dentinal tubules surface
    - ➢ It is a temporary solution
    - ➢ It is achieved by orange wood stick that is placed on the affected tooth
  - ○ Use of topical agents (occlude exposed tubules).
- ❑ Placement of restorations:
  - ○ Most common and effective restorative materials used here are:
    - ➢ Glass ionomer cements
    - ➢ Composite resins.
- ❑ Use of lasers:
  - ○ Carbon dioxide (CO_2) lasers
  - ○ Neodymium (Nd): 4AG, Erbium (Er): 4AG laser.

SHORT ESSAYS

Question 1

Write a short note on role of dentinal fluid, dentinal tubules and its permeability?

Answer

Dentinal Tubules

- ❑ It occupies 1% superficial to 30% deep space in the intact dentine. It continues as cell process of odontoblast
- ❑ Number of tubules innervated by pulpal nerves is 40% in coronal dentine over pulp horn
- ❑ Mid coronal dentine is 1% or below cemento enamel junction

  This is the reason why coronal dentine is more sensitive than root dentine. Because of the sensitivity it is the most challenging to treat. One needs to seal most of the tubules to prevent the sensitivity.

Dentinal Fluid

Free fluid occupies:
- ❑ 1% of superficial dentine
- ❑ 22% volume of deep dentine.

Definition

Dentinal fluid/hyper fluid is the fluid of dentine which appears on the surface of freshly cut dentine especially in young teeth. It is a transudate of extracellular fluid mainly cytoplasm of odontoblast process from the dental pulp via the dentinal tubules.

- ❑ It is an ultra-filtrate of blood in pulp capillaries
- ❑ If dentine becomes exposed a pressure gradient between pulp and oral cavity tends to be slow with outward flow
- ❑ The outward movement is accelerated by either dehydrating the surface of dentine with compressed or dry heat
  - ○ It is used as sink by which injured agents can diffuse into the pulp
  - ○ Acts as a vehicle for incursion of bacteria from necrotic pulp to peri-radicular tissue.

Dentine Permeability

Permeability increases as tubules decrease over the pulp, so fluid permeation is proportional to the tubule diameter and number.

- ❑ Permeability of radicular dentine is much lower than coronal dentine
- ❑ Dentine hypersensitivity directly related to dentine permeability. When the dentinal fluid movement stimulate the pulp as nociceptor it innervates dentinal tubules.

Question 1

Classify cast gold alloys. Discuss the cavity design for Class II cast gold restoration?

Answer

Classification of Cast Gold Alloys by American Dental Association (ADA)

- Type I alloys: Soft
- Type II alloys: Medium
- Type III alloys: Hard
- Type IV alloys: Extra hard.

Type I Alloys

- The gold content in this alloy is from 75–83%
- They are used to fabricate small inlays because they are subjected to low stress
- They can be easily burnished as they possess soft and low stress.

Type II Alloys

- The gold content ranges from 70–75%
- They are used for fabrication in moderate stress of inlays and onlays
- They possess medium strength and can be easily burnished.

Type III Alloys

- The gold content ranges from 65–70%
- They are used in high stress conditions, such as fabrication of onlays and crowns
- They cannot be burnished easily but can be heat treated.

Types IV Alloys

- The gold content is 60%

- They are used in crowns, bridges and also removable partial dentures
- They possess high strength and increased hardness
- They can be heat treated.

Cavity Design for Class II Cast Gold Inlay

- The outline form should be wider so that there is more of surface involvement and the cavity walls diverge occlusally
- The cavity width may increase up to 1/3rd of the intercuspal distance
- Using a bur number 271, 169 L cavity walls are diverged occlusally
- The cavosurface angle is 135–145°, which helps in achieving a lap, sliding fit with the inlay
- A steeper gingival bevel is given at 20–30° to prevent the cement line
- Undercuts should not be present at the time of preparation
- More clearance is required proximally
- Sub-gingival extension of gingival seat is indicated occasionally
- While restoration secondary retention is given by grooves, slots, internal boxes, skirts, collars and reverse bevels
- Primary and secondary flare should be seen at the proximal margins
- Well-defined internal angles
- Proximal outline is devoid of reverse curve
- To provide frictional retention bevels are placed at the occlusal and gingival cavosurface margins.

Question 2

Define inlay. Mention indications, contraindications, advantages and disadvantages of a cast gold restorations?

Answer

- Inlay: An inlay is an indirect intra-coronal restoration fabricated using the lost wax technique
- Class II inlay: This is an indirect restoration that caps one or more cusps of a posterior tooth but not all the cusps.

Advantages of Cast Gold Restorations

- Strength:
  - The cast gold alloys are very strong to replace and reinforce areas of high stress even in thin sections of 1 mm
  - They are ideally suited for inlays, onlays and crowns
  - They also possess high tensile strength.
- Accurate reproduction of contacts and contours:
  - Cast gold restorations can accurately reproduce precise form and minute details and can maintain them under function as they are fabricated by the indirect technique
  - They create ideal occlusal and axial contours and contacts.
- Biocompatibility: Noble and inert cast gold alloys are inert in the atmosphere, hence they are biocompatible and exhibit excellent longevity and durability
- Abrasion resistance: The wear rate of gold is similar to that of the enamel. So, the wear of the opposite tooth is very minimal
- Internal stresses: Cast gold restorations have minimal internal stresses and voids as they are built in bulk and not in increments, like amalgam or composite restorations
- Finishing and polishing: As cast gold restorations are finished and polished outside the oral cavity, they have excellent finishing and polishing. It can be done without even endangering the pulp.

Disadvantages of Cast Gold Restorations

- Microleakage: As cast gold restorations are indirect restorations, they are cemented into the prepared cavity using cutting cements. They are prone to microleakage at tooth-cement-casting junction due to several inter phase present
- Appointments: Cast gold restorations require more than one appointment and also the chair time is lengthy due to the need for impressions
- Need for temporary restorations: Before the cementation of cast restoration, temporary restorations must be placed between all the appointments
- Technique sensitive: Fabrication of cost gold alloy is a very meticulous· process. Any error during fabrication can cause defect in the restoration

- Cost: They are very expensive
- Aesthetic: They are aesthetically unexceptable in the anterior teeth and facial surfaces of the posterior teeth.

Indications of Class II Gold Inlays

They are mostly indicated primarily in extensive proximal caries that cannot be restored satisfactorily with silver amalgam.

- In cases where width of the cavity does not exceed $1/3^{rd}$ of the intercuspal distance
- Proximal caries which involve buccal and lingual line angles of the tooth that has become extensive
- In case the proximal margins extend gingivally as the polished gold alloys are compatible to periodontium
- In grossly carious tooth where one or more but not all the cusps need coverage
- Patients with low caries incidence and good oral hygiene
- When other gold casting are present in the mouth.

Contraindications of Class II Gold Inlays

- They cannot be used as abutment for a fixed or removable prosthesis because they are not strong enough
- In post-endodontic restorations, Class II inlays are contraindicated the reason being they can wedge and fracture the remaining tooth structure
- In young permanent teeth Class II gold inlays are avoided so there is no increased change for iatrogenic pulp exposure because of the high pulp horns present in the young permanent teeth
- Patients with high plaque and caries incidence. It should be avoided as there are greater chances for recurrent caries
- When adjacent and opposite teeth have dissimilar metallic restorations, prevent from galvanism
- When cost needs to be cut
- It is contraindicated in case of grossly destroyed teeth with weak cusps.

Question 3

Write in detail about casting defects?

Answer

Classification of Casting Defects

- Distortion
- Surface roughness and irregularities
- Discolouration
- Porosity
- Incomplete casting.

Distortion

- Distortion is a defect that is caused during fabrication where distortion of wax pattern occurs
- While it is not handled properly, the high co-efficient of thermal expansion of the inlay wax is responsible for the warpage of the pattern
- They are seen at the concave depression on the inner surface of the casting.
- **Causes:**
  - Dense modern investments used which are less porous
  - Fewer voids caused by vacuum investing
  - Improper wax elimination
  - Low casting temperature
  - Inadequate casting pressure
  - Short sprue resulting in more thickness between pattern and open end of the ring.
- **Prevention:**
  - Proper powder: Liquid ratio
  - Proper wax burnout
  - Use of vents
  - Adequate casting pressure
  - Use of porous investments.

Residual Air

Back pressure porosity: When the air in the mould cannot escape through the pores in the investment it causes back pressure porosity.

Surface Roughness and Irregularities

- Surface roughness: Surface roughness of the casting is caused by coarse silica particle in the investment.
  - It can happen with inadequate water: liquid ratio
  - Also by rapid heating of the investment leading to flaking of the investment
  - Prolong heating is the cause of disintegration of gypsum-bonded investment
  - Also by casting pressure being too high.
- Surface irregularities: They are nodules type of isolated imperfections. They are caused:
  - During investing air bubbles attached to the pattern
  - When sprue former is carelessly removed leading to bits of investment into the mould resulting in surface irregularities
  - A depression caused by molten alloy impacting on a weak portion.

Discolouration of the Casting

Removal of surface discolouration is done by a process called pickling.

- Under heating: Under heating of the investment leaves wax residues. A tenacious carbon coating is formed by carbon residues on the casting and thereby discolouring the casting
- Prolonged heating: Prolong heating can decompose the sulphur compound in the investment. This causes casting discolouration and makes it brittle
- High content of sulphur in the torch flame: The higher sulphur percentage in torch flame can also cause casting discolouration
- Use of mixture of different casting alloys: Mixture of different casting alloys discolour the cast by corrosion.

Porosity

- Porosity can be seen in both internal and external aspect of the casting surface
- With increase in the ambient temperature the warpage gets worse and the time lag between fabrication of the pattern and investing.

Classification of Porosity Defects

- Solidification defects:
  - Localised shrinkage porosity
  - Microeporosity.
- Trapped gases:
  - Pinhole porosity
  - Gas inclusion porosity
  - Subsurface porosity.

Solidification Defects

- Localised shrinkage porosity: This defect occurs if the molten alloy solidifies prematurely in the sprue before solidification
- Micro-porosity:
  - When the solidification is too rapid for the micro voids to segregate to the liquid pool. It is seen in fine grain alloy casting
  - They are small irregular voids
  - Porosity weakens the cast restoration
  - Cause: Sprue former diameter is too small.

Trapped Gases

- Pinhole porosity:
  - They are tiny spherical voids
  - Metals in the cast gold alloys like copper, silver, platinum and palladium are prone to dissolve oxygen or hydrogen when they are in the molten state
  - When they are solidified the gases are released causing pinhole porosities

- ○ Lack of reservoir in the sprue former
- ○ Improper sprue attachment, attachment at 90° to a broad surface gives a hot spot, where metal impinges first leading to solidification of the area after the alloy solidifies in the sprue
- ○ This produces suck-back porosity
- ○ This defect is prevented by choosing a sprue of sufficient diameter and length.
- ❑ Gas inclusion porosity:
  - ○ They are also spherical voids but are much larger than pinhole porosity
  - ○ They happen by mechanical entrapment of the gas by molten metal or due to gas inclusion during casting procedure
  - ○ Causes:
    - ➤ Poor adjustment of torch flame
    - ➤ If oxidizing zone is used instead of reducing zone of the flame.
  - ○ Prevention:
    - ➤ Correct adjustment and use of the torch flame
    - ➤ Use of graphite crucible for heating of the alloy
    - ➤ It is not a serious defect and can be prevented by:
      - » Increasing the melting temperature
      - » Increasing the casting temperature.

- ❑ Subsurface porosity:
  - ○ They can happen due to entrapped gases in the alloy.
  - ○ Causes: Simultaneous nucleation of solid grains and gas bubbles when alloy freezes at the mould walls.
  - ○ Prevention: Controlling the rate at which the molten enters the mould.

Incomplete Casting

When molten alloy has been prevented from filling the mould space completely.

Causes

- ❑ Improper venting of air from mould due to the back pressure
- ❑ Round margins created when improper burnout leaves wax residues
- ❑ Low powder to liquid ratio
- ❑ Inadequate heating of the alloy.

Prevention

- ❑ Proper venting of air from the mould
- ❑ Adequate heating of the alloy
- ❑ Use of porous investment
- ❑ Proper casting pressure
- ❑ Burning out of wax properly.

SHORT ESSAYS

Question 1

Write about sprue and sprue former?

Answer

Sprue Former

- ❑ Sprue former is a channel for the molten metal to flow into the mould space in an invested casting ring after the wax pattern has been eliminated
- ❑ A sprue former is attached to the wax pattern when it is still on the dye or the tooth
- ❑ It facilitates removal of the pattern for investing it.

Types of Sprue Formers

- ❑ Wax sprue formers
- ❑ Resin sprue formers
- ❑ Metal sprue formers.

Wax and Resin Sprue Formers

- ❑ These are the sprue formers that can be burnt during wax elimination as they do not require the removal

- ❑ Due to their low conductivity they do not stress the wax pattern
- ❑ They lack rigidity.

Metal Sprue Formers

- ❑ These sprue formers require removal after wax elimination
- ❑ They possess high thermal conductivity which can stress and distort the wax pattern
- ❑ They have good rigidity
- ❑ They can cause voids or incomplete details at the time of casting and at the time of removal and also loosen some investment.

Requirements of Sprue Former

Sprue Diameter

- ❑ Diameter of sprue former mostly depends on the size of wax pattern and the casting machine. Type of alloy that is used also decides the sprue diameter
- ❑ Ideally sprue former should be greater than the thickest portion of the wax pattern
- ❑ Diameter range: 8–18 gauge.

Sprue Former Length

- Sprue former length should be so that the end of the wax pattern is 1/8th to 1/4th of an inch away from the open end of the casting ring
- This will withstand the impact of the molten metal and also allows the mould gases to escape.

Site

Sprue former should be attached to the bulkiest portion of the wax pattern.

Reason Being

- It decreases the residual stress in the wax during attachment of the sprue former
- There will be better supply of the molten metal to fill all the thin sections of the mould
- Proximal area is the most preferred site for sprue former.

Angulation of Sprue Former

- Sprue former should be attached at an angle of 45° and to the bulkiest portion of the pattern
- This helps in the easy and efficient flow of molten alloy.

Placing Sprue Former at 90° and at Thin Surface Causes

- Hot spot at the first site of impact of the molten metal. This then leads to "suck-back" porosity in the casting
- A concavity is seen on the mould wall opposite to the point of sprue attachment.

Question 2

Write a note on suck-back porosity?

Answer

It can be classified as:

- Localised shrinkage shrink-spot/porosity
- Suck back porosity.

Localised Shrinkage Shrink-spot / Porosity

- This defect occurs as a result of cooling sequence which is incorrect and the sprue freezes before the rest of the casting
- Thus subsequent shrinkage produces voids or pits called as shrink-spot porosity
- They are usually found near the sprue-casting junction.

Suck Back Porosity

- It is an external void usually seen in the inside of a crown opposite the sprue. It is a variation of the shrink-spot porosity
- Hot spot is created by the hot metal impinging on the mould wall near the sprue
- This spot freezes in the end
- So, suck back porosity is caused when sprue has already solidified and no molten material is available and this results in shrinkage causing suck-back porosity
- It is avoided by reducing the temperature difference between the mould and molten alloy.

SHORT NOTES

Question 1

Write a short note on pickling?

Answer

Pickling is the process of removing the surface tarnish or the oxide layer on the casting surface.

Process

- Casting is placed in a test tube or a porcelain beaker
- A warm solution of 50% sulphuric acid or hydrochloric acid is poured over it
- After this, the acid is poured off and the casting is taken out and is washed.

Precautions

- Tweezers are used to remove casting, rubber-coated or Teflon tweezers are used
- Heated casting should not be dropped into the pickling solution because it can damage or distort the margins that are delicate in the casting
- Use of fresh solutions each time as old solution can contaminate the new casting.

CHAPTER 12

Minimal Interventional Dentistry

Question 1

Define minimal intervention dentistry (MID). Write about goals and concepts of MID?

Answer

Definition

It is defined as a philosophy of professional care, concerned with the first-occurrence, earliest detection and earliest possible care of disease on micro (molecular) levels, followed by minimal invasive and patient friendly treatment in order to repair irreversible damages caused by such disease.

Rational

- Emphasis upon educating and directing the patient towards self-care is minimal intervention
- The objective is to prevent or heal the disease firstly. Later the elimination or minimising the need for the surgery
- It is process that is a conservative process for the tooth structure and offers greater longevity for the tooth and dentition.

Goals

- To prevent the non-infective tooth structure
- Using of minimum restorative intervention
- Remineralisation for early lesions
- Use of chemical or mechanical methods to reduce cariogenic bacteria
- Repairing of defective restorations rather than replacing them
- Control of caries as infective communicable disease.

Concepts of MID (Tyas Et Al. 2000)

- Early caries diagnosis
- Classification of caries depth and progression
- Assessment of individual caries risk (high, moderate and low)
- Reduction in cariogenic bacteria to eliminate further progress of disease
- Remineralisation of early caries lesion
- Minimal surgical intervention of caries lesion
- Repair rather than replacement of defective restorations
- Assessment of disease management outcomes at intervals.

Question 2

Write about site and size classification. Write a short note about principles of minimal intervention dentistry?

Answer

New caries classification (Mount and Hume in 1997) based on the location and size of the carious lesions **(Table 12.1)**.

- According to their locations:
  - Site 1: Pits and fissures (occlusal and other smooth tooth surfaces)
  - Site 2: Contact area between two teeth
  - Site 3: Cervical area in contact with gingival tissues.
- According to various sizes:
  - Size 0: Carious lesion without cavitation can be remineralised
  - Size 1: Small cavitation, just beyond healing through remineralisation
  - Size 2: Moderate cavity not extending to cusps
  - Size 3: Enlarged cavity with at least one cusp undermined needing protection from occlusal load
  - Size 4: Extensive cavity with at least one lost cusp or incisal edge
  - Reflects the difference in caries progression in different locations and sizes of decay
  - Beneficial for the treatment, monitoring and intervention purpose of new carious lesions.

Table 12.1: New caries classification according to different location and sizes

Site (location)	Size			
	Minimal (1)	Moderate (2)	Enlarged (3)	Extensive (4)
Pit and fissure (1)	1.1	1.2	1.3	1.4
Contact area (2)	2.1	2.2	2.3	2.4
Cervical (3)	3.1	3.2	3.2	3.4

Principles of Minimal Interventional Dentistry (MID)

- Patient education:
  - Prevention through dietary and oral hygiene methods
  - Aetiology of dental caries
  - Visiting dentist.
- Modification of oral flora:
  - Plaque control
  - Reduction of carbohydrate and sugar intake
  - Control of infection.
- Minimal surgical intervention of lesion:
  - Operative procedure should only be implemented when:
    - Cavitation is such that lesion cannot be arrested
    - When there is need of aesthetic and functions.
  - It should focus on:
    - Removal of friable enamel and infected dentine
    - Extent of infected dentine rather than predetermined cavity design.
- Remineralisation of non-cavitated enamel and dentine lesions:
  - Assessment of saliva both qualitative and quantitative
  - White spots on enamel and non-cavitated lesions of dentine that can be reversed or stopped
  - Mineralisation of these lesions.
- Repair rather than replacement:
  - Replacement can cause high risk in the chance of tooth fracture.

Question 3

Describe chemomechanical techniques of minimal intervention dentistry?

Answer

Chemomechanical Methods

Caries detector dyes:

- Caries detector dyes are useful in detection of early enamel caries
- It also helps in the assessment of the depth of dentine caries
- They are protein based dyes.

Composition

- 1% acid red in propylene glycol
  - 0.5% basic fuchsine in propylene glycol.
- Carbolan green, coomassie blue and lissamine blue.

Caridex

It consists of two solutions:

- Solution 1:
  - Sodium hypochlorite.
- Solution 2:
  - Glycine
  - Aminobutyric acid
  - Sodium chloride
  - Sodium hydroxide
  - Tube 1 + Tube 2 mixed and applied on dentine.

Carisolv

Before the carisolv application, the carious lesion is dissolved in chemical medium followed by excavation of soft lesion using spoon excavators. Carisolv is available in two tubes:

- Tube 1:
  - Amino acids
  - Leucine
  - Lysine
  - Glutamic acid
  - Carboxymethyl cellulose
  - Sodium hydroxide.
- Tube 2:
  - Sodium hypochlorite
  - Mechanism of action:
    - Amino acids bind chlorine to form chloramines on mixing of gel at high pH
    - Chloramines bind to different proteinaceous areas in carious dentine
    - Departed collagen is porous mineral which is easily penetrated.

Advantages

- It is painless and comfortable to the patient
- It requires conservative cavity preparation.

Disadvantage

It is very time consuming.

Restorative Materials Used in MID

Properties of an ideal restorative material for MID:

- Material should contribute to the healing process of dentine which is demineralised
- They should be adhesive so as to conserve tooth structure as they should not require mechanical retention features.

Glass Ionomer Cement

Uses

- Atraumatic restorative treatment (ART)
- Tunnel/internal preparation for proximal lesions.

Advantages

- Good adhesion to tooth structure
- Release fluoride
- Recharge mechanism.

Disadvantages

- Technique sensitivity
- Opaqueness.

Giomer

It is a pre-reached glass ionomer technology. It is made by glass filler particles which are pre-reached with poly-acrylic acid.

Composition

- Bisphenol A-glycidyl dimethacrylate
- Triethyleneglycol-dimethacrylate (TEGDMA)
- Inorganic glass filler
- Aluminuoxide
- Silica
- Pre-reached glass ionomer filler
- Camphorquinone.

Composite Resins

- Combination of composite resin with sealant is called preventive resin restoration
- It is indicated when the carious lesion in a pit or fissures is small
- Flowable composite are preferred.

Disadvantages

- Low modules of elasticity
- Higher polymerization shrinkage
- Demineralised tissue is only removed from the cavitated part of the fissure.

Pit and Fissure Sealants

Used in pit and fissure caries to restrict the development of caries.

Sandwich Technique

Placement of composite resin followed by glass ionomer cement to get the properties of both the cements.

SHORT ESSAYS

Question 1

Define acid etching?

Answer

Definition

It is the process by which the enamel surface is etched with phosphoric acid so that the enamel which is covered with organic pellicle that makes bonding difficult because of its low reactivity is controlled by raising the critical surface tension, increasing the bonding area and roughness that allows the hydrophobic resins to penetrate the porosities of the dry etched enamel. 37% phosphoric acid is used.

Forms of Acid

- Liquid etchant
- Gel etchant.

Etching Time

- 15–30 seconds
- Increased in case of primary teeth and in teeth with fluorosis.

Mechanism

The smooth surface enamel after contact with phosphoric acid converts into a very irregular surface with high depth.

Three Types of Etch Patterns

1. Dissolution of the prism core leaving the prism peripheries intact
2. Dissolution of the prism peripheries leaving the prism cores intact
3. No prism structures are evident.

Rinsing

After etching, the enamel surface is thoroughly rinsed with a stream of water spray for 5–10 seconds, so that the acid is completely washed off the surface.

Drying

Drying is immediately followed by rinsing which produces a frosty, white appearance. Contamination of etched enamel can be prevented from saliva, moisture or blood.

Mechanism of enamel bonding is micromechanical in nature brought by formation of "resign tags" within the etched enamel.

The bond strength of composite to etched enamel is 15–25 MPa.

Question 2

Discuss pit and fissure sealants?

Answer

Definition

According to ADA, pit and fissure sealant is an adhesive material that is applied to pits and fissures of teeth in order to isolate from rest of the oral cavity.

Classification

- According to chemical structure of monomer used:
  - Methyl methacrylate (MMA)
  - Triethylene glycol dimethacrylate (TEGDMA)
  - Bisphenol dimethacrylate (BPD)
  - Bisphenol A-glycidyl methacrylate (Bis-GMA)
  - Propyl methacrylate urethane (PMU).
- According to generation:
  - 1st generation: light cured
  - 2nd generation: self-cured
  - 3rd generation: blue visible light
  - 4th generation: fluoride releasing.
- Based on filler content:
  - Unfilled
  - Filled.
- Based on colour:
  - White linted/opaque
  - Coloured.

Indications

- Adolescents and teenagers in high risk and adults for prevention of caries
- Incipient caries in enamel that are not extending to the dentino-enamel junction.

Procedure

- Isolate and dry the tooth surface
- Rubber dam application
- Cotton roll isolation and suctioning.

Etching the Tooth Surface

- Etch for 15–30 seconds for primary teeth and 15 seconds for permanent teeth
- Additional time is required for fluorosed teeth.

Apply Bonding Agent

Application of hydrophilic bonding agent before sealant application will improve retention with teeth, followed by curing.

Material Application

- Liquid etchants are preferred as they penetrate the enamel wall well
- With autopolymerising sealants, working time varies from 1 minute to 2 minutes and photoactive sealants 10–20 seconds for complete setting.

Rinse and Dry Etched Tooth Surface

- Rinse the etched tooth surface with air spray for 30 seconds
- Dry the tooth surface for 30 seconds
- Repeat the etching step if necessary
- Age range for sealant application:
  - 3–4 years: primary molars
  - 6–7 years: 1st permanent molar
  - 11–13 years: 2nd permanent molar and premolars.

SHORT NOTES

Question 1

Define extension for prevention?

Answer

It is defined as the tooth preparation for smooth surface caries. The restoration should be extended to areas that are normally self-cleansing so as to prevent recurrences of caries.

- It is necessary to remove remaining enamel defects, such as pits and fissures, by extension
- Prevention on smooth caries is eliminated because the relative caries immunity is provided by preventive measures like fluoride, proper diet, good oral hygiene

- Extension for prevention is restricted from full length inclusion of enamel fissures so as to conserve the tooth structure which is less prone to fracture and gives stability.

Question 2

Define air abrasion?

Answer

It is a powerful stream of focused narrow beam of aluminium oxide particles 20.5 microns in size sprayed at a pressure of 40–140 psi through a five angled nozzle.

- The force against the tooth structure abrades it and a conservative cavity is prepared
- It cuts enamel, dentine and cementum
- These cavities are well suited for composite restorations.

Advantages

- No anaesthesia required
- No noise, heat generation and vibration
- Conserve tooth structure
- Well tolerated by patient.

Disadvantages

- Does not remove soft caries
- Cavity preparation is limited
- Can damage adjacent teeth while Class II preparation
- Very expensive.

CHAPTER 13

Infection Control

LONG ESSAYS

Question 1

What is the importance of moisture control in operative dentistry? Discuss other methods of controlling moisture during operative procedures?

Answer

Moisture Control

To carry out an ideal operative dentistry in a saliva and blood field is a very difficult task.

Restorative materials and restorative procedures require clean and dry field to obtain their best properties.

- Proper isolation creates good conditions of the working area and improves the quality of treatment
- Isolation helps in
  - Eliminating saliva
  - Eliminating sulcular fluid
  - Eliminating gingival bleeding.

Goals of Isolation

- Moisture control
- Retraction
- Protection
- Improving treatment quality.

Methods of Isolation

- Indirect methods:
  - Relaxed patient position
  - Local anaesthesia (LA)
  - Drugs.
- Direct methods:
  - Rubber dam
  - Throat shields
  - Gingival retraction
  - Cotton rolls and cellulose waters
  - High volume evacuators and saliva ejector.

Indirect Methods

- Relaxed position of the patient: The objective of relaxing patient is to have control over the anxiety and unnecessary excess salivation
- Local anaesthesia: To eliminate the discomfort and also to control moisture, LA plays an important role
- Drugs: Suggested in patients with excessive salivation:
  - Atropine: 0.3–1 mg (1–2 hours before procedure)
  - Propantheline bromide: 7.5–15 mg (30–45 minutes before procedure).

Direct Methods

- Rubber dam: Rubber dam is the most preferred method in sterilisation. It ensures absolute moisture control. It is used to isolate one or more than one teeth in the procedure.
  - Indications:
    - Endodontic procedures
    - Restorations
    - Excavation of deep caries
    - Sub-gingival restoration
    - Bleaching
    - Composite restorations in anterior teeth
    - High-risk patient, e.g., human immunodeficiency virus (HIV), hepatitis.
  - Contraindications:
    - Unerupted teeth
    - Some third molars
    - Malpositioned teeth
    - Asthmatic patients
    - Patients with breathing problems
    - Patients with latex allergy
    - Uncooperative pediatric patients.
  - Rubber dam equipment:
    - Rubber dam material
    - Rubber dam frame

- ➤ Rubber dam retainers/clamps
- ➤ Rubber dam punch
- ➤ Rubber dam stamp
- ➤ Rubber dam clamp forceps
- ➤ Rubber dam napkin
- ➤ Rubber dam lubricant
- ➤ Other retainers
- ➤ Modelling compound.
- ❑ Throat shields:
  - ○ Used in recovering small objects
  - ○ Used as protection from aspirating or swallowing small objects
  - ○ It is done by using a gauge sponge which is unfolded and spread over the tongue and posterior part of the mouth.
- ❑ Gingival tissue retraction: It is the apical and lateral displacement of gingival tissue which helps in proper visibility and accessibility during sub-gingival tooth preparation and for the proper flow of impression material into the area. Methods of gingival tissue retraction:
  - ○ Physicomechanical method: It is done by mechanical forcing of gingival tissue away from tooth surface.

    Method used are:
    - ➤ Copper bands
    - ➤ Acrylic resin copings
    - ➤ Heavy weight rubber dam
    - ➤ Aluminium shell
    - ➤ Cotton twigs replacement in gingival sulcus
    - ➤ Use of ZOE pack. It should remain there for at least 48 hours.
  - ○ Chemical method: In this method chemicals are carried into gingival sulcus. For example,
    - ➤ Vasoconstrictors like epinephrine and norepinephrine
    - ➤ Biological fluid coagulants like alum, aluminium chloride, aluminium potassium sulphate, tannic acid
    - ➤ They coagulate blood and tissue fluids.
  - ○ Electrosurgical method: Electrosurgical methods produce have four actions:
    - ➤ Cutting
    - ➤ Coagulation
    - ➤ Fulguration
    - ➤ Desiccation.

    Mostly, cutting action is used in case of gingival tissue retraction.
  - ○ Surgical method: Using a sharp blade or surgical knife, surgical excision of interfering gingival tissue is done.

- ❑ Cotton roll isolation: Isolation with cotton roll for different teeth are specific.
  - ○ Maxillary teeth: Medium sized cotton roll is placed in facial vestibule
  - ○ Mandibular teeth: Medium size cotton rolls are placed in the facial vestibule and larger one is placed in between teeth and tongue
  - ○ Cotton rolls are replaced with new ones once they become saturated
  - ○ Dry cotton rolls are moistened before they are removed, so it does not pull back any epithelial covering.
- ❑ High volume evacuators and saliva ejectors:
  - ○ Evacuators are used to suck out the airotor water spray.
  - ○ It is high speed suction
  - ○ Tip is made of either plastic or steel
  - ○ Saliva ejectors just different from evacuators in a way that they work much slower.
    - ➤ Advantages:
      - » Very rapid water removal from operating site
      - » Rapid clearance of debris and shattered restorative materials
      - » Less pain in patients
      - » Precious metals are more readily salvaged
      - » Plastic ejectors are inexpensive and are easily moulded into the required shape at the time of procedure very easily.

Question 2

Write about methods of sterilisation. Discuss the importance of sterilisation of operative instrument?

Answer

- ❑ Sterilisation is the method of removal of all micro-organisms in the vegetative and spore forms
- ❑ It is important to clean and sterilise the instruments by different methods of sterilisation.

Methods of Sterilisation

- ❑ Steam pressure sterilisation (Autoclave)
- ❑ Dry heat sterilisation (Dri-clave)
- ❑ Chemical vapour pressure sterilisation (Chemiclave)
- ❑ Ethylene oxide sterilisation.

Steam Pressure Sterilisation (Autoclave)

- ❑ It is a double walled chamber to hold the instruments. Steam under high pressure is circulated inside it
- ❑ Superheated steam under pressure kills microorganisms by protein coagulation (**Table 13.1**).

Ideal Requirements of Proper Autoclaving

- Instruments should be wrapped in thin cloth, paper, perforated cassettes or steam-permeable plastic
- Instruments should be packed in such a way that it allows free circulation of the pressurised steam
- Fresh water should be used for each cycle
- Abstain tap water as it contains minerals that form deposits on the surface of autoclave
- To prevent carbon steel instruments and burs from corrosion they should be treated with 2% sodium nitrate which is a corrosion-inhibitor and then wrapped
- Only when autoclave reaches the appropriate temperature and pressure the sterilisation for adequate time is completed.

Types of Autoclaves

- Downward displacement autoclave
- High vacuum autoclaves.

- Downward displacement autoclaves:
  - They have low efficiency
  - There is a downward displacement of air as steam enters the top of the chamber.

- High vacuum autoclave:
  - They are rapid cycle autoclave
  - Air in this is evacuated by vacuum
  - Suction before the steam enters the chambers
  - They are most conventional autoclaves in dentistry.

Table 13.1: Sterilisation cycle

Cycle	Temperature	Pressure	Time
Standard	121°C	15 lbs	20 minutes
Flash	134°C	30 lbs	7–10 minutes

Advantages

- Most rapid and effective sterilisation process
- Does not dismantle cloth or cotton
- Penetration is very efficient
- Verification at the end of the cycle is possible.

Disadvantages

- Causes corrosion of carbon steel instruments
- Can cause damage to plastic or rubber items
- It dulls the improtective cutting edges of instruments.

Dry Heat Sterilisation (Dri-Clave)

- At 160°C, it effectively sterilises instruments at high temperature

- Dry heat from this kills microbes through oxidation
- It consists of heated chambers with dry heat over to allow air to circulate by gravity flow
- Instruments are placed at a distance of minimum 1 cm so that it helps in quick sterilisation
- Aluminium foil is used to warp the instruments
- Paper and cloth may form char **(Table 13.2)**.

Table 13.2: Dry Heat Sterilisation

Apparatus	Temperature	Time
Convention dry heat oven	160°C	90 minutes
Mechanical convection oven	320–370°C	6–12 minutes

Advantages

- Rapid cycles at high temperature
- Rusting of burs and carbon steel instruments are avoided
- Sterilisation can be verified
- Low cost.

Disadvantages

- Items like rubber and plastics can be destroyed
- At lower temperatures, sterilisation process is prolonged
- Crowding and overloading interferes with sterilisation process
- Inaccurate calibration and setting causes error.

Chemical Vapour Pressure Sterilisation

A mixture of formaldehyde, acetone, ketone alcohol and water employs chemical vapour when heated under pressure producing a gas that sterilises instruments **(Table 13.3)**.

- They kill microorganisms by destroying vital protein systems
- Instruments are packed in paper or steam permeable plastics
- Heat the steriliser before it becomes operational.

Table 13.3: Chemical Vapour Pressure Sterilisation

Temperature	Pressure	Time
132°C	20 lbs	20 minutes

Advantages

- It has a property of not corroding metal
- It has fast and good cycle time
- The load is dry when comes out.

Disadvantages

- High cost
- Foul smell of vapour; needs proper ventilation
- Manufacturer solution can only be used
- Cannot sterilise hand piece.

Ethylene Oxide Sterilisation

- ❑ An automatic device filled with ethylene oxide gas at temperature below 100°C is used to sterilise complex instruments and delicate materials
- ❑ Ethylene oxide is highly penetrable
- ❑ It kills microorganisms by chemically reacting with nucleic acids.

Advantages

- ❑ Gentle and sensitive sterilisation for hand pieces
- ❑ Operates even at low temperature.

Disadvantages

- ❑ High cost
- ❑ Long time for process

- ❑ Best for hospitals
- ❑ Ethylene oxide is carcinogenic and mutagenic.

Newer Methods of Sterilisation

Gamma-rays

Used to sterilise:
- ❑ Syringes
- ❑ Disposable needles
- ❑ Other heat sensitive items.

Ultraviolet Light

- ❑ It is used to purify the air in dental operatory
- ❑ Hydrogen peroxide vapour gas plasma sterilisation and lasers are still under process to be implicated.

SHORT ESSAYS

Question 1

Write in brief about OSHA. What are its regulations?

Answer

- ❑ **OSHA:** Occupational Safety and Health Act
- ❑ This act was passed by US Congress in the year 1970.
  - ○ Before this act was formed, term—standard operating procedures (SOPs) was used as regulations.

Regulations of OSHA

- ❑ It regulates universal precautions:
  - ○ Careful handling of shop instruments
  - ○ Using of the devices that reduce contamination risks, e.g., high volume suction, rubber dam.
- ❑ Provision of hepatis B vaccination
- ❑ Implication of protective equipments like masks, gloves and gowns
- ❑ Housekeeping provision which includes cleaning of:
  - ○ Instruments
  - ○ Operatory equipments
  - ○ Floors and walls

  - ○ Waste management
  - ○ Sterilisation procedures.
- ❑ Control of contamination production like spatter, mist or aerosol—use of rubber dam and high speed suctions are adviced and implicated
- ❑ Never hold any non-operating things with working gloves, e.g., phones, door handles, switches, pens, etc
- ❑ To avoid or minimise splashing, spattering or contact of bare hands with contaminated instruments:
  - ○ Use of brush by holding the instruments down at the sink is the method to do to avoid the mentioned hazards.
- ❑ Maintaining proper sterilisation of instruments and working area
- ❑ Provision of proper washing area like sink or basin after procedures
- ❑ Disposal of contaminated items like cotton rolls, bandages with blood and other sharp objects
- ❑ Proper laundering of garments, like apron and gowns
- ❑ Disposal of needles by mechanical methods and safe handling.

SECTION 2

ENDODONTICS

Clinical Diagnostic Aids in Endodontics

LONG ESSAYS

Question 1

Mention the various clinical diagnostic aids used in endodontics and write in detail about vitality tests?

Answer

Various Diagnostic Aids

- Visual and tactile inspection
- Mobility test
- Electric pulp vitality test
- Anaesthetic test
- Palpation and percussion
- Radiographic examination
- Thermal test
- Test cavity preparation.

Methods Used to Check the Vitality of the Teeth

- Electric pulp test (EPT)
- Thermal test:
  - Cold testing
  - Heat testing.
- Laser Doppler flowmetry (LDF)
- Pulse oximetry
- Liquid crystal testing
- Hughes probeye camera.

Electric Pulp Test

- Electric pulp test works on electric impulses which directly stimulate the nerves especially delta sensory nerves of the pulp
- Common EPT are:
  - Digitest
  - Neotest
  - Gentle pulse
  - Densitometer.

- It does not give the vascular supply or histological status of the pulp, it only shows responsive and non-responsive status.
- Disadvantages:
  - Adequate stimulus
  - Application method knowledge
  - Interpretation of the results.
  - It is technique sensitive
- Factors affecting electric pulp test response:
  - Thickness of enamel
  - Recently traumatized tooth
  - Anxiety level of patients
  - Cross-section area of probe tip
  - Interfering restorative material
  - Calcification of dentine
  - Use of medications like sedatives
  - Placement of probe.
- Procedure:
  - Patient should be briefed about the testing so as to reduce his/her the anxiety level
  - Tooth is isolated with cotton rolls
  - An electrical conductor or a toothpaste is applied to the tip of the electrode
  - The circuit is completed by placing patient's finger on the handle of the device or using a lip clip
  - Multirooted teeth may need to be tested by placing the electrode at more than one position in the crown
  - Most suitable electrode is placed to the dried enamel at middle third of the facial surface of the crown:
    - Current used: 5–20 MA.
  - The current is increased slowly till the tingling sensation turns to painful sensation
  - An average is taken after repeating the process 2–3 times.

- Precautions:
  - It is contraindicated in patients with cardiac pacemaker
  - It cannot be used against devices like desensitizers and electrosurgical units that can cause current leakage.
- False readings:
  - A false positive response means that pulp is necrotic
  - When patient feels sensation in tooth, it can be due to:
    - Gangrenous pulp present in the root canal
    - Anxiety
    - Metallic restoration
    - Multirooted teeth with necrotic pulp.
  - A false negative response means that pulp is vital. When patient does not complain about sensitivity it is due to:
    - Calcified pulp chambers
    - Restored teeth with base
    - Patients on sedations/alcohol
    - Low battery of electric pulp test
    - Psychotic disorder
    - Traumatized tooth
    - Tooth with incomplete root formation
    - Patients with high threshold to pain
    - Inadequate conductor media.

Thermal Tests

Thermal tests are based on the fluid flow in dentinal tubules. They can be done in two ways:
- Cold test
- Hot test.

Cold Testing

- Cold testing is the most common and reliable test
- It helps in distinguishing reversible pulpitis from irreversible pulpitis and also from necrotic pulp.

Cold Testing is Done with

- Air blasts
- Cold drink/water/air/ice stick
- Ethyl chloride spray
- Skin refrigerant spray:
  - This is known as endo ice
  - It has a temperature of –26.2°C
  - It is used with a cotton pellet and applied on the mid surface of the tooth.
- Frozen CO_2:
  - It is also known as dry ice
  - Temperature ranges from –56 to 98°C containing dichlorodifluoromethane
  - It is supplied in small plastic syringe

- It should not come in contact with soft tissue, as it can cause damage to it
  - No irreversible changes in pulp or enamel occur.
- Technique:
  - Isolation of teeth is done and ice stick is immediately applied on the middle third of the facial surface of the tooth
  - It should be kept for 5 seconds in contact with tooth or until the patient begins to feel pain
  - Cold test should start from most posterior tooth moving towards anterior tooth.
  - During testing:
    - If pain persists, after removal of stimulus— Irreversible pulpitis
    - If pain subsides, after removal of stimulus— Reversible pulpitis.

Heat Testing

- Heat testing is done by:
  - Heated Gutta percha stick
  - Hot green stick compound
  - Hot water
  - Heated burnisher.
- Technique:
  - Before heat testing, a thin coating of petroleum jelly is applied to prevent the warm Gutta perch sticking to tooth surface
  - Warm Gutta perch is applied on the middle third of the facial surface of the crown which leads to a response in less than 2 seconds
  - Rubber dam is used in case the hot water is used. Patient reaction is seen after 5 seconds.
- Thermal test response:
  - Non-vital pulp: No response
  - Normal pulp: Normal to moderate pain which subsides, once the stimulus is removed
  - Reversible pulpitis: Strong prolonged pain that subsides when the stimulus is removed
  - Irreversible pulpitis: Moderate to strong pain that does not subsides even after removal of stimulus.

Laser Doppler Flowmetry

- This is a method used to determine the blood flow in microvasculature system
- A laser beam of known wavelength is directed straight to the blood vessel within the pulp in the crown portion of tooth
- The movement of RBCs causes the frequency of laser beam to be doppler shifted

- The reflected light is detected by a photocell. Its output is proportional to the number and velocity of the blood cells
- If the tissue is static (necrotic pulp), there will be no change in frequency on passage through it.

Disadvantages

- Results may vary in patients who are on antihypertensive drugs and patients who are smokers. As this may affect the blood flow of the pulp
- Set up is expensive.

Pulse Oximetry

- This is highly used and common in past
- The oxygen saturation levels of blood are during the intravenous administration of anaesthesia
- It follows the principle that increased acidity and metabolic rate that is produced by inflammation causes haemoglobin deoxygenation which changes the oxygen saturation level of the blood.

Procedure

A probe that contains diode emits light of two different wavelenghts i.e., red light and infrared light.

- Red light: Emits 6,660 nm
- Infrared light: Emits 850 nm:
  - The light is received by a photo detector diode which is connected to a microprocessor
  - The ratio of the amplitude of the transmitted both lights is compared by the device
  - With the help of changes in oxygen saturation monitoring inflammation of the pulp or partial necrosis of vital teeth is detected.

Disadvantage

It is an expensive instrument.

Liquid Crystal Testing

- Cholestric liquid crystal is used
- It works on the temperature difference in tooth
- Vital pulps will have higher temperature
- Necrotic pulps will have lower temperature.

Hughes Probeye Camera

This device is capable of detecting temperature change that is as minimal as 0.1°C.

It is also been used to measure pulp vitality experimetry.

Question 2

Discuss the role and limitations of radiographs in endodontics. Write about radiovisiography?

Answer

Radiographs are most important diagnostic tool.

Uses of Radiographs in Endodontics

This can be divided into three phases:

1. Diagnosis
2. Different levels of treatment planning evaluation
3. Endodontic treatment.

Radiographs in Diagnosis

- To determine loss of hard tissue, calcification or alteration of tooth and periradicular structures
- To examine number of root canals, root curvatures and abnormal root morphologies
- To locate pulpal, bony or periapical abnormalities.

Various Treatment Steps in Radiographs

- To determine the working length
- Locating pulp that is calcified or receded
- Determining the change in angulation
- Extra canals
- Missed canals.

Radiographs for Evaluation after the Endodontic Treatment

- To access the quality of obturation
- Under-filled or over-filled canal
- Density of the filled canal
- Recall assessment of the patient.

Limitations

- Due to improper handling and technique variation there can be distortion in the image
- Many lesions can go undetected, e.g., in medullary bone
- Soft tissue lesions or periradicular lesions cannot be accurately diagnosed
- Histological verification is required for the perfect diagnosis.

Radiovisiography

Radiovisiography (RVG) is a computerized technique which can capture, view, enhance and store the radiographic images of multiple patients.

Parts of RVG

- Sensor
- Video monitor
- High resolution printer.

Sensor

- An intraoral sensor captures the image from the radiating source (X-ray)
- It is fluoroscopic with set of optic fibres that translate the image and an electronic signal is produced and displayed.

Video Monitor

- After the sensor displays an image, the monitor attached to it, transforms the signals into a digital image
- This image is displayed at the same moment into the monitor

- This image can be stored and viewed, when required.

High Resolution Printer

It transfers the image on a photographic paper.

Advantages

- No need of X-ray films
- Less exposure time, i.e., 1/100 of a second
- Image can be zoomed or coloured
- Educational Aid
- Instant display of image
- No distortion
- Enlargement up to four times the original size.

Disadvantage

Expensive.

SHORT ESSAYS

Question 1

What is percussion test?

Answer

- Percussion test is a type of test which determines the condition of the periodontium surrounding the tooth
- The handle of the instruments like mouth mirror and probe is used and the tooth is struck a quick, moderate blow initially with low intensity to determine the presence of absence of tenderness of tooth
- Test are done in order to eliminate any doubt however, the percussion test alone cannot help diagnose the condition
- One should change the direction of the blow from the vertical occlusal to the buccal or lingual surface of the crown and strike separate cusps in a different order
- Percussion is not done to a sensitive tooth beyond the patient's tolerance
- According to percussive sounds, a dull note signifies abscess formation, while a sharp note inflammation.

Question 2

Discuss radiography in endodontics? Limitations of radiographs?

Answer

Radiographs are one of the most important clinical tools in making a diagnosis:

Applications

- To arrive to a diagnosis and confirm the clinical findings
- To determine the loss of tooth structure
- To estimate the proximity of the lesions to the coronal pulp
- To identify pulpal pathosis such as pulp stone and periapical lesions
- To find out the length and the course of root canal
- To locate the size shape and direction of root
- To do working length estimation
- To locate apical foraminas
- To identify iatrogenic exposures, accident and mishaps
- To identify broken instruments
- To find out the periodontally involved lesions such as bone loss, furcation involvement, and widening of lamina dura periapically
- To identify fractures occurring under gingiva
- To identify impaction of foreign body into the soft tissue
- Evaluating the outcome of endodontic treatment.

Radiographs

- Radiography is a two dimensional representation of three dimensional object
- Initial lesions may go undetected as the translucency is only appreciated once the 30% of destruction has taken place
- This stage of pathosis remains unclear

❑ Super impositions of artefacts and over lapping structures may cloud the diagnosis
❑ Soft tissue lession may be difficult do diagnose and may require additional support such as histological examinations.

Question 3

What are the advantages and disadvantages radiovisiography?

Answer

❑ RVG is elaborated as radiovisiography and was introduced by Dr. Francis Mouyen in 1989
❑ It is a form of digital radiography that captures and stores images in a digital format
❑ The unit has an intraoral sensor that is available in two size that is adult and paediatric
❑ The sensor contains a set of optic fibres and the coupling device that produces an electronic signal and translates the image that is displayed.
❑ This sensor is connected to computer that converts this electronic signal into a digital image which can be then readily appreciated on to a screen

Advantages

❑ Minimal amount of exposure as compared to conventional radiography
❑ Exposure time is significantly decreased (1/100 of a second)
❑ Instant results and enhanced image with multiple option of zoom colour change etc
❑ Procedure is repeatable
❑ Easy to maintain records
❑ X-ray film is not used
❑ Useful for patient education.

Disadvantages

❑ Its not cost effective
❑ Difficult to maintain
❑ Some times difficult to use where patients have severe gag reflex and limited mouth opening.

Question 4

What is endometer?

Answer

❑ Endometer is also known as apex locater that is used to determine the length of a root canal that measures the impedance between the apical foramina and oral membrane
❑ It provides an accurate reading both in dry and wet condition
❑ The needle can be easily localized within the canal on the analogical screen
❑ If the needle crosses the physiological barrier and additional sound can be heard simultaneously.

Advantages

❑ Accurate
❑ Less time consuming
❑ Appropriate where radiographs are difficult to obtain
❑ Bleeps upon crossing apical foramina
❑ Avoids unnecessary exposure to radiation
❑ Decrease the treatment time.

Question 5

What is transilluminations in endodontics?

Answer

❑ Transillumination is a diagnostic test to detect cracks and fracture line of the permanent tooth
❑ It contains specialized fibreoptic wand, otoscope with fibreoptic attachment, a bore light of fibreoptic handpiece
❑ Additional applications are detection of inter proximal carries, occlusal carries, calculus and stained margins of composite
❑ Also known as FOTI i.e., fiber optic transilluminations that refers to thin cylindrical fibers of plastic or glass.

SHORT NOTES

Question 1

Define endometer?

Answer

❑ It is a device which is used to determine the root length
❑ It works on the principle of measuring electrical impedance between oral mucous membrane and the optical foramen
❑ The position of the needle in the root can be easily seen on the screen
❑ A sound of different tone and intensity is heard when the needle penetrates beyond the apical foramen.

Advantages

- Useful in those conditions where radiographs are not easy to be captured
- Penetration of needle beyond the apical foramen
- Prevents the radiation exposure to both patient and the doctor
- Accuracy maintained despite of any technical or mechanical issues.

Question 2

What is glass bead sterilizer?

Answer

- Glass bead sterilizer is the most common form of sterilization used in endodontic practice
- It has many small glass beads ranging from 1.2-1.5 mm in diameter at a very high temperature between 220° to 240° C
- It is usually used for around 45 seconds to inactivate micro organisation.

Disadvantage

Only small instruments can be sterilized.

Question 3

Explain thermal test?

Answer

- Thermal tests are usually conducted to determine the vitality of the pulp
- There are usually two types of thermal test i.e., cold and heat.

Cold Test

- Frozen CO_2
- Endo ice
- Ethyl chloride
- Ice sticks.

Heat Test

- Heated GP
- Hot water
- Hot green stick compound
- Hot burnisher.

Question 4

Endodontic triad?

Answer

- Endodontic triad refers to a three step procedure that consists of biomechanical preparation, microbial control and complete obturation of the canal space
- The ultimate goal of the treatment is to create an environment in which the body will heal itself.

Question 5

Enumerate diagnostic aids used in endodontics?

Answer

Various diagnostic aids used commonly for endodontic practice are:
- Visual and tactile inspection
- Palpation and percussion
- Mobility test
- Test cavity preparation
- Anaesthetic test
- Electric pulp vitality test
- Thermal test
- Radiographic examination.

Question 6

What are the methods to check pulp vitality?

Answer

Methods Used to Check the Vitality of the Teeth

- Electric pulp test (EPT)
- Thermal test:
    - Cold testing
    - Heat testing.
- Laser Doppler flowmetry (LDF)
- Pulse oximetry
- Liquid crystal testing
- Hughes probeye camera.

Question 7

What is laser doppler flowmetry?

Answer

Laser Doppler Flowmetry

- This is a method used to determine the blood flow in microvasculature system
- A laser beam of known wavelength is directed straight to the blood vessel within the pulp, in the crown portion of tooth
- The movement of RBCs causes the frequency of laser beam to be Doppler shifted

❑ The reflected light is detected by a photocell. Its output is proportional to the number and velocity of the blood cells
❑ If the tissue is static (necrotic pulp), there will be no change in frequency on passage through it

Question 8

Define endodontic triad?

Answer

Endodontic triad consists of:
❑ Biomechanical preparation
❑ Microbial control
❑ Complete obturation of the canal space:
  ○ Endodontic triad is the ultimate goal of the treatment
  ○ It is the base of endodontic treatment.

CHAPTER 15

Diagnosis and Treatment Planning

Question 1

Describe the role of various radiographic techniques in diagnosis and treatment planning?

Answer

Classification

- Conventional methods:
  - Intraoral periapical radiograph (10 Pa)
  - Occlusal and panoramic radiographs
  - Bitewing radiographs
  - Xeroradiographs.
- Advanced methods:
  - Digital imaging [Radiovisiography (RVG)]
  - Complicated image analysis
  - Subtraction radiography
  - Tuned aperture computed tomography
  - Magnetic resonance micro-imaging.

Indications

- History of pain
- Swelling
- Mobility of the tooth
- Sinus tract or fistula
- Trauma
- Missing teeth
- Bleeding or sensitive tooth
- Deep caries
- Malpositioned or impacted tooth
- Evidence of foreign objects
- Tooth anomalies.

Types of Radiographs

Conventional Methods

Bitewing radiographs:
- Detecting interproximal caries
- Patient education

- Saves time
- Diagnosis of restoration contour and cervical margin integrity
- Elimination of X-ray film.

Disadvantages:

- Expensive
- Needs computer knowledge to operate.

Xeroradiography

- It contains rigid aluminium/selenium coated photo-receptor plate
- Electrically charged plate is placed in waterproof cassette which is then positioned in the mouth and then exposed to X-rays
- Plates can be recharged and used several times
- This image is transformed to visible image with pigmented deposition particles called toner
- The image formed is transferred to a paper or laminated between the translucent and transparent sheet of plastic
- The image is than viewed under referred light.

Advantages:

- Sharp image
- Radiation exposure is less
- Better resolution
- Superior contrast.

Digital Subtraction Radiography

- They are used to detect progress of caries from incipient lesion
- Measuring changes in the lesions
- The method used is taking a conventional radiograph and digitalising it
- Pulp size, calcification can be seen
- Status of existing restoration
- Location of calculus
- Alveolar crest height.

Intraoral Periapical Radiographs

- Periapical area of the tooth
- Supporting bone and periodontal membrane
- Detect crown-root ratio
- Periapical pathology
- Root curvature and length
- For post and core canal angulation.

Panoramic Radiographs

- Gives overall inclusive view of teeth, its associated structures and the temporomandibular joint (TMJ)
- Mostly used in patients having gag problems with intraoral radiographs as they are extraoral
- Major disadvantage bring the expensive costing of it.

Advanced Methods

Radiovisiography

It consists of:
- Intraoral sensor which captures the image
- Extraoral radiation source.

Advantages:
- Instant display of image on computer
- Can be stored for future records
- Less error in diagnosis
- Images can be printed for records
- High quality imaging.

Cone Beam Computed Tomography

- It is used in determination of buccolingual and mesiodistal width of the teeth
- Used for observing:
  - Carious lesions
  - Extension of maxillary sinusitis
  - Proximity of root apices.
- Used for three-dimensional (3D) reconstruction of root canals.

Tuned Aperture Computed Tomography

It uses digital radiographic images and has software that correlates the individual image of an object by layering of images which are viewed as slices.

Disadvantages:
- Slices are too thick
- 1.25 mm
- Cannot detect small lesions.

Question 2

Discuss in detail about pulp vitality test. Discuss the recent advancements?

Answer

They are the sites to monitor the state of health of the dental pulp, mostly needed after traumatic injuries.

Types

- Electric pulp testing
- Thermal testing:
  - Cold testing
  - Heat testing.
- Test cavity
- Anaesthesia testing
- Bite test
- Laser Doppler flowmetry
- Pulse oximetry
- Liquid crystal camera
- Hughes probeye camera
- Dual wavelength photometry.

Electric Pulp Testing

It is an instrument that uses the gradation of electric excitations of neural elements within the pulp (A-delta fibres):
- Positive response indicate that pulp is vital
- Negative response indicates necrosis/non-vital pulp.

Factors Affecting the Response of the Pulp

- Enamel thickness
- Trauma
- Placement of the probe
- Calcification of the denture
- Anxiety level
- Sedatives
- Restorative material interference.

Contraindication

- Patients with pacemakers
- Patient with electrosurgical units or desensitizers.

Procedure

- Isolation and drying of tooth is done
- Complete the circuit by placing the patient's finger on the Probe handle
- Electrode should be placed on the facial surface of the tooth
- Increase the current till the time tingling sensation becomes painful
- It should be done for 2–3 times to eliminate any chance of false reading.

False Reading

It is of two types:
- False positive response
- False negative response.

False positive response:

This response means necrotic pulp and patient feels sensation in the tooth.

False negative response:

This response means that pulp is vital but patient does not complain of any sensation.

Thermal Testing

It is done in two ways:
- Cold testing
- Heat testing.

Cold Test

It is done with:
- Ice sticks
- Dry ice (frozen CO_2)
- Endo ice
- Ethyl chloride.

Procedure

- Isolation of tooth is done
- Cold air is sprayed directly on the facial middle third surface of the teeth
- This is the most common method, easy to implicate and no specific instruments used in this method.

Other Methods

- Use of cotton pellet saturated with ethyl chloride, dry ice, endo ice or ice sticks
- Dry ice (Frozen CO_2) tens P: –56°C–98°C
- Endo ice (temp): –26.2°C
- Any of the cold stimulus is applied for 5 seconds
- It should start from the posterior most tooth and then advanced towards the anterior teeth
- If there is pain even after stimulus is removed: Irreversible pulpitis
- If pain subsides after the stimulus is removed: Hyper sensitivity or reversible pulpitis.

Heat Test

It is done with:
- Hot burnisher
- Heated Gutter-percha
- Hot water.

Procedure

- Teeth are needed to be protected with petroleum jelly to deal with thermal trauma and isolation is done
- Heated Gutta-percha sticks is the most common method for heat testing
- It is applied at the middle third of the facial surface of the teeth
- Heated Gutta-percha is applied for 2–5 seconds.
- Heat test is not usually called as vitality test. It starts if there is an abnormal response to heat, it indicates the presence of pulpal or periapical pathology which requires endodontic treatment.

Test Cavity

It is a method that is done when diagnostic tests have failed, which need endodontic treatment trauma to the tooth in which nerve supply to the pulp is damaged but the blood supply is intact.

Procedure

A small test cavity is prepared with high speed, till it reaches the dentinoenamel junction (DEJ) in the unanaesthetised tooth.

- Patient is asked to respond to any painful sensation at the time of drilling
  - Positive response: Pulp vitality
  - Negative response: Necrotic pulp.
- A probe with diode is used that emits light of two wavelengths:
  - Red light
  - Infrared light.
- The diode is connected to a micro-processor
- The device compares the ratio of amplitudes of transmitted lights
- Its monitor changes in oxygen saturation
- Also used in the detection of pulp inflammation or partial necrosis in the vital teeth.

Laser Doppler Flowmetry

It is a process in which the laser beams of known wavelength that is directed through the crown of the tooth to the blood vessels within the pulp.

- The red blood cells in the pulp frequently causes the laser beam to be shifted to Doppler
- The light which is shattered back is detected by photocell on the tooth surface that is proportional to the number of velocity of blood cells.

Advantages

- This is the objective measurement of pulp vitality and its health
- Useful in patient who are non-responsive.

Anaesthesia Test

It is done when patient is unable to point out the site of pain and when other pulp testing techniques are inconclusive.

Procedure

In this method individual tooth is considered:
- Single tooth at a time is anaesthetised until the pain disappears
- The procedure should start from the most posterior tooth in the quadrant
- Till the source of pain is pointed, it should carry on to the anterior line in the quadrant
- This test should be preferred over the test cavity test.

Recent Advancements

The recent advancements are more specific and more prominent for the vitality tests.
- Pulse oximetry
- Laser Doppler flowmetry
- Liquid crystal testing
- Hughes probeye camera
- Dual wavelength spectrophotometry
- Gas saturation
- Electromagnetic flowmetry.

Pulse Oximetry

This technique is used for recording, blood oxygen saturation levels during administration of intravenous anaesthesia.
- Most useful in the cases with children and old age
- Also can be used in depressed and nervous patients.

Disadvantages

- Expensive
- Shows inaccurate results in patients who are on specific drugs, e.g., anti-hypertensive drugs
- Also patients who are smokers.

Liquid Crystal Testing

They are used to distinguish between the vital and necrotic pulp.
- Teeth with vital pulp: Have higher temperature
- Teeth with necrotic pulp: Have lower temperature.

Hughes Probeye Camera

They detect the pulp vitality by detecting the temperature variation. They can detect variations even as small as 0.1°C.

Dual Wavelength Spectrophotometry

- This method is used to detect oxygenation changes in the capillary and not the blood vessels
- The diagnosis does not depend on the pulsatile blood flow.

CHAPTER 16

Instruments

Question 1

Classify and discuss handcutting, rotary instruments used in operative dentistry?

Answer

There is a numeric formula that describes angles and dimensions of the working end of a hand cutting instrument.

Given by GV Black

It consists of three units:

1. Unit blade width: It is the width of the blade expressed in $1/10^{th}$ of an mm.
2. Unit blade length: It is the length of the blade in mm.
3. Unit blade angle: It is the angle of blade relative to the long axis of the instrument handle in centigrade.
   (a) 1 centigrade = $1/100^{th}$ of a circle.
   (b) 1 centigrade = 3.6°.
      P = F/A (F: force, A: area, P: pressure).

Heat

It is produced by the combination of pressure, speed, and area with contact of tooth, and surface with the cutting tool.

Vibration

Vibrations causes:

- Fatigue to the operator
- Annoys patient
- Excessive wear of instrument.

Patient Reaction

- The aim is to minimise patients' fear and discomfort
- To minimise tissue damage.

Source of Power

Turbine which is electrically operated.

Instrument Design

- Handpiece
- Cutting tool.

Rotary Instruments

It is defined as instrument that turn on an axis to perform the work and are used on the patients as well as in pre-clinicals.

Types

- Rotary cutting: Dental burs which are used for the removal of tooth structure
- Rotary abrasive: Diamond abrasive stone which are used for shaping, finishing and polishing.

Features of Rotary Instruments

- Speed: It is the surface feet per unit time of contact that instrument makes with the tooth structure measured in rpm
- Pressure: It is the result of two factors which are under the control of operator.

Other Cutting Instruments

- Files: Used to trim excess restorative material at gingival margins
- Knife: Used to trim excessive restorative material on gingival, facial and lingual margins at proximal region. Also to trim contour on Class V restoration
- Discoid-cleoid instrument: Used to trim inlay-onlay margins. Also carving of occlusal area in amalgam restoration.

Enamel Hatchet

- It is a type of chisel which has a blade that is heavier, larger and bevelled on just one side

- ❑ Used for cutting undermined enamel in the proximal cavity
- ❑ They come in two forms:
  - ○ Smaller enamel hatchet—used in anterior region
  - ○ Larger enamel hatchet—used in posterior region.

Gingival Marginal Trimmer (GMT)

- ❑ It is smaller than enamel hatchet
- ❑ Blade is curved
- ❑ Primary cutting edge is at the angle to the axis of the blade
- ❑ Used to bevel walls of the gingival enamel margins of proximal occlusal preparations
- ❑ It has two pairs of instruments for both left and right sides.

Binangle Chisel

It has two angles between the shank and cutting blade.

Triple-angled Chisel

It is three-angled and its usually used to flatten the floor.

Wedel Steads Chisels

They are used for carving undermined enamel while shaping the wall.

Triangular Chisel

It has a triangular blade with base away from the shank.

Angle Former

It has a primary cutting edge at the blade angle:
- ❑ Used for placing bevels on the enamel
- ❑ Cutting action is by lateral scraping.

Spoon Excavators

- ❑ They are made in pairs with one cutting blade to the right and another curved to the left
- ❑ Used for removing caries and carving of the amalgam on direct wax pattern.

Chisels

Primarily used for cutting enamel.

Types

- ❑ Straight: Has a shank and blade in the line angle. Bevel of the blade is at right angle to the shank.
- ❑ Monoangle: Cutting blade placed at an angle to the shaft.

Miscellaneous Instruments

- ❑ Mouth mirrors
- ❑ Explorers
- ❑ Probes
- ❑ Scissors
- ❑ Pliers
- ❑ Others.

Commonly Used Hand-cutting Instruments

They are used to cut hard and soft tissues of the mouth.

Excavators

Used for caries removal and refinement of the internal parts of the cavity.

Types

- ❑ Ordinary hatchets: Single-planed bi bevelled cutting action is by pushing and putting in the direction of blade
- ❑ Hoe excavators:
  - ○ Cutting edge of the blade is perpendicular to the long axis of the shank
  - ○ Used to cut mesial or distal wall of premolars and molars.
- ❑ Plastic instruments:
  - ○ Spatulas
  - ○ Carriers
  - ○ Burnishers
  - ○ Packing instruments.
- ❑ Finishing and polishing instruments:
  - ○ Hand
    - ➤ Orange wood sticks
    - ➤ Polishing points
    - ➤ Finishing strips.
  - ○ Rotary
    - ➤ Finishing burs
    - ➤ Mounted brushes
    - ➤ Mounted stones
    - ➤ Rubber cups
    - ➤ Impregnated discs and wheels.
- ❑ Isolation instruments:
  - ○ Rubber dam
  - ○ Saliva ejector
  - ○ Cotton roll holder
  - ○ Evacuating tips and equipment.

Question 2

Discuss root canal instruments?

Answer

Root Canal Instruments
- ❑ ADA No. 28—Root canal files and reamers of 0.02 mm tip
- ❑ ADA No. 58—Hedstrom files

- ADA No. 63—Rasps and Broaches
- ADA No. 71—Spreaders and Condensers
- ADA No. 78—Obturation points
- ADA No. 95—Mechanical root canal enlargers
- ADA No. 101—Root canal insruments not covered in No. 28.

Classification: ISO Grouping

According to Method of Use

- **Group I:** Hand use only (**Fig. 16.1A and B**)
  Files, Reamers, Broaches, Pluggers, Spreaders
- **Group II:** Engine Driven Latch type
  Same design as Group I but can be attached to handpiece; includes paste carriers
- **Group III:** Engine Driven Latch type
  Drills or Reamers, Gates Glidden drill, Piezo reamers, A.D.O.KO,T,M—type reamers, Kurer root facer
- **Group IV:** Root Canal Points
  Gutta-percha, Silver, Paperpoints.

According to Cohen Pathways of Pulp

- **Group I:** Hand and finger operated instruments, such as barbed broaches and K, H-type instruments
- **Group II:** Low speed latch type of instruments. Gates Glidden drills, piezo reamers
- **Group III:** Engine driven of same as Group I. However, handles are latch type. NiTi rotary files.

According to Grossman's Endodontics

Classified according to their function:

- **Exploring instruments**, e.g. smooth broach, endodontic explorer.
- **Debridement**, e.g. barbed broach.
- **Shaping**, e.g. reamers, files.
- **Obturating**, e.g. pluggers, spreaders, lentulospirals.

Standardization

- Before 1958, endodontic instruments were manufactured without benefit of any established criteria (**Fig. 16.2**)
- Put forward by Ingle and Levine
- Points put forward by them are:
  - Formula for diameters and taper in each size instrument and filling material
  - A formula for a graduated increment in size from one instrument to the next was developed
  - A new instrument numbering system based on instrument metric diameter was established.

Original recommendation for standardized instruments:

- Cutting blades 16 mm in length are of the same size and numbers as standardized filling points

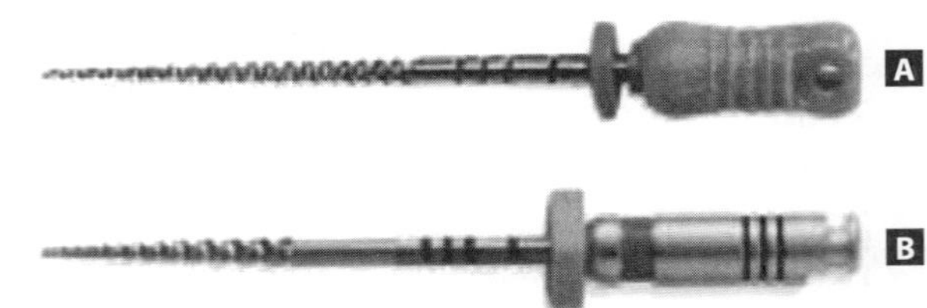

Fig. 16.1A and B: Root canal instruments: (A) Hand root canal instrument and (B) Rotary root canal instrument

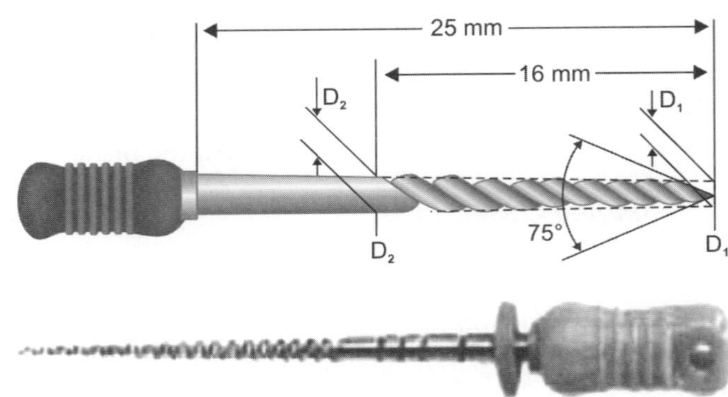

Fig. 16.2: Standardization of root canal instruments specification

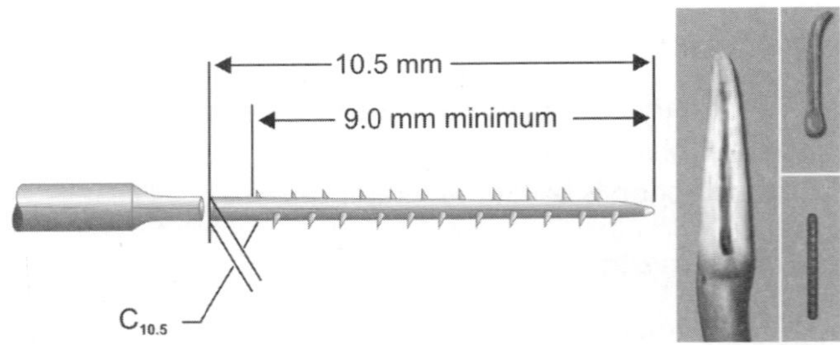

Fig. 16.3: Broaches

- The number of the instrument is determined by diameter size at D1 in hundredths of millimeters
- Diameter 2 (D2) is uniformly 0.32 mm greater than D1.

Two modifications were:

- Additional measurement at D3, 3 mm from D1
- Tip angle of an instrument should be 75°± 15°.

Other modifications are:

- Instrument sizes of tip should increase by 0.05 between No. 10-60 and increase by 0.1 mm from No. 60-150
- Instrument handles have been coloured for easier recognition.

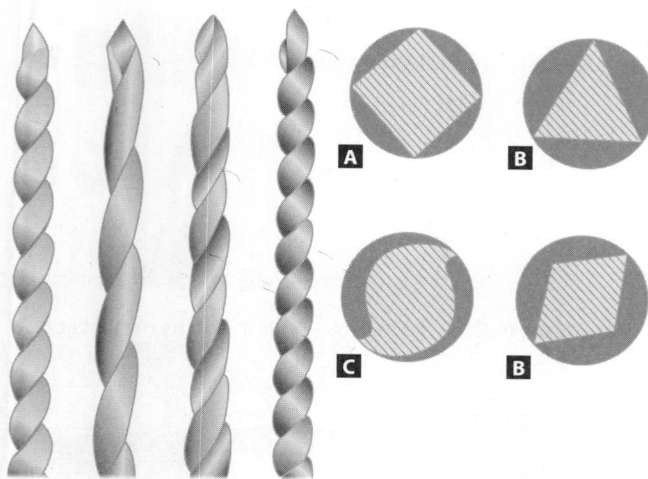

Fig. 16.4A to D: K-type file and its modification and cross-section of file

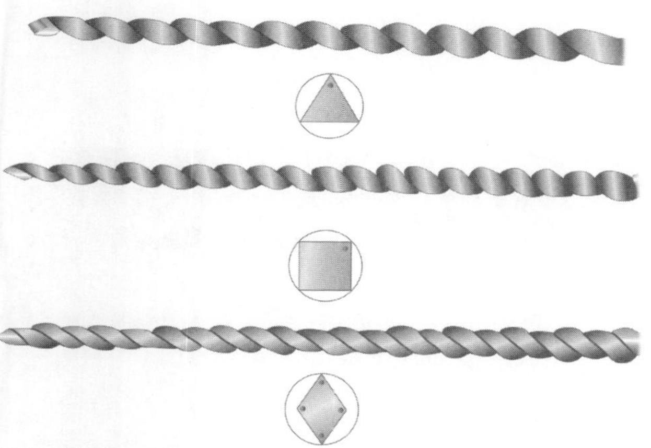

Fig. 16.5: K-type modification

Barbed Broach and Rasps

- Barb height for broaches should be half the core diameter, whereas rasps have barbs equal to 1/3rd the diameter of tip
- Greater depth of cut in broaches they are more fragile instruments **(Fig. 16.3)**
- Taper of broach 0.007 mm/mm is slightly less than that of rasp (0.015)
- Broaches are used for removing intact pulp and paper points.

Files and Reamers

- The clinician should understand the importance of differentiating endodontic files and reamers from drills
- Drills are used for boring holes in solid materials, such as gold, enamel, and dentin

- Files, by definition are used by rasping
- Reamers, on the other hand, are instruments that ream—specifically, a sharp-edged tool for enlarging or tapering holes
- Traditional endodontic reamers cut by being tightly inserted into the canal, twisted clockwise one quarter to one-half turn to engage their blades into the dentin, and then withdrawn—penetration, rotation, and retraction. The cut is made during retraction
- Reaming is the only method that produces a round, tapered preparation, and this only in perfectly straight canals
- The heavier reamers, however, size 50 and above, can almost be turned with impunity
- The tighter spiral of a file establishes a cutting angle (rake) that achieves its primary action on withdrawal, although it will cut in the push motion as well
- The cutting action of the file can be effected in either a filing (rasping) or reaming (drilling) motion
- To summarize the basic action of files and reamers, it may be stated that either files or reamers may be used to ream out a round, tapered apical cavity but that files are also used as push-pull instruments to enlarge by rasping certain curved canals as well as the ovoid portion of large canals.

K-type Instruments

Made from steel that is ground to tapered square or triangular cross-section **(Fig. 16.4A to D)**.

- The wire is twisted in clockwise direction to produce spiral flutes
- There are twice the number of flutes in files compared to reamer
- Instrument with triangular blank has thicker cutting edge removing more dentin and also because of more space between flutes
- K-type and modifications fracture during clockwise motion after plastic deformation
- Square blanks resist fracture more efficiently, therefore smaller instruments are of square blanks
- Reamer manufactured from triangular blank and file from square blank.

K-type Modifications

K-flex File

- Cross-section is rhomboid-or diamond-shaped **(Fig. 16.5)**
- Cutting edges of high flutes are formed by two angle (acute) of rhombus which give increased cutting efficiency
- Low flute formed by obtuse angles gives more area for debris removal
- Increases flexibility and decreases danger of compacting dentinal filings.

Triple-flex File

- More number of flutes than reamer but less than files
- Made from triangular blank.

Hedstrom Files (H-file)

- Cutting spiraling flutes into the shaft of a round, tapered, stainless steel wires
- Similar to screw cutting machine
- Cuts only in retraction
- More cutting efficiency but more fragile (**Fig. 16.6A to C**).

H-file Modifications

- These files were designed with two spirals for cutting blades, a double helix design
- In cross-section, the blades presented an "S" shape rather than the single-helix tear drop cross-sectional shape of the true Hedstrom file
- Other modifications Hyflex file, S-File
- Safety Hedstrom (Sybron Endo/Kerr; Orange, Calif.), which has a non-cutting side to prevent ledging in curved canals.

U-file

- The U-files cross-sectional configuration has two 90° cutting edges at each of the three points of the blade
- The flat cutting surfaces act as a planning instrument and are referred to as radial lands
- Heath pointed out that the new U shape adapts well to the curved canal, aggressively planning the external convex wall while avoiding the more dangerous internal concave wall, where perforation stripping occurs
- A non-cutting pilot tip ensures that the file remains in the lumen of the canal, thus avoiding transportation and zipping at the apex
- Files are used in both a push-pull and rotary motion and are very adaptable to nickel-titanium rotary instruments.

GT Profiles

- Developed by Buchanan in the U design, are unusual in that the cutting blades extend up the shaft only 6–8 mm rather than 16 mm
- The tapers start at 0.06 mm/mm (instead of 0.02), as well as 0.08 and 0.10, tapered instruments
- They are made of nickel titanium and come as hand instruments and rotary files. GT instruments all start with a non-cutting tip ISO size 20.

Characteristics of Files and Reamers

Motions used in cleaning and shaping are:
- Filing

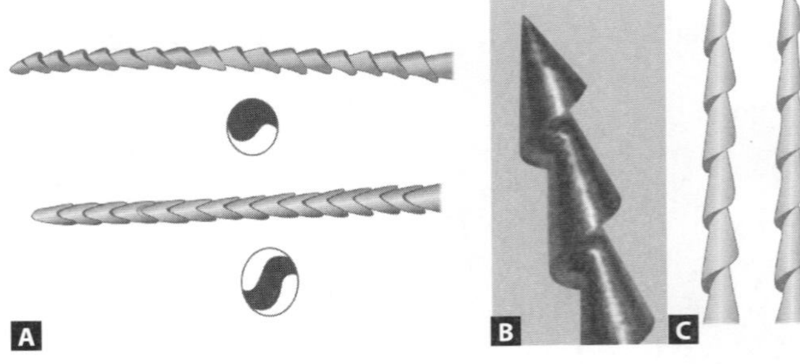

Fig. 16.6A to C: H-file its cross-section and its modification

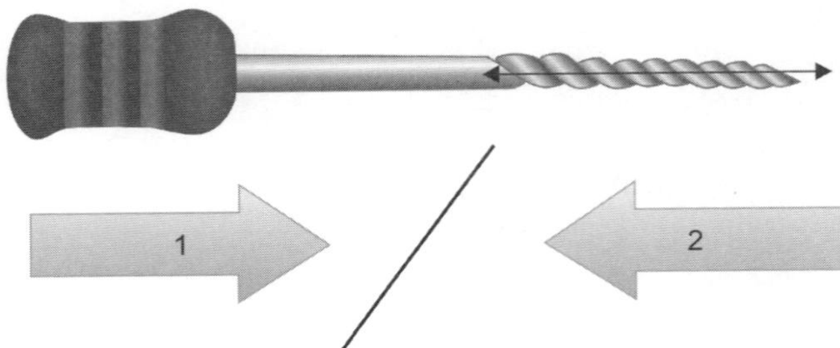

Fig. 16.7: Filing motion

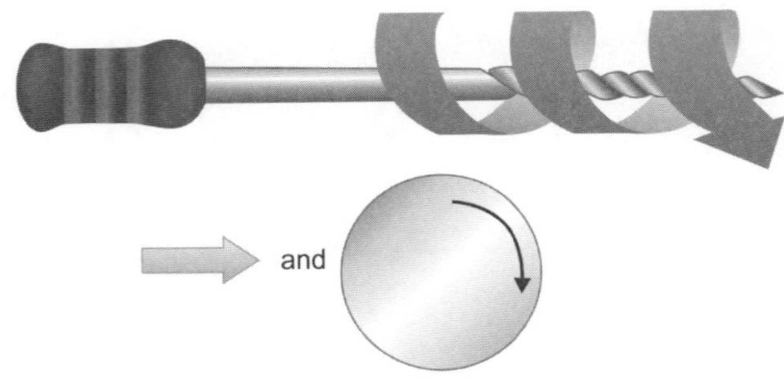

Fig. 16.8: Reaming motion

- Reaming
- Watch winding
- Balanced force instrumentation.

Filing

- Push and pull motion with instrument (**Fig. 16.7**)
- Inward passage of file can lead to canal damage
- Efficient with hedstrom file.

Reaming

- Clockwise rotation of an instrument
- Best used with reamers because of their cutting angle axial orientation (**Fig. 16.8**)
- As the instrument is rotated, it penetrates into the canal deeper
- Usually, rotation is limited to quarter to half turn.

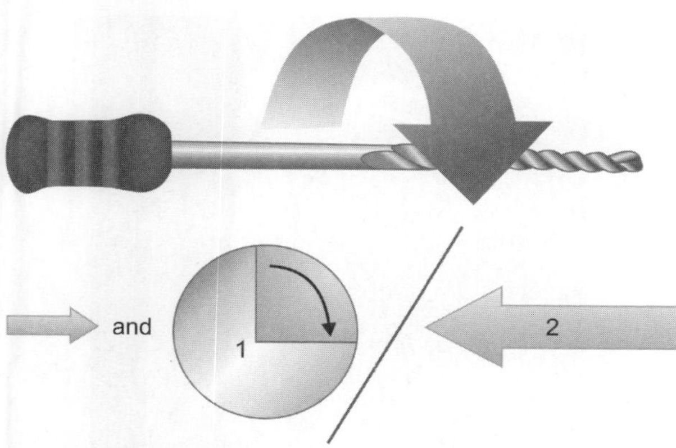

Fig. 16.9: Turn and pull motion

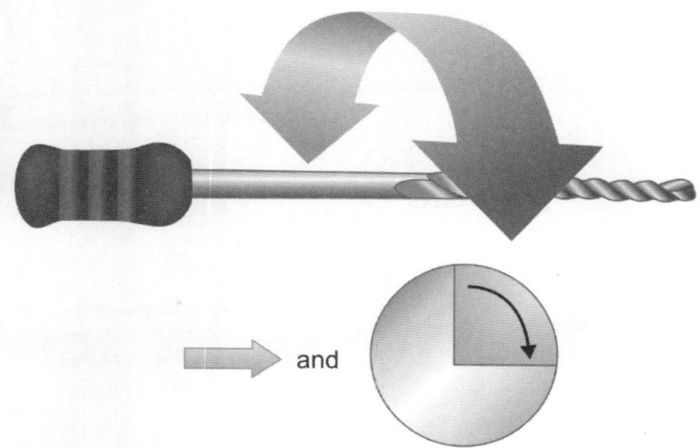

Fig. 16.10: Watch winding motion

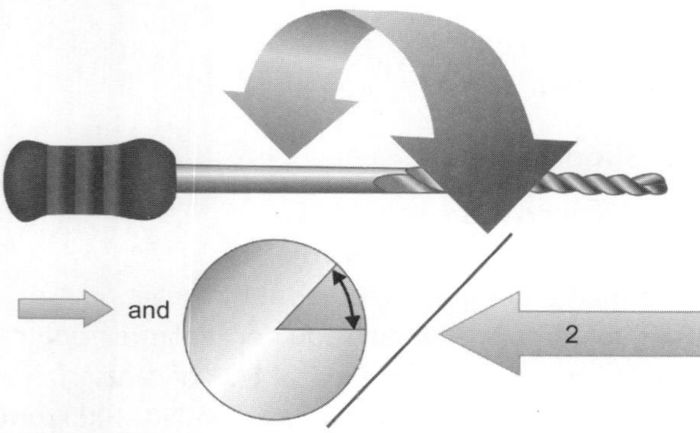

Fig. 16.11: Watch winding and pull motion

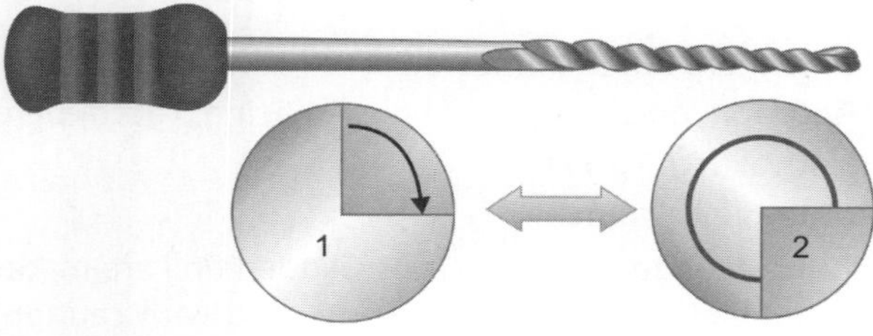

Fig. 16.12: Balance force technique

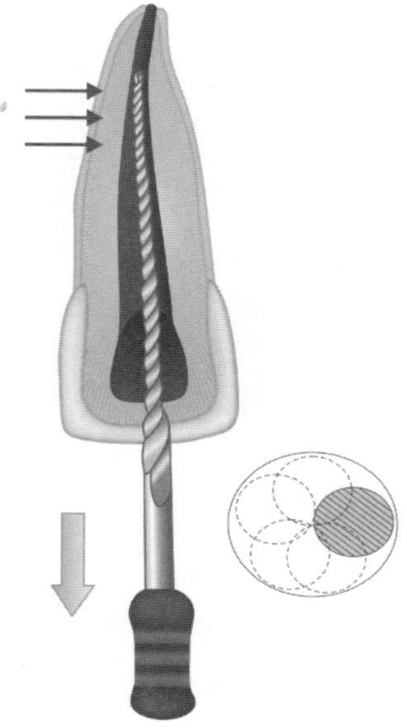

Fig. 16.13: Circumferential filing

Turn and Pull

- It is a combination of filing and reaming motion **(Fig. 16.9)**
- It is detrimental to prepare apical stop with this technique (Weine et al).

Watch Winding Motion

- It is back and forth oscillation of file (30-60°) right and (30-60°) to the left
- This is an efficient technique to remove dentin from root canals **(Fig. 16.10)**
- Each cut opens space and frees the instrument for deeper insertion with the next clockwise motion
- This technique is predecessor to balanced force technique
- It is effective with all types of K-files.

Watch Winding and Pull

- This technique is used with H-file as wriggling motion alone cannot cut dentin **(Fig. 16.11)**
- Cutting action is initiated only during pulling out action.

Balanced Force Technique

- Most efficient way to cut dentin
- Used with Flex R-file **(Fig. 16.12)**
- This technique extrudes no debris, better canal centering ability, specifically designed for K-type file and modifications not with H-type files
- It involves quarter turn clockwise along with inward pressure to insert the canal
- Next, it is rotated counter clockwise at least 1/3rd of revolution with gentle inward pressure maintained.

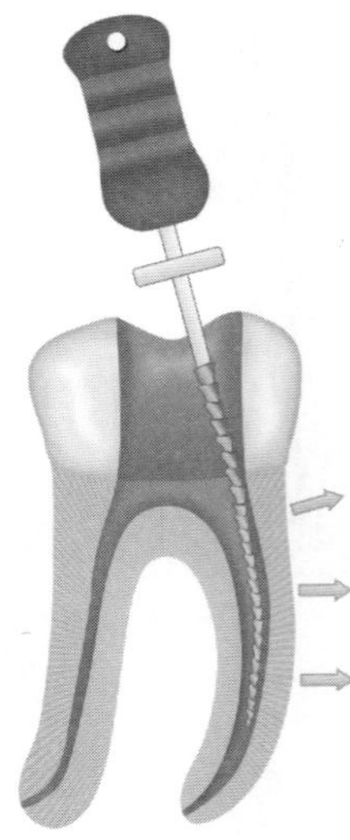

Fig. 16.14: Anticurvature filing

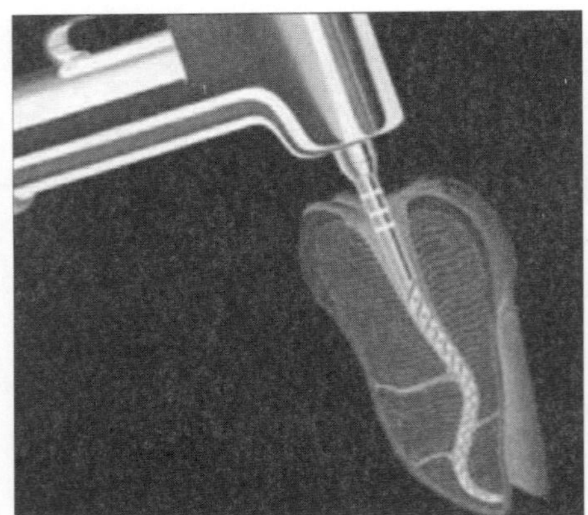

Fig. 16.15: Rotary instrument

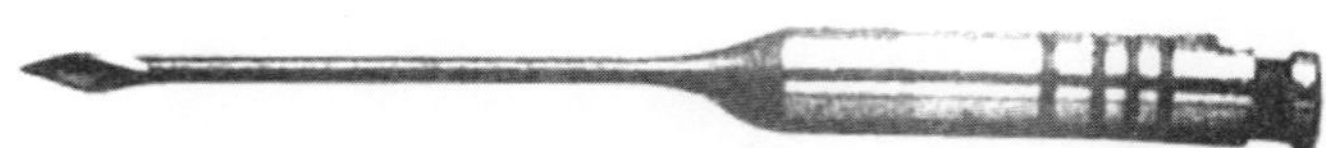

Fig. 16.16: Gates glidden drill

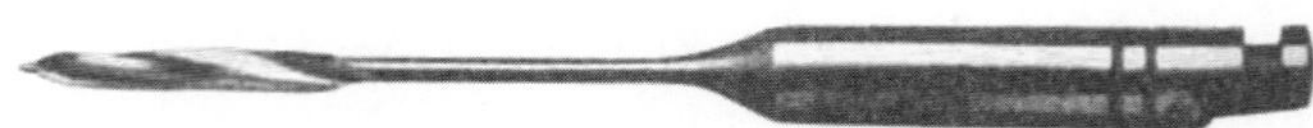

Fig. 16.17: Peeso reamer

Circumferential Filing

Used in flaring coronal access and ovoid canals (**Fig. 16.13**).

Anticurvature Filing

- Applying instrument pressure that shaping will occur away from inside of root curvature (**Fig. 16.14**)
- Abou Raas, Frank, Glick recommended it.

Question 3

Write a note on mechanical instrumentation?

Answer

Classification

Rotary

16:1 gear reduction, e.g. NiTi Mac (**Fig. 16.15**).

Reciprocal

- Contrarotates through 90°, e.g. Giromatic, Endo Cursor
- Kerrs endolift has in addition a vertical motion.

Vertical

Canal Finder System, Canal Leader.

Random

W and H handpiece—Excalibur.

Disadvantages

- Loss of tactile sensation
- Ledge formation
- Extrusion of debris out of apical foramen.

Power Driven Instruments

- Gates Glidden drill
- Piezo reamer.

Gates Glidden Drill

- Flame-shaped head with safe tip
- Flame cuts laterally (**Fig. 16.16**)
- Long shaft is designed to break at the neck
- Used to remove lingual shoulder, enlarge root canal orifices, clean and shape cervical 1/3rd of canals
- Used in brushing strokes at a speed of 750–1000 rpm
- Available in 32 mm and 28 mm length.

Piezo Reamer

- Long, sharp flutes connected to a thick shaft
- Used for preparation of post-spacing, gutta-percha removal (**Fig. 16.17**)
- It is a stiff instrument.

Both piezoo reamer and Gales Glidden drill are made of hardened carbon steel and must be used with caution to avoid over instrumentation and perforation.

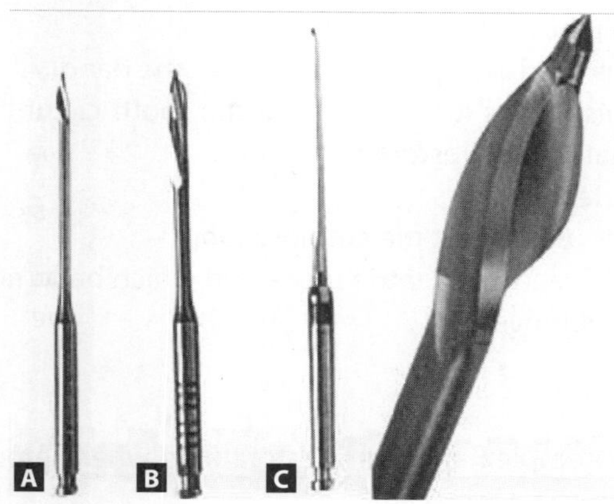

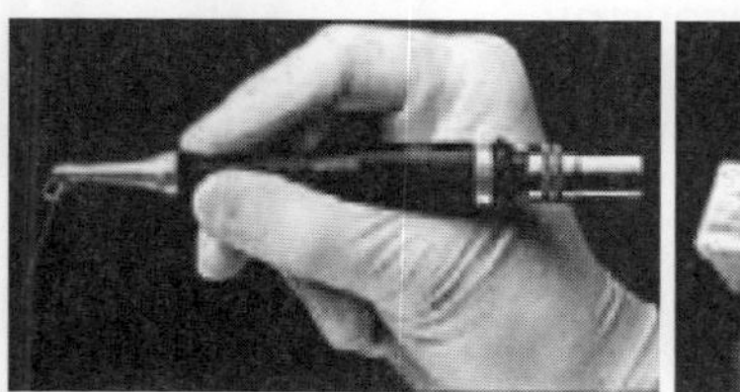

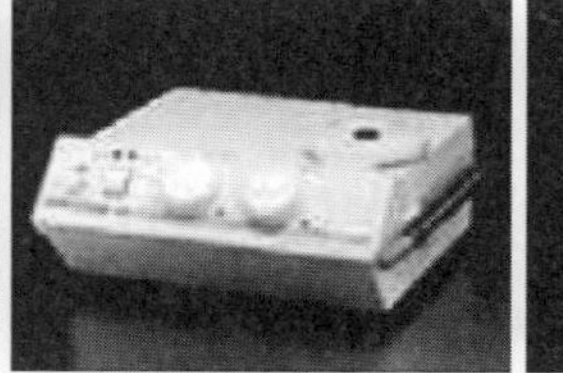

Fig. 16.18A to C: Gates Glidden modification

Fig. 16.19: Sonic and ultrasonic instruments

Gates Glidden Modification

- A hand instrument also designed for apical preparation is the Flexogates, Handygates (Dentsply/Maillefer; Tulsa, Olka)
- A safe-tipped variation of the traditional Gates Glidden drill, the Flexogates **(Fig. 16.18)**.

Sonic and Ultrasonic Instruments

Sonic Vibration

- Vibration wave introduced in shank changes from vertical motion when constrained by root canal walls **(Fig. 16.19)**
- Rispi files—coronal 2/3rd
- Shaper files—apical 1/3rd.

Fig. 16.20: Rotary NiTi instruments

Ultrasonic Instrument

Piezoelectric and Magnetostrictive

- Piezoelectric units are more powerful and no water coolant required
- Sodium hypochloride used as irrigant
- Files used are K-files and diamond files
- Main advantage is in cleaning of canals rather than shaping.

Nickel Titanium Instruments

- Discovered in 1960's by Buchler and Wang as NiTiNol (US Navy Ordinal Lab)
- NiTi (56% Ni and 44% Ti)
- Zero degree residual deformation compared to 10–18°in stainless steel file.
- Eight percent strain can be sustained by NiTi compared to less than 1% by stainles steel
- NiTi instruments cannot be produced by twisting but can be only machined
- Cutting efficiency is low
- Torsional strength is low
- Superelasticity due to change in crystalline form from austentite to martensite.

Rotary NiTi Systems Available are

- Profile **(Fig. 16.20)**
- Protaper
- Quantec series
- GT
- Light speed
- Hero RACE.

SHORT ESSAYS

Question 1

Discuss matrices and different types of matrices?

Answer

Matrix: It is a device which is used during restorative procedures so that it holds the restorative material within the tooth while setting.

Ideal Requirements of a Matrix

- Easy to use: It should be simple in design and easy to apply
- Comfort: The retainer or its handle should not interfere with the condensation of the restoration and also patients comfort
- Easy to remove: After the restoration has hardened, it should come out easily without any type of tissue injury or faulting the hardened restoration

- Rigidity: It should be firm and rigid so as in case of pressure it should be rigid to withstand its position and does not gets displaced easily from its position
- Providing proper proximal contact and contour: It should be ingenuous enough to provide desired proximal contours at different conditions
- Non-reactive: It should not react or bind to the restorative material and to the surroundings
- It should not be expensive.

Functions

- To withstand and restrain the restoration material until it hardens
- Establishing optical contact and contours for the restorations
- Prevents gingival overhanging of the restoration
- Providing acceptable surface texture for the restoration.

Parts of Matrix

- Band
- Retainer.

Materials used in Class II

- Automatrix
- Tofflemire matrix
- Pre-contoured matrix
- T-shaped matrix band
- Ivory matrix no. 1 and 8
- S-shaped matrix band.

Tofflemire Matrix

This is also called universal matrix. It is widely preferred in Class II amalgam restoration.

Two sizes are available as:

1. Standard: Adult
2. Small: Primary.

Indications

- Class I cavities with buccal or lingual extensions
- Class II in posterior tooth.

Automatrix

It has three parts:

1. Automatrix bands
   Thickness: 0.0013–0.002 inch
   Width
   Narrow: 3/16th inch
   Medium: 1/4th inch
   Wide: 5/16 inch.

2. Automate II tightening device:
   (a) It is used in adjusting the loop of the band
   (b) This makes it adjustable to the tooth circumference that is to be restored.
3. Shielded nippers:
   (a) It is used to cut the autolock loop
   (b) It is needed after the process in which band needs to be removed.

Indication

Used in complex amalgam restorations where more than one cut is to be replaced.

Write a note on speed in dentistry?

Classification

According to sturdvant:

- Low/slow speed: 13,000 rmp
- Medium/intermediate speed: 12,000–2,00,000 rpm
- High/ultra speed: Above 2,00,000 rpm.
  (Rpm is the rotation per min of an instrument used for cutting)

High Speed Dentistry

- A high speed device holds the rotating instrument, gives power supply and used for intra-oral positioning
- The rational speed is measured in rpm
- High speed gives 2,00,000–4,50,000 rpm
- Hand piece in dentistry is considered most reliable to control and to regulate the speed. It helps the operator to obtain optimal speed, type and size of rotating instruments accordingly at any point of time while the procedure is still in progress.
- Uses Mostly used for tooth preparation
- Used in removal of old restorations
- Used in the crown preparation for tooth reduction.

Advantages

- Patients are more comfortable with the quickness of the treatment
- It gives operator a better control
- Need for lot other cutting instruments is not required
- Removes tooth structure faster with less heat generation and pressure.

Disadvantages

- Sound and vibration makes patient uncomfortable
- Air-water spray can impair the visibility of operator
- Adjacent tooth may be scarred during the procedure
- Over cutting of tooth is a possibility
- Injury to hard and soft tissues.

Hand Piece

Hand piece is a device for holding rotating instruments, transmitting power to them and for positioning them intraorally.

Classification

According to driving mechanism:
- Gear driven hand piece
- Water driven hand piece
- Belt driven hand piece
- Air driven hand piece.

According to Angulations

- Straight
- Contra-angled
- Right-angled.

According to Speed

- Low speed
- Medium speed
- High speed.

Parts of Dental Hand Piece

- Head: It is the end that holds the rotary instruments, e.g. burs, polishing stones
- Shank: It is the handle portion of the hand piece
- Connecting end: The part connected to the power source of the unit.

Criteria to be used for hand piece evaluation:

Friction

- It occurs in the parts that are movable in hand piece
- Heat should be prevented from friction so that there is no harm in oral cavity
- Ball bearings, glass and resin bearings are therefore used
- Tongue: It is the ability of hand piece to withstand the pressure while the tool is revolving without any impact on its speed and cutting efficiency.

It depends on

- Bearings used
- Energy applied to the hand piece.

Vibration

It is caused by excessive wear of the turbine bearing that causes eccentric running resulting in vibration.

It depends on:

- Speed
- Bearings.

SHORT NOTES

Question 1

Write a short note on instrument formula?

Answer

According to GV Black, operative instruments can be classified based on their use. They are:
- Cutting instruments
  - Hand instruments
    - Hatchets
    - Chisels
    - Excavators
    - Others.
  - Rotary instruments
    - Burs
    - Stones
    - Discs
    - Others.
- Condensing instruments
  - Pluggers
    - Hand
    - Mechanical.
- Mostly there is a three-numbers formula for instruments, but a fourth unit is added for instruments, like gingival marginal trimmer and angle former because they have the cutting edge other than at right angles to the blade
- Unit primary cutting edge angle:
  - It is the angle between the cutting edge and the long axis of the handle in centigrade
  - This fourth unit is placed second in the code in instrument formula with four units.

CHAPTER 17

Materials in Endodontics

LONG ESSAYS

Question 1

Classify root canal sealers. Write about zinc oxide-eugenol containing sealers?

Answer

Classification

- Based on absorbability:
  - Absorbable:
    - Grossman's sealer
    - Kerr sealer (Rickert)
    - Roth root canal cement
    - Tubliseal, Tubliseal EWT
    - Sealapex.
- Non-absorbable:
  - Ketac-Endo (glass-ionomer based)
  - Diaket (polyvinyl resin)
  - AH Plus (epoxy-type resin).
- Based on composition:
  - Gutta-percha-based root canal sealers
  - Zinc oxide-eugenol (ZOE) based root canal sealers
  - Calcium hydroxide [$Ca(OH)_2$] based root canal sealers
  - Formaldehyde-based root canal sealers
  - Glass-ionomer-based root canal sealers
  - Resin-based root canal sealers
  - Silicon-based root canal sealers.

Zinc Oxide-eugenol-based Root Canal Sealers

- These were introduced as alternate to gutta-percha based sealers
- Initially entire root canals were used to be filled by them
- Zinc oxide containing sealers:
  - Kerr root canal sealers
  - Tubliseal
  - Roth's sealers
  - Wach's cement

- Nogenol
- Medicated ZOE cements.

Kerr Root Canal Sealer

Composition is based on the powder and liquid content.

- Powder
  - Zinc oxide
  - Silver
  - Oleoresin (white resin)
  - Thymol iodide.
- Liquid
  - Clove oil
  - Canada balsam.
- Properties
  - They are germicidal and have adhesive properties
  - They are radiopaque
  - They resorb periapical tissues over a certain period of time.

Disadvantages

- It stains the tooth
- In the presence of heat and humidity it sets very quickly
- Increased microbial leakage is seen
- There is tissue irritation from the extruded material periapically.

Tubliseal

- It is prepared in the form of a paste. Two ingredients are base and catalyst
- Mix contains:

Zinc oxide	–	57.4%
Oleoresin	–	21–25%
Bismuth trioxide and oils	–	7.5%
Thymol iodide	–	3.75%
Modifier	–	2.60%

Roth's Sealer

It is available as Roth's 80% or as m/p root canal sealer.

Wach's Cement

- It is supplied by manufactures
- It is zinc oxide-based cement.

Nogenol

- It is available as base and catalyst paste
- It is non-irritating and provides neutral substrate to the adhesion of composite resin
- Base contains:
  - Zinc oxide
  - Barium sulphate
  - Vegetable oils
  - Catalyst contain
  - Hydrogenated rosin
  - Methyl agitate
  - Tannic acid
  - Chlorothymol, salicylic acid.

Medicated Variants of ZOE Cements

It consists of nitrogen (N_2) and endomethasone. N_2 is not used now because of its toxic and carcinogenic property.

Question 2

Classify and describe the various intracanal medicaments in root canal treatment?

Answer

- They are antiseptic agents which are in chemical form and are applied to the walls of the canal with the objective that it will eliminate microorganisms present even after the cleaning and shaping and also after irrigation is done in the canal
- This process is done to disinfect the canal when the cleaning and irrigation is done and there can be bacteria present.

Disinfection

Disinfection is the destruction of pathogenic microorganisms that presuppose to adequate removal of pulp tissue and debris clearing of enlarging of the canal by biomechanical method followed by irrigation.

- Four factors that predispose tooth infection:
  - Trauma
  - Devitalised tissue
  - Dead spaces
  - Accumulation of exudate.

- The microorganism invade periapical tissue and destroy the periodontium including bone
- The intracanal medication reduces or eliminates the microbial flora in root canal.

Functions

- Disinfecting root canal
- Reduces inflammation
- Facilitates periapical heating.

Basic Requirements of Intracanal Medicament

- Should be germicidal and fungicidal
- Should have prolonged antimicrobial effect
- Should have low surface tension
- Should be non-irritating to the tissues
- Should not interfere with the periapical healing
- Should have adequate shelf life
- Should have easy access to the canal
- Should have low surface tension.

Functions

- Flushes root canal debris
- They should have antimicrobial property
- Should penetrate in inaccessible area
- Should act as lubricant during instrumentation
- Should have bleaching effect.

Commonly Used Root Canal Irrigants

- Physiologic saline solution
- Proteolytic enzymes
- Urea peroxide
- Ultrasonic irrigation
- Sodium hypochlorite (NaOCl)
- Huddle solution
- Iodine-based irrigants
- MTAD
- Electrochemically activated water.

Hydrogen Peroxide (H_2O_2)

- It is always used in conjugation with NaOCl
- H_2O_2 produces nascent oxygen that caries loose debris to the access opening that restrict and kills anaerobes
- H_2O_2 irrigation should be followed by NaOCl because nascent oxygen causes gaseous pressure in closed cavity that produces pain, swelling or emphysema.

Chlorhexidine Gluconate (CHx)

- It is a biguanide in chemical form
- Available commercially as oral rinses.

Composition:

- CHx with water: 0.12%
- Alcohol: 11.6%
- Glycerine
- Flavouring agents
- Saccharine.

Advantages:

- It has longer antimicrobial action, more than calcium hydroxide [$Ca(OH)_2$].
- It is used with NaOCL.
- Concentration between 0.2–2%.
- It is biocompatible.

Disadvantages:

- It does not dissolve pulp tissue.
  - NaOCl.
- It is a clear, straw coloured reducing agent which has chlorine in concentration of 5%
- Used as lubricant during instrumentation
- Acts as solvent of vital and non-vital pulp tissue
- Have good antimicrobial properties
- Removes smear layer along with chelation agents
- In expensive
- Long shelf life.

Bis-dequalinium Acetate (BDA)

- It is a disinfectant, chemotherapeutic agent
- Low toxicity and good lubricant
- It has low surface tension
- Excellent chelating properties
- Used in patient allergic to NaOCl, e.g., solvidont.

Organic Acids

- They can be used as endodontic irrigants as they have the ability to soften denture and enlarges the canal

- 20–30% citric acid is used to remove smear layer which is followed by NaOCl irrigation
- They effect periradicular tissue because of their toxic matrix.

Instruments Used

- Close-end needles with side-vent:
  - Prorinse
  - Max-I: probe.
- Open-end meddles without side vent:
  - Monojet endodontic needles
  - Stropko irrigator.

Method

- Irrigants should be always used in disposable syringe and needle
- Gauge size of needle 21–30 should reach 2 mm short of working length or apex
- Should be flexible to be bent at an obtuse angle for access
- Special needles with closed tips and needles having lateral openings are used sometimes
  - Example: Maxi probe, pro rinse probes
  - They help to prevent solution from extruding beyond apex.
- The syringe is filled with solution. The needle is then attached and placed into the canal
- Needle should not bind into the root canal ways as it should be loose enough to let the solution flow
- Gauze sponge is placed near the access opening when solution plunges back
- Paper points are used to dry the canal
- Intracanal medicaments are than placed after canal is dried and is restored with temporary restorative materials.

SHORT ESSAYS

Question 1

Discuss Gutta-percha?

Answer

Gutta-percha commonly known as GP is the most used and common obturating material.

- GP exits in alpha and beta forms
- Recent advancement provides low viscosity alpha form of GP, i.e., thermophile, densfil, microseal.

Composition

- GP: 19–22%
- Zinc oxide: 60–75%
- Metal salts: 1–7%
- Wax or resin: 1–4%.

Gutta-percha is Supplied As

- Sticks
- Points

- Cones
- Syringe materials, e.g., alpha seal
- Coating on metal or plastic cone, i.e., thermophile
- GP pellets/bars, i.e., obtura system
- GP sealers, i.e., chlorpercha, eucapercha.

Properties

- The cones are colour-coded which are exact match with the instrument size
- They are generally used as master concentrations
- Convention points (non-standardised cones) are:
    - More tapered
    - Extra fine
    - Fine-fine
    - Medium fine
    - Fine medium
    - Large
    - Extra large.
- GP is disinfected with 2% glutaraldehyde and 5.25% chlorhexidine
- Should be stored in cool and dry area
- Exposing to high causes oxidation and make it brittle.

Advantages

- It adapts to irregularities
- Can be made plastic and softened by heat or solvent
- It is inert and dimensionally stable
- It is tissue tolerant
- Radiopaque
- Tooth structures are not discoloured.

Disadvantages

- Lacks adhesive properties
- It lacks rigidity
- It can be easily displaced by even a soft pressure.

Question 2

Explain the role of calcium hydroxide as intracanal medicament?

Answer

Intracanal medicaments are defined as antiseptic agents in the chemical form which are applied to the walls of the canal with the objective of eliminating microorganisms present even after cleaning and irrigation of the root canal.

Types

- Essential oils
- Aldehydes
- Biocides
- Medicated gutta-percha
- Phenolic compounds
- Heavy metal salts
- Halogens
- Antibiotics and corticosteroids
- Calcium hydroxide [$Ca(OH)_2$]
- Chlorhexidine Gluconate.

Calcium Hydroxide

- $Ca(OH)_2$ is superior to all the intracanal medicaments in posing antibacterial activity
- Because of its high alkalinity and tissue dissolving property, it is commonly used.
- Gram-positive and gram-negative bacteria are commonly found in infected root canals so the antimicrobial property makes it the choice of material used
- $Ca(OH)_2$ alters biological properties of bacterial lipopolysaccharide (LPS) to stimulate antibody production of B lymphocytes
- Glycerine, polyethylene glycol is mixed with $Ca(OH)_2$ and also propylene glycol as they play an important role in achieving max antibacterial effect.
- $Ca(OH)_2$ is also available in unstable form than can also be used conveniently.

Biological Properties

- $Ca(OH)_2$ is biocompatible due to low solubility in water
- It also inhibits root resorption and stimulates periapical healing.

Uses

- It is used as direct and indirect pulp capping agent in pulpotomy
- It is used in the treatment of phoenix abscess
- In apexification, it is used as sealer at the time of obturation
- Used in weeping canals
- Also used in treatment of resorption.

Question 3

What are root-end filling materials?

Answer

Root-end Filling Materials

- Zinc oxide-eugenol (ZOE) cements [retrograde materials (RM) and super ethoxybenzoic acid (EBA)]
- Glass-ionomers
- Composite resins (retroplast)

- Resin-ionomer hybrids
  - Composes
  - Geristore.
- Mineral trioxide aggregate (MTA).

Less Commonly Used Materials

- Amalgam
- Gold foil
- Polycarboxylate cements
- Zinc phosphate cements.

Properties

- ZOE cement [intermediate restorative material (IRM)]
  - It releases more eugenol
  - It is more soluble and has low compressive strength.
- Glass-ionomer cement (GIC)
  - It has chemical adhesion to the tooth
  - The sealing properties are better than amalgam
  - Excellent tissue compatibility
  - The only drawback is the moisture contamination increases the solubility which reduces bone strength
- MTA
  - It is most widely used and best root-end filling material
  - Available as:
    - Grey MTA
    - White MTA.

Composition

- Calcium silicate (Ca_2SiO_4).
- Bismuth oxide (Bi_2O_3)
- Calcium carbonate ($CaCO_3$)
- Calcium sulphate ($CaSO_4$)
- Calcium aluminate ($CaAl_2O_2$)
- MTA is mixed with sterile water to form colloidal gel that solidifies and forms crystals
- Calcium oxide is amorphous matrix
- White MTA release tetra calcium alumina ferrite.

Advantages

- Helps in regeneration of cementum
- It gives apical double seal
- PH: 9–12
- It is radiopaque
- Pressure of moisture/blood does not alter the property of MTA.

Disadvantage

- Setting time is high: 2.3 hours
- Need special carrier to place the material.

Question 4

Write in detail about Obturating Points?

Answer

- Geometric isomer, which means that it can have different structural arrangements despite having the same composition
- Cis-isoprene, is known as natural rubber trans-isoprene polymer is commonly referred to as gutta-percha.
- In the cis form, the hydrogen atom and methyl group prevent close packing such that the natural rubber is amorphous and consequently soft and highly flexible, whereas the gutta-percha crystallises, usually about 60% crystalline, forming a hard rigid polymer
- Gutta-percha is a thermoplastic material and softens at 60–65°C and will melt at about 100°C, so it cannot be heat-sterilized
- If necessary, disinfection can be carried out in a solution of sodium hypochlorite (5%)
- The use of solvents, such as acetone or alcohol should be avoided, as these are absorbed by the gutta-percha, causing it to swell. Eventually, the gutta-percha will return to its unswollen state, thus compromising the apical seal
- On exposure to light, gutta-percha oxidises and becomes brittle
- The gutta-percha is able to take up two distinct conformations
- At high-temperature, the gutta-percha chains take on an extended conformation, which can be preserved if cooled rapidly so that it forms the crystalline β-phase, whereas when the gutta-percha is cooled more slowly, the denser phase is formed

Table 17.1: Composition of gutta-percha points

Constituent	Amount (%)	Purpose
Gutta-percha	19–22	Rubber
Zinc oxide	59–75	Filler
Heavy metal salts	1–17	Radiopacifier
Wax or resin	1–4	Plasticiser

- The B-phase gutta-percha has better thermoplastic characteristics and is therefore preferred for use in hot gutta-percha application systems (**Fig. 17.1**)
- An alternative approach is to dissolve the gutta-percha in a chemical solvent, such as chloroform or xylene. This softens the gutta-percha and allows it to be adapted closely to the canal wall and duplicate the intricate canal morphology

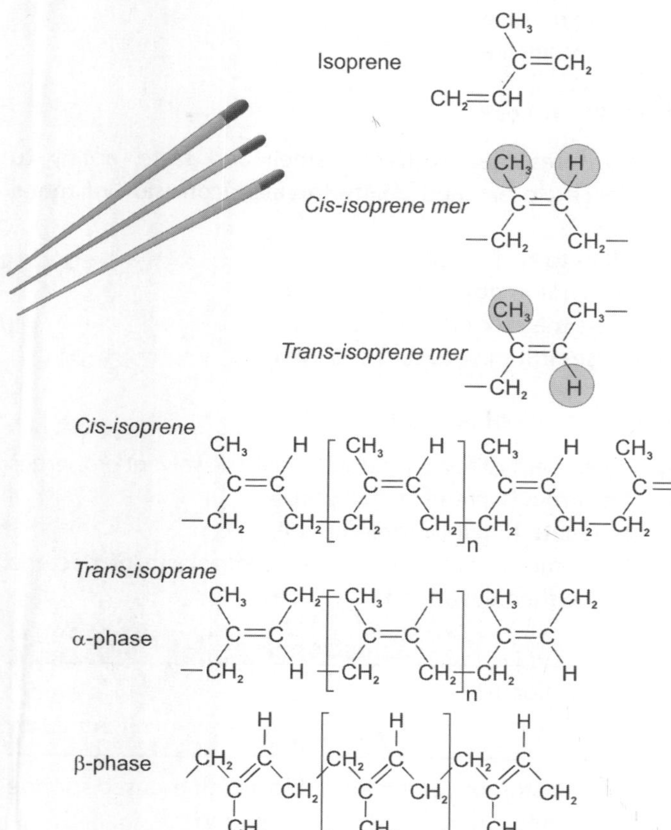

Fig. 17.1: Structural arrangement of various forms of isoprene

- However, as the solvent is lost, so the dimensional stability may be compromised and concerns have been expressed regarding the possible cytotoxic effects of using these solvents
- The composition of commercially available gutta-percha obturating points (also as pellets) will vary from product to product
- The additional ingredients are added to overcome the inherent brittleness of the rubber and to make it radiopaque
- Gutta-percha points are available in standardized sizes from 15-140 and non-standardized cones available as fine, extra fine, fine-fine as auxillary cones.

Advantages

- Bioinert
- Non-irritating
- Easily inserted or removed
- Dimensionally stable
- Radiopaque
- Unaffected by moisture
- Does not discolour tooth.

Disadvantages

- Cannot be sterilized
- Does not sufficiently seal root canal so a sealer is required
- Cannot be inserted in narrow canals because of lack of rigidity.

SHORT NOTES

Question 1

Write about mineral trioxide aggregate?

Answer

Mineral trioxide aggregate (MTA) is an alternative to calcium hydroxide [$Ca(OH)_2$].

It is available in powder form.

Composition

- Tricalcium silicate
- Tricalcium aluminate oxide
- Silicate oxide
- Bismuth oxide
- Calcium: 33%
- Phosphate: 49%
- Water is used to make it thick, graining paste

- PH: 10.2–12.5 in 3 hours on hydration which is on higher alkaline pH and determines the mechanism of action of MTA
- Setting time: 3–4 hours
- Compressive strength: 76 mpa
- It has excellent solubility
- It has low solubility
- In pulpotomy it produces good results because of its low solubility property
- It is biocompatible because of less cytotoxic and non-mutagenic properties
- MTA releases cytokines, such as interleukin-1 alpha, interleukin 1-beta, interleukin-6
- This help in bone metabolism
- Osteoblasts are stimulated through biologically active substrate of cells.

Question 2

Write a short note on camphorated paramonochlorophenol?

Answer

Camphorated paramonochlorophenol (CMCP):
It is the most common endodontic medicament.

Composition

- Parachlorophenol and three parts of gum camphor
- Camphor acts, like a diluent to suppress the irritating effect of parachlorophenol
- It prolongs antimicrobial action
- CMCP is most toxic and irritating followed by cresatin.

Question 3

Discuss ethylene diamine tetra acetic acid?

Answer

- Ethylene diamine tetra acetic acid (EDTAA).
- Nygaard-ostby first used EDTA.

Composition

- Disodium salt of EDTA
- Distilled water
- Sodium hydroxide
- EDTA is commercially available as REDTA.

Uses

- It is conjugated with sodium hydrochlorite as a chelating agent
- Liquid EDTA removes the smear layer of the dentine which increases the permeability of the dentinal tubules
- Working time: 15 minutes.

Question 4

What are advantages and disadvantages of sodium hypochlorite in endodontics?

Answer

Sodium hypochlorite is the most commonly used root canal irrigant: 5%–chlorine, which is clear, straw coloured reducing agents.

It is a clear, straw coloured.

Advantages

- It dissolves organic substances present in the root canal system
- Has higher antimicrobial property

- Not expensive
- Good shelf life.

Disadvantages

- It is presented with foul smell and taste, ability to bleach clothes and ability to cause corrosion of metal objects
- It fails to kill bacteria
- Does not remove all smear layer
- Alters the properties of dentine
- Causes irritation to skin and eyes.

Mechanism of Action

- It posesses both antimicrobial and tissue solvent properties
- It destroys bacteria by two phases:
    1. Penetration into bacterial cell
    2. Chemical combination with protoplasm of bacteria and then destroys it.

Question 5

What is Gelfoam?

Answer

It is hard, restorable, water insoluble gelatine-based sponge as it becomes soft with contact with blood.

- It stimulates intrinsic clotting pathway which results in platelet disintegration and release of thromboplastin
- At first inflammation is shown but later it possess good bone healing.

Question 6

What are the ideal requirement of irrigants and its importance?

Answer

Requirement of an Ideal Irrigant

- It should be good tissue or debris solvent
- It should have antimicrobial properties
- It should remove smear layer
- It should have good shelf life
- It should be biocompatible
- It should be least toxic
- It should possess good lubricating properties
- It should easily neutralize the canal.

Importance of Irrigant in Endodontic Treatment

- It helps in flushing out the root canal debris
- It describes the bacterial count
- It acts as a lubricant during instrumentation
- It has a bleaching effect

- ❏ It penetrates in inaccessible areas
- ❏ It removes intracanal medicament in the subsequent visit.

Question 7

What is Hank's balanced salt solution?

Answer

Hank's balanced salt solution is a storage media that is used in avulsed tooth.

Composition

- ❏ Sodium dichloride ($NaCl_2$)
- ❏ D Glucose
- ❏ Potassium chloride (KCl)
- ❏ Sodium hydroxide (NaOH)
- ❏ Calcium chloride ($CaCl_2$)
- ❏ Potassium hydroxide (KOH)
- ❏ Magnesium chloride ($MgCl_2$).

Question 8

What are ideal requirement of root canal sealers?

Answer

- ❏ It should be easy and quick in application
- ❏ It should be easily introduced into root canal
- ❏ It should be odourless and tasteless
- ❏ It should be chemically intact
- ❏ It should inhibit bacterial growth
- ❏ It should not irritate the periradicular tissues
- ❏ It should be pliable and moldable
- ❏ It should seal laterally and apically

- ❏ It should be radio-opaque and durable
- ❏ It should not shrink.

Question 9

Discuss Diaket?

Answer

It is supplied as powder and liquid.

Powder

- ❏ Zinc oxide
- ❏ Bismuth phosphate.

Liquid

- ❏ 2, 2 dihydroxy, -5, 5'dichloro-diphenyl methane
- ❏ Propionyl according to phenone
- ❏ Triethanolamine
- ❏ Caprylic acid
- ❏ Copolymers of vinyl acetate vinyl chloride
- ❏ Vinyl isobutyl ether.

Properties

- ❏ Good adhesion
- ❏ Low solubility
- ❏ It sets quickly
- ❏ It has good tensile strength.

Disadvantages

Have tendency towards fibrous encapsulation if extruded.

CHAPTER 18

Principles and Rationale of Endodontic Treatment

Question 1

Elaborate the rationale of endodontic treatment?

Answer

There can be many changes that occur after the injury to pulp due to either caries, trauma or chemicals.

- Multiplication of microorganisms in the root canal grows out of the root canal or by the root canal flora toxins and they may diffuse into periradicular area
- When there is decline in the host defence, these microorganisms are virulent and they destroy polymorphonuclear (PMN) leucocytes which than leads to chronic abscess
- Dead PMN releases proteolytic enzymes that produce pus.

Changes Occurring from Diseased Pulp

- Periapical infection
- Periapical radiolucency seen at the apex
- Infiltration of lymphocytes, macrophages, phagocytes, fibroblasts, PMN lymphocytes and osteoclasts is seen
- Endodontic treatment is a must treatment to remove toxins from the root canal
- Endodontic treatment will heal, repair and establish the tooth function and structure.

Fish Zones

- In an experiment by Fish, he established foci of infection in the jaws of guinea pig
- The bone of guinea pig was drilled and packed with wool
- Fibre saturated with a broth culture of microorganisms.

There were four well-defined zones of reaction:

1. Zone of infection
2. Zone of contamination
3. Zone of irritation
4. Zone of stimulation.

Zone of Infections

- Characteristic feature is PMN leukocytes
- Infection can be seen at the centre of the lesion.

Zone of Contamination

- Characterised by round cell infiltration (RCI)
- There was cellular destruction around the central zone which is not bacterial but from the toxins discharged from the central zone
- Appearance of empty lacunar resulting from dead bone cells causing autolysis
- Lymphocytes are seen shattered.

Zone of Irritation

- It is characterized by the pressure of macrophages and osteoclasts
- There is irritation further from the central lesion as the toxins become more diluted
- Phagocytic cells digest the collagen frame work
- Osteoclasts destroy one tissue
- There is also some repair that can be seen histopathologically.

Zone of Stimulation

- Fibroblasts and osteoblasts are present
- The toxins are mild enough to be a stimulant at the periphery
- Due to the response by stimulation, collagen fibres are laid down by fibroblasts. They both act as a defence wall around the zone of irritation and also as scaffolding in which new bones were built by osteoblasts
- Irregular bone formation is seen.

CHAPTER 19

Biomechanical Preparation

Question 1

Describe in detail cleaning and shaping of root canal. Write about step back and step down preparations?

Answer

- The removal of all the contents of the root canal system, like micro flora, organic substrates, pulp stones, bacterial by products, food debris, root canal fillings and dentinal filling is called as root canal cleaning
- Cleaning allows access to files and irrigants during the shaping process
- Shaping is the removal of all contents from root canal system. This process is done inside the canal which creates a smooth, tapered opening to the terminus to the three-dimensional obturation material which will favour periapical healing.

Methods of Cleaning and Shaping

- Corono-apical techniques:
  - Step-down preparation
  - Crown-down pressureless technique.
- Apico-coronal techniques:
  - Step back preparation
  - Standardised technique.
- Other techniques:
  - Lasers
  - Endosonics.
- Balanced force technique
- Non-instrumentation technique (NIT)
- Hybrid technique of canal preparation.

Step-back Preparation

- It is also known as serial technique / telescope preparation
- In this technique, preparation starts at apex with fine instrument and working one's way back up or down the canal with progressively larger instrument

- This helps in the instrument transportation in the apical third of the canal.

Objectives

- The apical portion of preparation should be as small as possible
- There should be an increasing taper throughout the remaining canal
- The final apical preparation should be at or close to the original canal preparation
- This creates a smooth flow and more tapered preparation from the apical portion to the coronal portion.

Technique

It is divided into two phases:

- **Phase I**: Apical preparation starting at the apical constriction
- **Phase II**: Remaining canal is prepared by gradually stepping back while increasing the size.

Phase I

- Apical preparation should start at the apical constriction
- Lubricating the canal and explored using a file $< no \neq 10/15$
- The initial apical file is the one that fits the apical constriction first
- A clockwise counter motion is used till the instrument becomes loose and this is than followed by irrigation
- Size 20 is then used to the same working length (WL) in the same motion till this also becomes loose and irrigation is done
- Apical portion is enlarged up to 25.30 size instrument.

Phase II

- Instrumentation is completed by successively using larger instruments and it should be remembered that each larger instrument should be kept 1 mm shorter than the previous instrument **(Fig. 19.1)**

- Step back manner preparation of the remainder of the root canal is done with larger number files **(Fig. 19.2 to 19.4)**
- Till the straight mid-canal is reached preparation is done using step back manner, that time the instrument will no longer fit tightly
- At last apical instrument is used to smoothen all the walls with push-pull motion followed by irrigation.

Advantages

- It facilitate in removal of more debris
- Periapical trauma is at low risk
- Lateral and vertical condensation of gutta-percha is easy by the greater flare caused by instrumentation
- Development of apical matrix and overfilling of root canal can be achieved
- It can fill lateral canals by giving greater condensation pressure which can be exerted.

Disadvantages

- This process requires special instruments and they are large in number
- Tactile control is limited when the preparation of apical region is done

- There is risk of pushing debris back in the canal and it becomes difficult to remove all the debris
- There is ledge formation in coronally tight canal by straight instrument
- Accumulation of dentinal mud leads to foramen blockage as it holds minimal volume of irrigant
- The coronal constriction is removed in the end which changes the WL.

Step Down Technique

- It is also called as crown down pressure less technique **(Fig. 19.5)**
- This is the technique that involves cleaning and shaping from coronal third of the canal to the apical third **(Fig. 19.6)**
- Apical third is approached only after the coronal two thirds preparations.

Technique

- Coronal preparation is done in two ways:
  - By Gates-Glidden (GG) drill **(Fig. 19.7)**
  - By larger files.

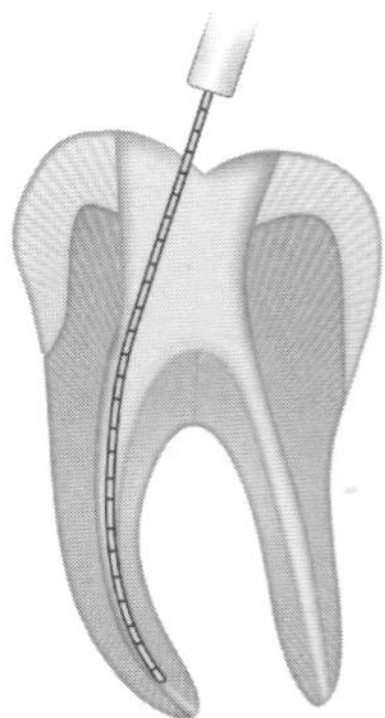

Fig. 19.1: No. 30 file 1 mm short of working length

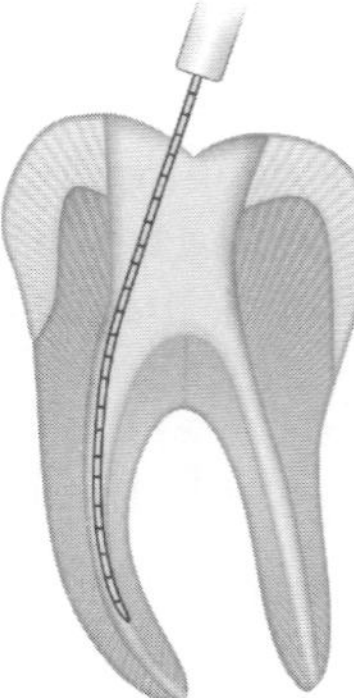

Fig. 19.2: No. 40 file 3 mm short of working length

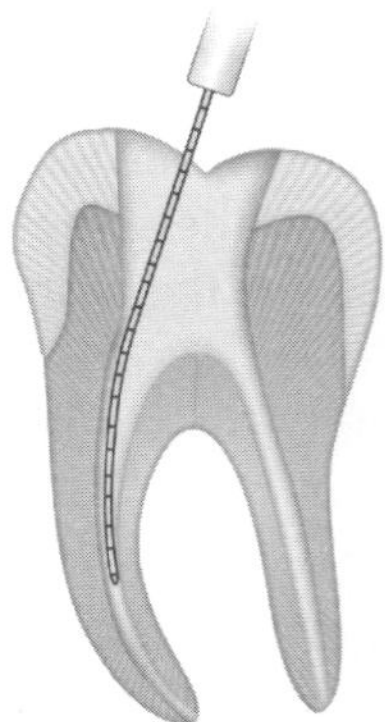

Fig. 19.3: No. 45 file 4 mm short of working length

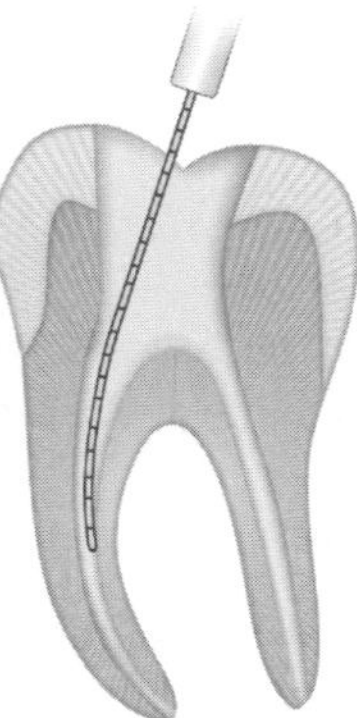

Fig. 19.4: No. 50 file for canal preparation

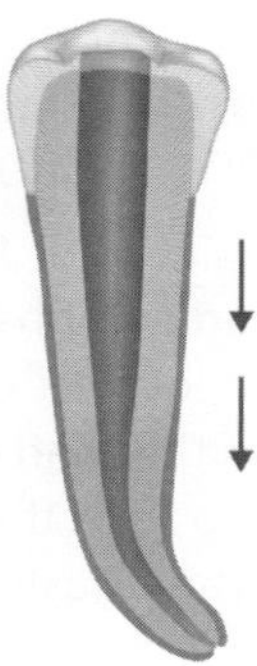

Fig. 19.5: Crown-down technique

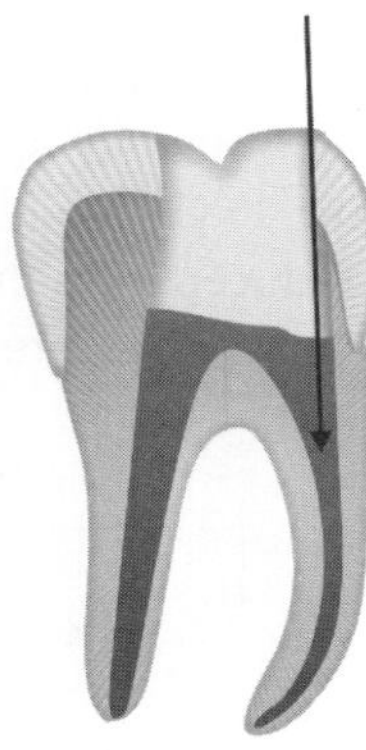

Fig. 19.6: Straight line access to root canal system

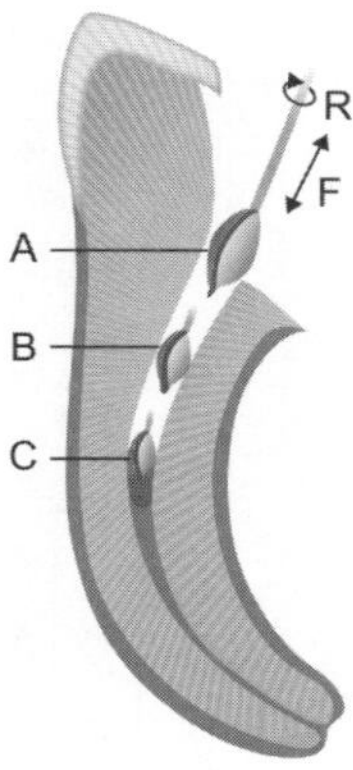

Fig. 19.7: Use of Gates-Glidden for preflaring

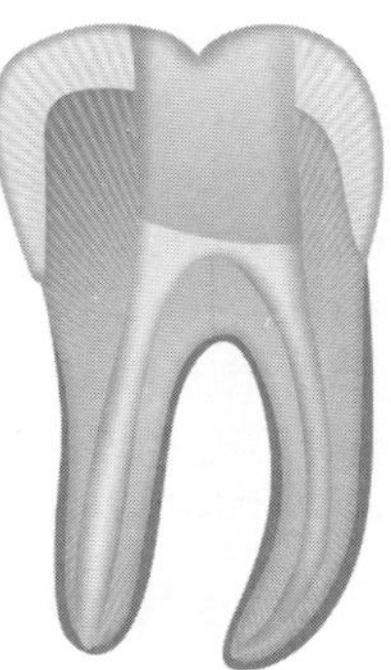

Fig. 19.8: Filling the chamber with irrigant solution

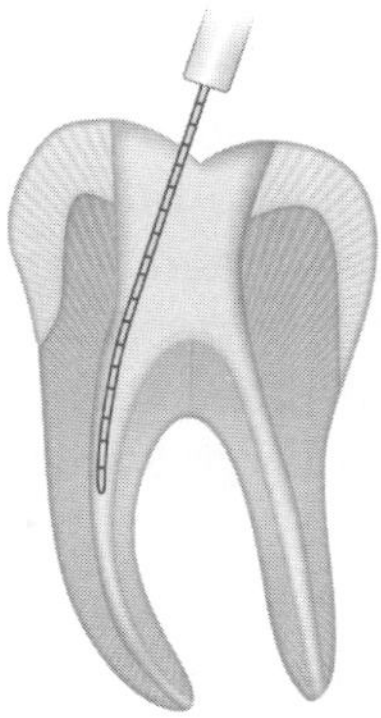

Fig. 19.9: Use of larger files to prepare coronal third

- The drilling is done in the apical direction till the desired length is reached
- Fill the access cavity with an irrigant and start preflaring of the canal orifices **(Fig. 19.8)**
- Final apical preparation is prepared and finished along with frequent irrigation of the canal system **(Fig. 19.9).**

Coronal and Mild Root Preparation

- Firstly, the determination of WL is done
- Coronal area is prepared using:
  - 16 mm H files
  - GG drill 15–40 size.
- Each larger file should be inserted shorter to the predecessor by approximately 1 mm.

SHORT ESSAYS

Question 1

What is apical preparation?

Answer

The objective of apical preparation is to enlarge the apex by 2–3 times the size from the first file that binds apically.

Advantages

- It eliminates the debris and microorganisms from the most coronal part of the root canal which prevents the inoculation of apical tissues with contaminated debris
- Coronally placed interferences is eliminated which might adversely influence instrumentation

- There is early movement of large volume of irrigant and lubricant to the apical part of the canal
- In early preparation, coronal curvature is eliminated; hence, there is accurate working length (WL) determination
- WL is unlikely to be changed
- As it accepts larger files into apical 1/3rd, determining foramen becomes easy in radiographs
- There is less chance of instrument fracture.

Question 2

What are the various methods of determining working length in endodontics?

Answer

- Working length (WL) is defined as the length measured from a coronal reference point to the point at which canal preparation and obturation should terminate
- The distance from a coronal reference point to the point at which canal preparation and obturation should terminate (glossary of endodontics).

Methods

1. Radiographic methods:
   a. Grossman's method
   b. Ingle's method
   c. Xeroradiography
   d. Radiovisiography (RVG)
   e. Subtraction radiography.
2. Non-radiographic methods:
   a. Paper point method
   b. Audiometric method
   c. Endometric probe method
   d. Electrical resistance method
   e. Apical periodontal sensitivity.

Radiographic Methods

- Grossman's method
- Instrument extending to the apical constriction is placed in the root canal which can be determined by digital tactile sense and radiograph is taken
- Stopper is placed at the level of incisal or occlusal reference point
- Measurement is then taken of the length of X-ray of both, the tooth and measuring instrument and also the actual length of the instrument in the canal.

Formula

- A: Actual length of the tooth (**Fig. 19.10A to D**)
- B: Actual length of instrument
- C: Radiographic length of tooth
- D: Radiographic length of instrument in tooth.

Ingles Method

- Firstly pre-operative radiographs are taken
- Approximately length of the root canal is found by +6lusal rubber stop on the shaft of the file
- 1 mm length is reduced from this by moving the rubber stopper on the shaft. This is just a safety measure
- Radiographs are taken with the instrument in position
- On the X-ray, the difference between the tip of the root and tip of the instrument is added to safety measure if it is short of the apex
- If the instrument has gone beyond the apex, the measurement that is obtained is subtracted from the original measurement
- In the end, 1 mm is reduced from the final measurement so that the tip of instrument corresponds to the apical foramens

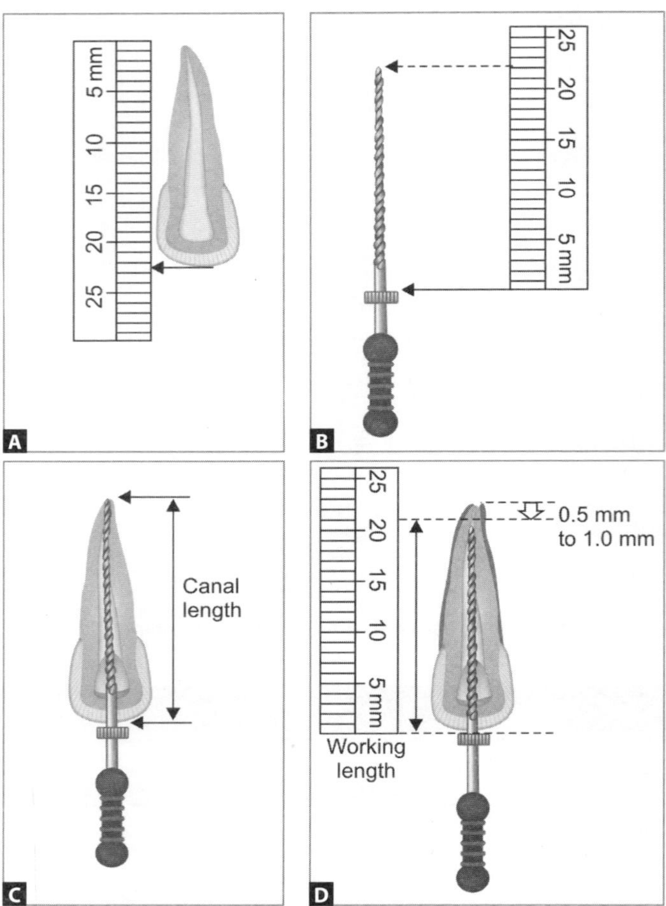

Fig. 19.10A to D: Radiographic method of working length determination

❑ It is assumed in this method that apical foramen is 0.5 mm away from the radiographic root tip.

Wein's Modification for Ingle's Method

This method states that if radiographically there is no resorption of the root end or the bone, the length should be shorten by standard 1 mm (**Fig. 19.11A to C**).

❑ If there is periapical bone resorption the length is shorten by 1.5 mm
❑ If both root and bone resorption is present shorten the length by 2 mm
❑ The reason being, if there is root resorption the apical constriction is probably destroyed.

Radiographic Grid

❑ In this method, a millimetre grid is superimposed on the radiographs which overcome the need for calculation
❑ For the easy reading of radiograph every 5 mm interval is darker.

Disadvantage

❑ If radiograph is bent during exposure, correct reading is unlike
❑ It may be correctly oriented to the file for easy measurement
❑ May obscure the tip.

Endometric Probe

❑ There are graduations on diagnostic file which are visible on the radiographic grid
❑ They are etched at millimetre increments.

Disadvantages

The smallest file size is no ≠ 25.

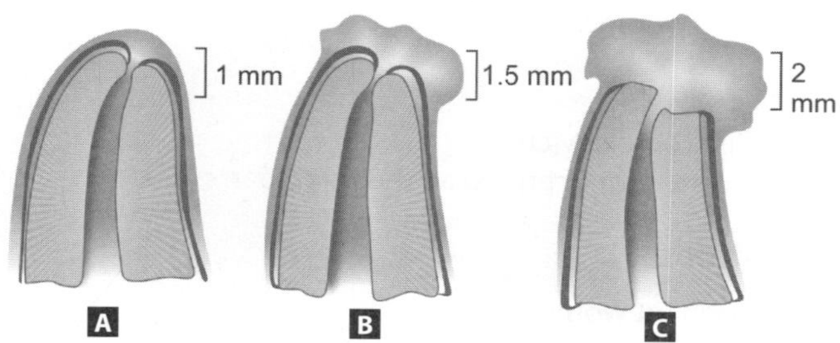

Fig. 19.11A to C: Modification in length by subtraction in case of resorption

Non-radiographic Methods of Working Length

❑ Digital tactile sense:
  ○ The WL is determined by radiographic or electronic method
  ○ It is based on the experience if the coronal portion of the canal is not constricted there will be increase in resistance as file approaches the apical 2–3 mm.
❑ Apical periodontal sensitivity:
  ○ It is based on patient's pain perception.

Disadvantage

It is very rarely accurate while determining the WL.

Measurement Using Paper Point

❑ Paper point is one of the reliable methods in determining WL
❑ After anaesthesia is administered, paper point with blunt end is inserted in the canal with open apex
❑ WL is determined by the moisture or blood on paper point when it passes beyond the apex
❑ It may not give accurate reading if the pulp is not completely removed.

SHORT NOTES

Question 1

What is Recapitulation?

Answer

It is the reintroduction and reapplication of instruments that are previously used throughout the process of cleaning and shaping in order to create a well-designed smooth, unclogged and stepless root canals.

Question 2

What are Electronic apex locators?

Answer

❑ The electronic apex locator determines the working length for canal preparation in reference with the radiographs
❑ They work on the direct or altering current which determines the apical constriction

- Part of apex locator:
  - Lip clip
  - File clip
  - Electronic device
  - A cord connecting to all the three parts.

Indications

- In pregnant women
- In heavily sedative patients
- In children

- Patients with complain of gag reflex
- When there is obstruction in the apical portion, e.g., infected teeth
- Excessive bone density
- Overlapping roots.

Contra Indications

- Patients with cardiac pacemakers
- Tooth with open apices.

CHAPTER 20

Obturation of Root Canal

Question 1

Classify obturation methods. Elaborate lateral condensation method?

Answer

Obturation

It is a three-dimensional (3D) filling of an entire root canal system as close to the cemento-dentinal junction so as to obtain an impermeable seal at the apex.

Objectives

- To create a favourable environment at the periapical region for healing of tissue
- To seal the root canal to stop the bacterial movement
- To eliminate leakage from periradicular tissue into root canal.

Material Used for Obturating Root Canal

- Plastics
  - Gutta-percha (GP)
  - Resilon.
- Metal core/solids
  - Silver points
  - Stainless steal
  - Gold
  - Tantalum titanium
  - Iridium platinum.
- Cements and pastes
  - Hydrogen calcium
  - Resorcinol
  - MTA
  - Calcium phosphate
  - Gutta flow.

Classification of Various Methods of Obturating Techniques

There are two basic procedures:

1. Lateral compaction of cold GP.
2. Vertical compaction of warm GP.

Ingle's Classification of Various Obturating Techniques

- Solid-core GP with sealants
  - Cold GP points
    - Lateral compaction
    - Variations of lateral compaction.
  - Chemically plasticised cold GP
  - Essential oils and solvents
    - Eucalyptol
    - Chloroform
    - Halothane.
  - Canal warmed GP
    - Vertical compaction
    - System B compaction
    - Sectional compaction
    - Lateral/vertical compaction
      - Endotec II.
    - Thermomechanical compaction.
      - Micro seal system, Engine Plugger, Maillefer condenser
      - Hybrid technique
      - IS-Quick-fill
      - Ultrasonic plasticising.
  - Thermoplasticized GP
    - Syringe insertion
      - Obtura
      - Inject-R-fill, backfill

- ➤ Solid-core carrier insertion.
  - » Thermafil and Densfil
  - » Soft core
  - » Silver points.
- ❑ Apical third filling
  - ○ Light-speed simplifill
  - ○ Dentine chip
  - ○ Calcium hydroxide.
- ❑ Injection or spiral filling
  - ○ Cements
  - ○ Pastes
  - ○ Plastics
  - ○ Calcium phosphate.

According to Cohen

- ❑ The cold compaction of GP:
- ❑ The compaction of GP that has been heat-softened in canal and cold compacted
- ❑ The compaction of GP that has been thermoplasticised, injected into canal and cold compacted
- ❑ The compaction of GP that has been placed in canal and softened through mechanical means.

Lateral Condensation Technique for Obturating Root Canal

Lateral Condensation Technique

It encompasses first placing a sealer lining in the canal, followed by a measured primary point that in turn is compacted laterally by a spreader used with lateral pressure, to make room for additional accessory points.

Significance

It is a preferred technique for most of the canals as most teeth present wide canals or flares that cannot be densely filled with the single cone technique.

Technique

This is a procedure where additional auxiliary cones are inserted and condensed laterally around the primary cone. Tapered preparation is necessary (**Fig. 20.1**).

Selection of Master Cone

- ❑ GP cone is inserted to the working length and should fit snugly and resist to removal or "tug back" (**Fig. 20.2**)
- ❑ A radiograph is taken to determine the apical and lateral fit of the primary cone (**Fig. 20.3**)
- ❑ Cone is fitted in canal short of 1 mm from the apex. Once the primary cone is accurately fitted in the root canal, it is removed to dry the canal (**Fig. 20.4**)

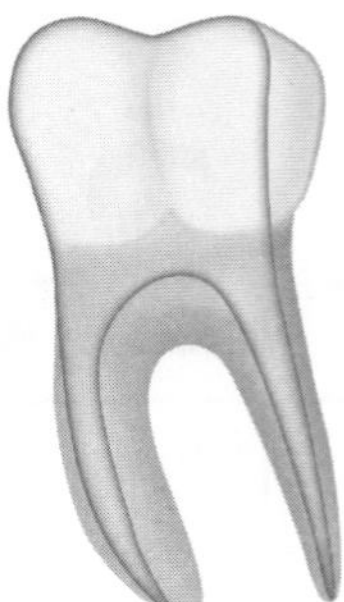

Fig. 20.1: Tapered preparation of root canal system

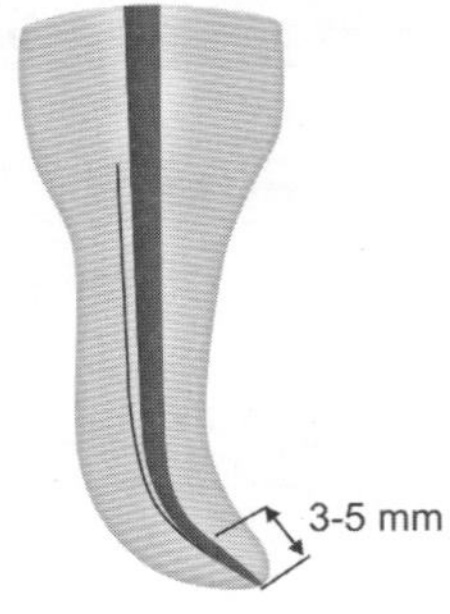

Fig. 20.2: Tugback with master gutta percha cone

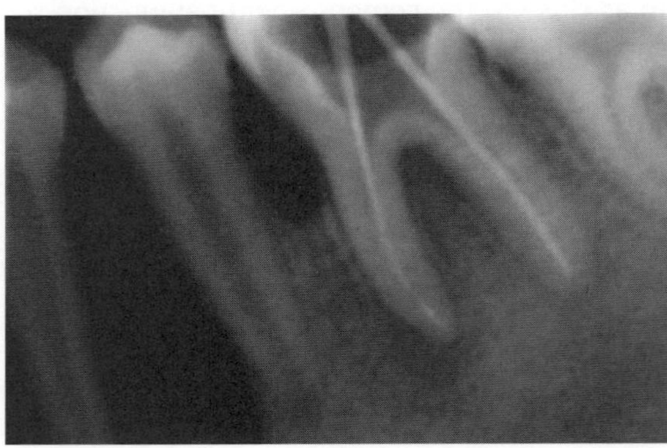

Fig. 20.3: S-shaped appearance of cone in mesial canal shows that cone is too small for the canal, replace it with bigger cone

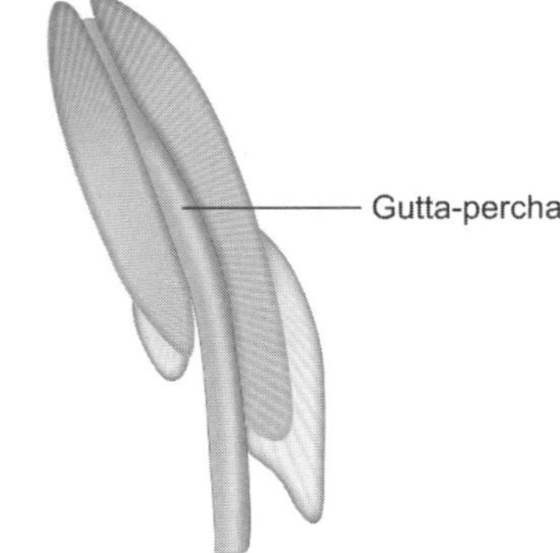

Fig. 20.4: Gutta-percha showing tight fit in middle and space in apical third

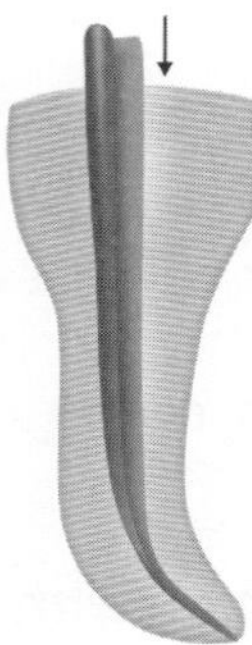

Fig. 20.5: Placing accessory cone along master cone

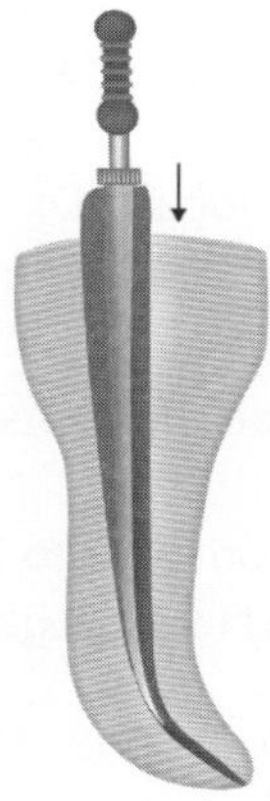

Fig. 20.6: Compaction of gutta-percha using spreader

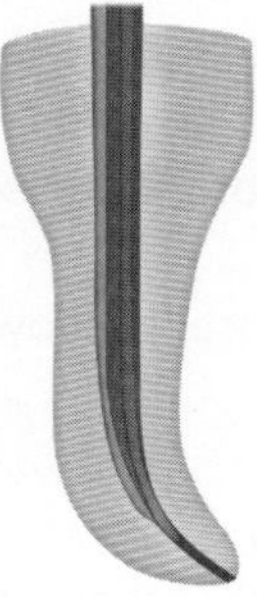

Fig. 20.7: Use of more accessory cones to complete obturation of the canal

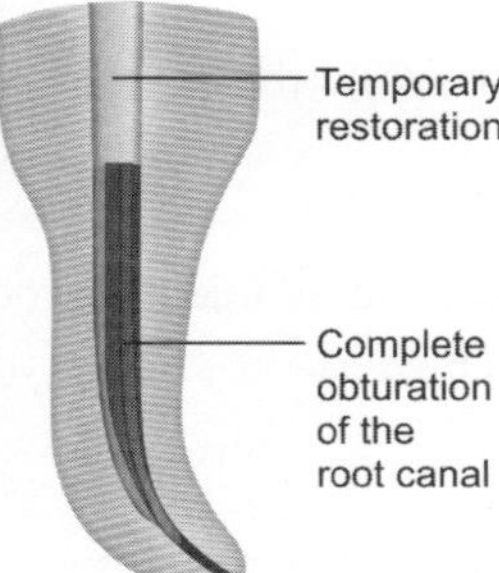

Fig. 20.8: Cut the protruding gutta-percha points at orifice with hot instrument and place temporary restoration over it

- ❑ Walls are coated with thin layer of cement. Cementing is not necessary for accessory canals (**Fig. 20.5**)
- ❑ Now the selected master cone is inserted and condensed with spreader (**Fig. 20.6**)
- ❑ If gap is present then accessory cone is inserted and condensed. The process continues till the canal is filled completely (**Fig. 20.7**)
- ❑ After verifying the canal by radiograph, the battened of GP in the pulp chamber is cut off with a hot instrument (**Fig. 20.8**)
- ❑ The chamber is cleaned and temporary restoration is placed in the access cavity.

Advantages

- ❑ Faster
- ❑ Simplicity and ease
- ❑ During compaction of GP, it provides length control, thereby prevent overfilling.

Disadvantages

- ❑ Cannot adapt to canal wall irregularities
- ❑ Does not achieve a dense homogenous mass
- ❑ Filling of lateral and accessory canals not achieved
- ❑ Chances of stress development and fracture especially in roots with less mesio-distal dimensions like premolars.

Question 2

Write in brief about gutta-percha in obturation?

Answer

Obturation is a three-dimensional (3D) filling of an entire root canal system as close to the cementodentinal junction so as to obtain an impermeable seal at the apex.

Gutta-percha (GP)

- ❑ GP is the most common obturating material
- ❑ It is a hydrocarbon that resembles a rubber
- ❑ Alpha and beta form of GP is used. GP in pure form is not used
- ❑ Low-viscosity alpha forms of the GP are: Thermafil, Densfil, and Microseal.

Composition

- ❑ *Zinc oxide*: 66%
- ❑ *GP*: 20%
- ❑ *Heavy metal surfaces*: 11%
- ❑ *Waxes of resins*: 3%.

Gutta-percha Available in Different Forms

- GP flow
- GP points
- GP sealer
- GP syringes
- GP pellets/bars
- Pre-coated core carrier GP.

Standardized / Core Points

- Standardise sizes are co-ordinated with the 150 sizes of root canal files
- They are primarily used as the main core material for the obturation.

Non-standardised / Auxiliary Points

- They are more tapered from the tip to top. They are used as secondary and auxiliary cones
- They are designed as:
  - Extra-fine
  - Fine-fine
  - Medium-fine
  - Fine-medium
  - Medium
  - Medium-large
  - Large
  - Extra-large.
- GP comes in pellet form and also in cannulas for injectable thermoplastic obturation techniques
- For thermo mechanical technique they are available in heatable syringes
- Medicated GP point are available that contain iodoform which enhances the antimicrobial properties.

Properties

- The standardised cones are colour coded which match the instrument size
- They are used as master cone
- They are stored in cool and dry area
- It is disinfected with 2% glutaraldehyde and 2% chlorhexidine.

Advantages

- GP is tissue tolerant or non-allergic
- GP does not discolour tooth structure
- GP is least toxic, inert and radiopaque
- GP does not shrink after insertion
- GP can be easily removed from root canal when required
- GP being a plastic adapts and seals better with irregularities of canal.

Disadvantages

- Becomes brittle with age
- Can be displaced with pressure
- It is used with a sealer as it lacks adhesive qualities
- Lacks rigidity
- Cannot be placed in narrow canals and canals with extreme curvature.

Technique of Obturation with Gutta-percha

- Use of beta phase:
  - Obtura
  - Obtura II.
- Use of alpha phase:
  - Ultra three-dimensional (3D).

Using Obtura II

- GP is heated externally followed by the placement in canal
- Temperature range from 160° to 200°
- Needle size is reduced to 2023 gauze.

Method

- The temperature control panel has a temperature display and temperature control
- GP gun has a flexible needle attached to the gun
- The needle should be pre-fitted in the canal and should be 3.5–5 mm short of the apex
- Sealers, like AH plus or seal apex are used and filled the canal slowly
- GP is compacted vertically followed by a radiograph.

Advantages

- Filling of all accessory canals
- Used in obturating C-shaped canals with internal resorption.

Disadvantage

The GP might flow beyond the apex.

Ultrafil 3D

- This is a thermoplastic GP injection technique
- 70° temperature is used.

Types

- Regular set which has low viscosity—sets in 30 minutes
- Firm set which has low viscosity—sets in 4 minutes
- Endo set which has higher viscosity—sets in 2 minutes.

SHORT ESSAYS

Question 1

What is vertical compaction technique of obturation?

Answer

Procedure

- Canal is dried with paper point
- Three vertical pluggers are pre-fitted:
  - **First:** Widest plugger reaching 10 mm depth from the orifice
  - **Second:** Middle plugger reaching 15 mm depth from the orifice
  - **Third:** Apical plugger: 3–4 mm short of apical terminus.

A root canal sealer is used to obtain impervious seal and is used with core obturating material.

- Master GP cone is selected which fits 0.5–1.0 mm short of working length
- GP is placed with sealer in the canal
- Cone is cut as incisal reference point.

Heat Transfer Instrument

Touch 'n' heat 5004 is heated at temp 42–52°C till it turns to cherry red. It is then placed in coronal third of root canal for 2–3 seconds. It is then withdrawn in slightly circular motion to remove a portion of the GP.

- Wide pluggers are used to compact the warmed GP
- Introducing the heat carrier back for 2–3 seconds and 3–4 mm of the GP is removed
- Mid-size coated pluggers are used to obturate mid root lateral canal with vertical and lateral pressure
- Third heat wave is used for 2–3 seconds and 3–4 mm of GP is removed
- GP is compacted with small pulggers into apical preparation
- Accessory canal is then obturated.

Question 2

What is lateral condensation technique?

Answer

Two basic procedures of obturatory techniques are:
1. Lateral compaction of cold GP.
2. Vertical compaction of warm GP.

Lateral Condensation Technique for Obturating Root Canal

- This is the most used obturating technique

- In this process, root canal is coated with sealer followed by the placement of measured point which is laterally compacted by spreader
- A hot instrument is used at the canal orifice and vertical compaction is done using large plugger.

Procedure Follows Five Steps

- Primary point size selection
- Spreader size and length
- Drying of canal
- Mixing and placement of the sealer
- Accessory point selection and placement.

Primary Point Size Selection

- This is caused as master cone selection
- This size matches the size of last instrument used at the apical constriction.

Selection of Spreader Size and Length

- The spreader sizes should be loose and reach 1 mm within the working length. It should not penetrate beyond the apex
- The force applied by spreader should be against GP, so that GP absorbs the force and there is no stress on the wall as it may fracture the tooth.

Drying of Canal

- Paper points are used to dry the canal. Air syringe should not be used
- Mixing and placement of sealer:
  - Sealant should be mixed in glass slab
  - It should be of creamy consistency
  - This gives clinician extra time to work.

Placement of Sealers

- GP can be used as spreaders
- File or reamer should be used anticlockwise and in a pumping action
- Centuro spirals
- Ultrasonic file without coolant
- Spreader of appropriate taper.

Accessory Point Selection and Placement

- Accessory point should be of same size or smaller in diameter than spreader size
- It is placed in obturating canal to obtain cohesive filling.

Advantages

- Simple method
- There is no need of special instrument.

Disadvantages

- Canal irregularities cannot be filled
- Does not produce homogenous mass.

SHORT NOTES

Question 1

What is sectional method of obturation?

Answer

This method is used where the tooth requires post and core:

- A pre-fit plugger which fits loosely in the canal and extends within 3 mm of working length
- Master cone is fitted within 1.0 mm of the working length and radiograph is taken
- Gutta-percha (GP) is cut so that only apical 3–4 mm of GP is left
- GP is warmed and coated with sealer
- Warm GP is placed and packed into place
- Radiograph is taken to confirm apical filling
- It has a disadvantage that it has a poor control on small section of GP which results in unpredictable outcomes.

Question 2

What are silver points?

Answer

- They are introduced when two-dimensional sealing of root canal is started
- They are used in solid core metallic filling material.

Indications

- It is used in mature teeth with small calcified canal
- In round, straight and curved canals.

Contraindications

- Open apex
- Large avoid canals.

CHAPTER 21

Endodontic Emergencies

Question 1

Classify endodontic emergencies. Write about phoenix abscess?

Answer

Classification of Endodontic Emergencies

- Before treatment:
  - Acute pulpitis:
    - › Acute reversible pulpitis
    - › Acute irreversible pulpitis.
  - Acute abscess:
    - › Alveolar abscess
    - › Periodontal abscess.
  - Acute pulpitis with apical periodontitis
  - Traumatic injury.
- During treatment:
  - Hot tooth
  - Inter-appointment flare-up.
- After treatment:
  - Post-endodontic pain
  - Vertical root fracture.

Phoenix Abscess

- It is also known as recrudescent abscess
- It is an acute exacerbation of chronic lesion
- They are mostly inflammatory reactions which are superimposed on the existing chronic lesions, like cyst or granuloma
- They are characterised by the formation and retention of pus in the alveolar bone around the root apex present on the tooth with non-vital pulp along the extension of the infection which is through apical foramen into the periapical tissues.

Aetiology

- The periradicular tissue reaction to noxious stimuli from a pulp that is infected is in a state of equilibrium cyst or a granuloma is formed
- An acute inflammatory response is initiated with necrotic product or bacteria from the diseased pulp.

Symptoms

- The tooth which is affected will be over sensitive to any touch
- There will be tenderness on percussion
- Asymmetry of face due to swelling in oral mucosa around the teeth is involved
- Redness and swollen mucosa is seen over the radicular area
- Affected tooth may be elevated in its socket and most of the time it becomes mobile
- Surface tissue appears tightly stretched and inflamed. There is pus discharge from beneath the tooth
- Fever, malaise, nausea, dizziness, lymphadenopathy can be seen.

Diagnosis

- Radiographs are the diagnostic tools to reveal periradicular radiolucency indicating a lesion
- Pulp testing will not be a diagnostic option as the tooth will not respond to it.

Histopathology

- Local anaesthesia is contraindicated
- Treatment is done in two phases:
  - Pulp debridement
  - Incision drainage.
- Medicament of calcium hydroxide in the intracanal is the choice of treatment

- If there are systemic symptoms antibiotic therapy should be initiated
- To control pain: non-steroidal anti-inflammatory drugs (NSAIDs)
- Root canal treatment.

Question 2

Write in brief about endodontic emergencies?

Answer

Classification of Endodontic Emergencies

- Before treatment:
  - Acute pulpitis:
    - Acute reversible pulpitis
    - Acute irreversible pulpitis.
  - Acute abscess:
    - Alveolar abscess
    - Periodontal abscess.
  - Acute pulpitis with apical periodontitis
  - Traumatic injury.
- During treatment:
  - Hot tooth
  - Inter-appointment flare-up.
- After treatment:
  - Post-endodontic pain
  - Vertical root fracture.

Acute Irreversible Pulpitis

Clinical Features

- Pain is spontaneous
- Pain is exaggerated with hot and cold stimulus that lasts even when it is removed
- Involved tooth will have extensive caries or restoration
- Pain aggravates at the time of lying down
- Extra-oral examination findings will be tender, enlarged lymph nodes and tender on palpation.

Radiographic Findings

Widening of the periodontal ligament (PDL) is seen.

Treatment

- Initial pain is treated by simple analgesics
- In case of inflammation for long, medicine will be far less effective
- Last choice of treatment is pulpotomy and pulpectomy.

Procedure

- Rubber dam application on the tooth after anaesthesia is administered

- Access opening is done
- Removal of pulp and debridement and irrigation is done
- Root canal orifice is located and the root canal is explored
- Working length is determined and cleaning and shaping of the canal is done
- Dry the canal with sterile adsorbent points
- Sealing of the access cavity is done
- Analgesic and antibody therapy is used if required
- Obturation is then done after the endodontic restoration.

Acute Reversible Pulpitis/Hyperaemia

Acute reversible pulpitis is caused when there is increased blood flow in the pulp.

Clinical Features

- Tooth become sensitive to thermal changes
- Especially with cold stimulus and it disappears after the stimulus is removed
- The sharp pain produced is because of the a-delta fibres
- Dull lasting pain is caused by heat application which stimulates c-fibre.

Treatment

- Palliative procedures is the treatment of acute reversible pulpitis, which uses zinc oxide-eugenol (ZOE) cement as a temporary sedative filling
- Contouring all the high spots that will relieve the pain and allows the pulp to recuperate
- If pain does not eliminate the pulp; extirpation is done.

Other Treatment

- Resin adhesive varnish as a protective insulating base under any metallic restoration. This will eliminate chances of hypaeremia
- Placement of a pulp protective base under all restorations which avoids marginal leakage, and reduce occlusal trauma
- Contouring all restorations and avoiding pulp injury which prepares or polishes a metallic restoration.

Acute Periapical Abscess

- It is also known as acute alveolar abscess (AAA)
- It is a localised collection of pus in the periradicular tissue following death of the pulp due to extensive infection through apical foramen.

Aetiology

- Chemical irritation
- Bacteria and its by-products
- Trauma.

Symptoms

- First symptom is tenderness on percussion
- Tooth can be mobile and slightly extruded
- There can be localised swelling
- Swelling can become cellulitis if left untreated which leads to asymmetric face of the patient
- General symptoms are fever, malaise and lymphadenopathy.

Diagnosis

- On examination, the tooth is tender and slightly mobile
- Necrosis is shown in vitality test
- Radiographs show:
  - Defective restoration
  - Widened PDL
  - Break down of bone in apical region.

Treatment

- Mostly fair
- In case of extreme periodontium, destruction prognosis can be poor.

Periapical Cyst

It is also known as radicular cyst or "dental root end cyst" or "apical periodontal cyst".

- It is classified as inflammatory odontogenic cyst
- It is a sequel associated with bacterial invasion and death of the dental pulp.

Clinical Features

- They are most common in maxillary incisor region
- It has male predominance
- Tooth involved is mostly non-vital and asymptomatic
- Large lesions produce a slow enlarging bony hard swelling of the Jaw with cortical plate being expanded
- Secondary cyst will lead to the formation of abscess and is called "cyst abscess"
- Pus formation in the cyst will lead to sinus or pus discharge.

Treatment

- Treatment depends on if it is reversible or irreversible pulpitis
- Any restoration that is associated with loose cusp should be removed and restored to the shape and size of the cavity
- Pulp extirpation
- Randomized controlled trial (RCT).

Apical Granuloma

- Inflamed granulation tissue growth in the PDL as a result of pulpal death due to bacteria and its toxin from root canal
- It is asymptomatic
- Can be diagnosed with radiographic examination
- Does not respond to electric stimulation
- Size varies from millimetres to centimetres.

Treatment

- RCT
- If lesion does not resolve then surgical approach is used

Acute apical periodontitis:

It is a painful inflammation of the periodontium as a result of trauma, irritation and infection through the root canal in spite the pulp is vital or non-vital.

Aetiology

- Vital tooth:
  - Occlusal trauma
  - Blow to the teeth
  - Wedging between the restoration and teeth extending beyond occlusal plane.
- Non-vital teeth:
  - Sequelae of the pulpal disease.

Radiographic Features

- PDL is thickened
- Pulpless teeth may show periapical rarefaction.

Treatment

- Vital: relieving the symptoms
- Non-vital: RCT.

Question 3

Describe the various causes of pulp diseases and describe the clinical features and management of irreversible pulpitis?

Answer

Various causes of pulp diseases are as follows:

According to Grossman

Physical

Mechanical

- Trauma-accidental and iatrogenic dental procedures
- Pathologic wear
- Crack through the body of tooth

- Radiation
- Restorations
- Barodomalgia.

Thermal Injuries

- Heat produced during cavity preparation
- Exothermic heat during setting of cement
- Frictional heat during the polishing of restorations
- Conduction of heat and cold through deep restorations without a protective base.

Electrical Injuries

Galvanic shock.

Chemical

- Dental erosion (acids)
- Phosphoric acid, acrylic monomer, etc.

Bacterial

- Direct invasion of pulp from caries or trauma
- Toxins associated with caries
- Anachoresis
- Fractures.

According to Ingle

Bacterial Causes

Coronal Ingress

- Caries
- Non-fracture trauma
- Fracture-complete and incomplete
- Anomaous trackt.
  - Dens invaginatus
  - Dens evaginatus.

Radicular Ingress

- Caries
- Haematogenic
- Cariogenic infection-periodontal pocket and periodontal abscess.

Traumatic Causes

Acute

- Coronal fracture
- Radicular fracture
- Vascular stasis
- Luxation
- Avulsion.

Chronic

- Adolescent female bruxism
- Traumatism
- Attrition or abrasion
- Erosion.

Iatrogenic Causes

- Cavity preparation: Includes depth of preparation, Heat produced on preparation, dehydration, pulp exposure and pulp hemorrhage
- Restoration: Includes force of insertion, cementing, heat of polishjng and either complete and incomplete fracture of restoration
- Intentional extirpation and root canal filling
- Intubation for general anaesthesia
- Rhinoplasty
- Electro surgery
- Periodontal and periapical curettage
- Orthodontic movements.

Chemical Causes

- Restorative materials, e.g., plastics. cements, cavity liners, etching agents
- Erosion, e.g., phenol, silver nitrate. sodium fluoride
- Desiccants, Alcohol, ether, etc.

Idiopathic Causes

- Ageing
- HIV and AIDS
- Internal resorption
- External resorption.

Irreversible Pulpitis

Irreversible pulpitis is defined as a persistent inflammatory condition of the pulp, which may be symptomatic or asymptomatic caused by a noxious stimuli.

Aetiology

- Chemical, thermal or mechanical causes
- Reversible pulpitis may deteriorate into irreversible pulpits
- Bacterial invasion through dental caries is most common.

Types

- Acute irreversible pulpitis
- Chronic irreversible pulpitis.

Clinical Features

Early Stage

- There is intense, continuous and prolonged pain due to pressure of secondary irritants
- Pain is due to change in temperature
- Pain is posteriorly which is radiated to ear and temporal area
- No external stimulus is required.

Later Stage

- If inflamed, involved PDL-percussion test is positive, or else it will be normal
- Normal to elevated response
- Pain relieved by cold occasionally
- Acute pain.

Diagnosis

- On examination, a deep cavity/caries exposes the pulp
- Radiograph reveals exposure of pulp
- Thermal and electrical tests elicit pain that persist even after the removal of stimulus.

Treatment

- Pulpectomy
- Pulpotomy for posterior tooth as an emergency procedure
- Extraction of the tooth if it is unrestorable.

Question 4

Classify the pulp diseases. Give aetiology, signs and symptoms, differential and treatment of acute pulpitis?

Answer

Classification of Pulpal Diseases

According to Ingle

Inflammatory Changes

- Hyper-reactive pulpalgia
  - Hypersensitivity
  - Hyperaemia.
- Acute pulpalgia
  - Incipient
  - Moderate
  - Advanced.
- Chronic pulpalgia
- Hyperplastic pulpitis
- Pulp necrosis.

Retrogressive Changes

- Atrophic pulposis
- Calcific pulposis.

According to Grossman

Based on clinical features.

Pulpitis (Inflammation)

- Reversible
  - Symptomatic (acute)
  - Asymptomatic (chronic).
- Irreversible.
  - Acute
    - ➤ Abnonnal response to cold
    - ➤ Abnormal response to heat.
  - Chronic.
    - ➤ Asymptomatic with pulp exposure
    - ➤ Hyperplastic pulpitis
    - ➤ Internal resorption.

Pulp Degeneration

- Calcific
- Others.

Necrosis

Acute Pulpitis

Acute pulpitis can be reversible and irreversible:

Acute Reversible Pulpitis Hyperemia

Reversible pulpitis is mild-to-moderate inflammatory condition of the pulp caused by noxious stimuli in which the pulp is capable of returning to the normal state following removal of stimuli.

Etiology

Trauma

- Accident or occlusal trauma
- Thermal injury
- While tooth preparation with dull bur without coolant
- Overheating during restoration and polishing
- Long exposure of bur in the same area
- Chemical exposure from sweet or sour foodstuff.

Diagnosis

- Pain is sharp but of brief duration, ceasing when irritant is removed. It is usually caused by cold, sweet and sour stimuli
- Radiographic examinations reveal caries, traumatic occlusion and undetected fracture
- Percussion test shows negative response
- Vitality test shows pulp responds readily to cold stimuli.

Treatment

- ❑ The best treatment of reversible pulpitis is prevention
- ❑ Endodontic treatment is not needed for this condition.

Acute Irreversible Pulpitis

It is a persistent inflammatory condition of the pulp, symptomatic or asymptomatic, caused by a noxious stimulus.

Etiology

- ❑ Bacterial involvement
- ❑ Chemical, thermal and mechanical injuries
- ❑ Diagnosis
- ❑ On inspection, one may see deep cavity involving pulp
- ❑ Radiographs show depth and extent of caries
- ❑ Tooth is tender on percussion (due to increased intrapulpal pressure as a result of exudative inflammatory tissue)
- ❑ Cold tends to relieve pain because of its contractile effect on vessels, reducing the intrapulpal pressure.

Treatment

- ❑ Pulpectomy
- ❑ Root canal treatment.

Question 5

Classify periradicular lesions/diseases. Write in detail the causes, symptoms, diagnosis, differential diagnosis, treatment and prognosis of acute alveolar abscess?

Answer

Classification of Periradicular Lesions

- ❑ Acute Periradicular Lesions
  - ○ Acute apical periodontitis:
    - ➤ Vital
    - ➤ Non-vital.
  - ○ Acute alveolar abscess
  - ○ Phoenix abscess.
- ❑ Chronic Periradicular Lesions
  - ○ Chronic alveolar abscess
  - ○ Granuloma
  - ○ Cysts.
- ❑ Condensing osteitis
- ❑ External root resorption
- ❑ Disease of periradicular tissues of non-odomogellic origin.

Ingle's Classification

Apical Periodontitis

- ❑ Acute apical periodontitis (AAP)

  - ❑ Chronic apical periodontitis (CAP).
    - ○ Periradicular granuloma
    - ○ Radicular cyst
    - ○ Condensing osteitis.

Apical Abscesses

- ❑ Acute apical abscess (AAA)
- ❑ Chronic apical abscess (CAA)
- ❑ Phoenix abscess.

Non-endodontic Periradicular Lesion

Odontogenic Cysts

- ❑ Primordial cyst
- ❑ Dentigerous cyst
- ❑ Lateral periodontal cyst
- ❑ Odontogenic keratocyst
- ❑ Residual apical cyst.

Non-odontogenic Cyst

- ❑ Nasopalatine duct cyst
- ❑ Traumatic bone cyst
- ❑ Median palatine cyst
- ❑ Globulomaxillary cyst.

Fibro-osseous Lesions

- ❑ Periradicular cemental dysplasia
- ❑ Osteoblastoma and cementoblastoma
- ❑ Cementifying and ossifying fibroma.

Odontogenic Tumours

Ameloblastoma.

Non-odontogenic Tumours

- ❑ Central giant cell granuloma
- ❑ Exostosis.

Acute Alveolar Abscess

It is a localized collection of pus in the alveolar bone at the root apex of the tooth, following the death of pulp with extension of the infection through the apical foramen into periradicular tissue.

Etiology

- ❑ Most common cause is invasion of bacteria from necrotic pulp tissue
- ❑ Trauma, chemical or any mechanical injury resulting in pulp necrosis
- ❑ Chemical and mechanical treatment causing periapical tissue irritation during root canal treatment.

Features

- Patient may have systemic symptoms like fever, increased WBC count
- Tooth is nonvital
- Rapid onset of pain
- Slight tenderness to intense throbbing pain
- Marked pain to biting
- Swelling
- Mobility
- No change to large periapical radiolucency.

Diagnosis

- Pulp vitality tests give negative response
- Tenderness on percussion and palpation
- Tooth may be slightly mobile and extruded from its socket
- Radiographs shows bone destruction at root apex.

Treatment

- Drainage of the abscess should be initiated as early as possible
- Incision and drainage
- Extraction.

Pathophysiology of Apical Abscess Formation

Flowchart 21.1 : Pathophysiology of Apical Abscess Formation

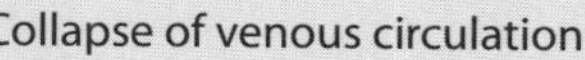

SHORT ESSAYS

Question 1

Define barodontalgia?

Answer

It is also known as aerodontalgia. It is a condition that is seen in people flying in high altitudes and also seen with deep-sea divers.

Classification

- Class I: In acute pulpitis, sharp momentary pain is seen on ascent
- Class II: In chronic pulpitis, dull throbbing pain is seen on ascent
- Class III: In necrotic pulp, dull throbbing pain is seen on descent and symptomatic on ascent
- Class IV: In periradicular abscess or cyst, severe persistent pain is seen on both ascent and descent.

Treatment

- Use of zinc phosphate cement, with a sub-base of zinc oxide-eugenol (ZOE) in deep caries
- Lining of the cavity with a varnish.

Question 2

What is cracked tooth syndrome?

Answer

It is the incomplete fracture through the body of the tooth that may cause pain of apparently idiopathic origin.

- Most effected teeth are mandibular molars
- Pain is localised, form an unidentified posterior tooth on biting or cold stimuli
- Clinically and radiographically, caries might not be detected, and the offending tooth may be heavily restored
- Affected tooth responds to electrical stimulation
- Hairline cracks can only be seen with careful examination with the intraoral light
- Pain is detected by asking patient to bite a cotton roll with opposite tooth
- If this process fails, cold stimuli in the form of ice may be applied on the tooth and the hypersensitive response will indicate the offending tooth.

Principle

The crack contains bacteria whose toxins pass down the dentinal tubules to cause pulpal inflammation.

When it is made to chew or bite there is a fluid movement in the crack and the communicating tubules will elicit pain in the tooth that is already sensitive.

Question 3

Describe pulpal necrosis and its management?

Answer

- Pulp necrosis or death is a condition following untreated pulpitis
- The pulpal tissue becomes dead and if the condition is not treated, noxious materials will leak from pulp space forming the lesion of endodontic origin
- It is the death of the pulp which can be either partial or total.

Causes

Necrosis is caused by noxious insult and injuries to pulp by bacteria, trauma, and chemical irritation.

There are two types of pulpal necrosis:

1. Coagulation necrosis.
2. Liquefaction necrosis.

Coagulation Necrosis

- In this type of necrosis protoplasm of all cells becomes fixed and opaque
- Cell mass is recognizable histologically intracellular details are lost.

Liquefaction Necrosis

- In this type of necrosis, the entire cell outline is lost
- The liquefied area is surrounded by dense zone of PMNL and chronic inflammatory cells.

Signs and Symptoms

Symptoms

- Discoloration of tooth is the first indication of pulp death
- Tooth can be asymptomatic.

Diagnosis

- There is no pain in complete necrosis
- Patient's history is recorded to find if there was trauma in past and history of pain
- Radiograph shows a large cavity or restoration
- Tooth may not be responding to any vitality tests but some multirooted teeth may show mixed response because only one canal may have necrotic tissue
- Tooth shows colour change like dull or opaque appearance due to lack of normal translucency.

Treatment

Complete removal of pulp followed by restoration or extraction of nonrestorable tooth.

Question 4

Describe pink tooth?

Answer

- It is also known as Pink tooth of mummery
- Resorption begins centrally within the tooth which is initiated by peculiar inflammatory hyperplasia of pulp.

Aetiology

- Persistent chronic pulpitis
- History of trauma
- Idiopathic.

Clinical Features

- There are more than one tooth involved
- Hyperplastic vascular pulp tissue filling which is pink hued area on crown of the teeth has tissue filling in the resorbed area showing the remaining overlying substance
- Resorbed dentine is replaced by granulomatous tissue which is seen through enamel giving a pink tooth appearance in the pulp chamber.

Radiographic Features

Round/ovoid radiolucent area in central portion of tooth associated with the pulp but not with external surface of tooth.

Treatment

Root canal therapy or extraction of tooth depending on the condition of the tooth.

Question 5

What is reversible pulpitis/acute reversible pulpitis?

Answer

Reversible pulpitis is mild-to-moderate inflammatory condition of the pulp caused by noxious stimuli in which the pulp is capable of returning to the normal state following removal of stimuli.

Etiology

- Trauma
- Accident or occlusal trauma
- Thermal injury
- While tooth preparation with dull bur without coolant
- Overheating during restoration and polishing
- Long exposure of bur in the same area
- Chemical exposure from sweet or sour foodstuff.

Diagnosis

- Pain is sharp but of brief duration, ceasing when irritant is removed. It is usually caused by cold, sweet and sour stimuli
- Radiographic examinations reveal caries, traumatic occlusion and undetected fracture
- Percussion test shows negative response
- Vitality test shows pulp responds readily to cold stimuli.

Treatment

- The best treatment of reversible pulpitis is prevention
- Endodontic treatment is not needed for this condition.

Question 6

What is acute irreversible pulpitis?

Answer

It is a persistent inflammatory condition of the pulp, symptomatic or asymptomatic, caused by a noxious stimulus

Etiology

- Bacterial involment
- Chemical, thermal and mechanical injuries
- Diagnosis
- On inspection, one may see deep cavity involving pulp
- Radiographs show depth and extent of caries
- Tooth is tender on percussion (due to increased intrapulpal pressure as a result of exudative inflammatory tissue)
- Cold tends to relieve pain because of its contractile effect on vessels, reducing the intrapulpal pressure.

Treatment

- Pulpectomy
- Root canal treatment.

Question 7

What is acute alveolar abscess?

Answer

It is a localized collection of pus in the alveolar bone at the root apex of the tooth, following the death of pulp with extension of the infection through the apical foramen into periradicular tissue.

Etiology

- Most common cause is invasion of bacteria from necrotic pulp tissue
- Trauma, chemical or any mechanical injury resulting in pulp necrosis

- Chemical and mechanical treatment causing periapical tissue irritation during root canal treatment.

Features

- Patient may have systemic symptoms like fever, increased WBC count
- Tooth is nonvital
- Rapid onset of pain
- Slight tenderness to intense throbbing pain
- Marked pain to biting
- Swelling
- Mobility
- No change to large periapical radiolucency.

Diagnosis

- Pulp vitality tests give negative response
- Tenderness on percussion and palpation
- Tooth may be slightly mobile and extruded from its socket
- Radiographs shows bone destruction at root apex.

Treatment

- Drainage of the abscess should be initiated as early as possible
- Incision and drainage
- Extraction.

Pathophysiology of Apical Abscess Formation

Increase in pulpal pressure

Collapse of venous circulation

Hypoxia and anoxia of local tissue

Localized destruction of pulp tissue

Formation of pulpal abscess because of breakdown of PMNs, bacteria and lysis of pulp remnants

Question 8

Define cracked tooth syndromes?

Answer

- The crack tooth syndrome means incomplete fracture of a tooth with vital pulp
- The fracture commonly involves enamel and dentin but sometimes pulp and periodontal structure may also get involved
- It is seen in those teeth with large and complex restorations.

Diagnosis

- It is diagnosed by taking proper history of the patient, regarding dietary and parafunctional habits and any previous trauma
- During tactile examination, pass the tip of sharp explorer gently along the tooth surface, so as to locate the crack by catch
- Patient is asked to bite on Orange wood stick, rubber wheel or the tooth sloth. The pain during biting or chewing especially upon the release of pressure is classic sign of cracked tooth syndrome.

Treatment

- Treatment of cracked tooth involves the immediate reduction of its occlusal contacts by selective grinding of tooth at the site of the crack
- Preserving the pulpal vitality by providing full occlusal coverage for cusp protection
- Full coverage crown if fracture involves crown portion only
- Endodontic treatment if fracture involves pulp
- In case the fracture extents to the root extraction is done.

Question 9

Define barodontalgia?

Answer

Clinical Features

- It is pain experienced in a recently restored tooth during low atmospheric pressure
- Pain is experienced either during ascent or descent
- Chronic pulpitis which appears asymptomatic in normal conditions, may also manifests as pain at high altitude because of low pressure
- It is generally seen in altitude over 5000 feet but more likely to be observed in 10,000 feet and above.

Treatment

- Varnish the lining of the cavity
- A sub base of zoe cement in deep cavities
- Base of zinc phosphate cement after sub base in deep cavities.

SHORT NOTES

Question 1

Write a short note on nerve fibres of pulp?

Answer

- Pulp contains myelinated a-delta fibres and also unmyelinated c nerve fibres
- The activations of both these fibres have different actions
- On activation of a-delta fibre a sharp localized pain is felt
- On activation of c fibre a dull localized pain is seen
- The response helps in the diagnosis of pulp vitality.

Question 2

Discuss accessory canals?

Answer

- They are also called as lateral canals
- Accessory canals may exist anywhere on the root surface, though majority of them are found in apical third and furcation area of the root
- The accessory canals percentage is up to 40 percent in teeth
- The Accessory canals are exposed to oral cavity when there are periodontal diseases present which progress down the root
- Radiographs can hardly identify these canals
- They are identified by isolated defects on the lateral surface of roots or by post obturation radiographs showing sealer puffs.

Question 3

Define anachoresis?

Answer

- Anachoresis refers to the attraction of blood borne bacteria in the areas of inflammation
- Pulp is a idea place for this process when it goes under necrosis
- It is a process by which microorganisms are transported in the blood to an area of inflammation where they establish an infection.

Question 4

What is root resorption and classify them?

Answer

Resorption is defined as a condition associated with either a physiologic or a pathologic process that result in loss of substance from a tissue, such as dentine, cementum or alveolar bone is known as root resorption (American Association of Endodontics).

Classification

Based on the Nature

- Pathological root resorption
- Physiological root resorption.

Based on Inflammatory Response

- Inflammatory resorption
  - Internal root resorption
  - External root resorption.
- Non-inflammatory resorption
  - Pressure
  - Transient
  - Replacement.

Question 5

Define hyperaemia of pulp?

Answer

This is the first stage where the pulp is symptomatic. There is a sharp hypersensitive response to cold, but the pain subsides when stimulus is removed.

Etiology

- Trauma
- Accident or occlusal trauma
- Thermal injury
- While tooth preparation with dull bur without coolant
- Overheating during restoration and polishing
- Long exposure of bur in the same area
- Chemical exposure from sweet or sour foodstuff.

Diagnosis

- Pain is sharp but of brief duration, ceasing when irritant is removed. It is usually caused by cold, sweet and sour stimuli
- Radiographic examinations reveal caries, traumatic occlusion and undetected fracture
- Percussion test shows negative response
- Vitality test shows pulp responds readily to cold stimuli.

Treatment

- The best treatment of reversible pulpitis is prevention
- Endodontic treatment is not needed for this condition.

Question 6

Define periapical cyst?

Answer

The radicular cyst is an inflammatory cyst which results because of extension of infection from pulp into the surrounding periapical tissues.

Etiology

- Caries
- Irritating effects of restorative materials
- Trauma
- Pulpal death due to development defects.

Findings

- It is asymptomatic
- It is found in periapical radiographs of tooth with nonvital pulp
- Mostly found in anterior maxilla
- It is slowly enlarging swelling, sometimes attains a large size.

Treatment

- Endodontic treatment
- Apicoectomy.

Question 7

Define clinical management of apical granuloma?

Answer

- Apical granuloma is one of the most common sequelae of pulpitis
- It is usually described as a mass of chronically inflamed granulation tissue found at the apex of nonvital tooth
- Mostly discovered on radiographic examination
- Thickening of periodontal ligament at the root apex is seen
- Lesion may be well circumscribed or poorly defined
- Size may be from small to more than 2 cm in diameter.

Treatment

- In restorable tooth, root canal therapy
- In non-restorable tooth, extraction followed by curettage of all apical soft tissue.

Question 8

Define barodontalgia?

Answer

- Barodontalgia is also known as aerodontalgia
- It is seen in people flying in high altitudes and also is seen in deep-sea divers.

Classification of Aerodontalgia

- Class I: In acute pulpitis, sharp momentary pain is seen on ascent
- Class II: In chronic pulpitis, dull throbbing pain is seen on ascent
- Class III: In necrotic pulp, dull throbbing pain is seen on descent and a symptomatic on ascent
- Class IV: In case of periradicular abscess or cyst, persistent pain with both ascent and descent.

Question 9

Describe weeping canal?

Answer

In few cases after root canal treatment tooth shows constant clear or reddish exudation associated with periapical radiolucency. Tooth can be asymptomatic or tender on percussion. When opened in next appointment, exudates stops but it again reappears in next appointment. This exudation is termed as weeping canal.

Treatment

- Dry the canals with sterile absorbent paper points
- Calcium hydroxide is placed in the canal
- Call for follow up
- The canal will be ready for obturation.

Question 10

Define acute apical periodontitis?

Answer

- Acute apical periodontitis is defined as painful inflammation of the periodontium as a result of trauma, irritation or infection through the root canal, regardless of whether the pulp is vital or nonvital
- It is an inflammation around the apex of a tooth.

Etiology

- In vital tooth, it is associated with occlusal trauma, high points in restoration, wedging or forcing object between teeth
- In nonvital tooth it is associated with sequelae to pulpal diseases.

Signs and Symptoms

- No swelling
- Pain on biting
- Tooth is tender on percussion
- Dull, throbbing and constant pain
- Pain occurs over a short period of time
- Negative or delayed vitality test
- Cold may relieve pain or no reaction.

Treatment

- Endodontic
- Analgesics are prescribed post treatment
- Antibiotics to control the infection
- Extraction.

LONG ESSAYS

Question 1

Define intentional replantation. Give indications, contra-indications and techniques of intentional replantation?

Answer

Replacement: Replacement of a tooth in the socket with its objective of attaining reattachment when the tooth has been completely avulsed from it socket by an accident.

Intentional replantation: It is defined as an act of deliberately removing a tooth and repair returning the tooth to its original socket.

Indications

- Failed apical surgery
- Anatomic limitations
- Accidental avulsion unintentional replantation
- Persistent chronic pain
- Perforation in accessible areas
- When apical surgery creates defect
- Deciduous teeth needing space maintenance.

Contraindications

- Non-removable teeth
- Curved and flared canals
- Severe periodontal diseases
- Missing interseptal bone.

Management

- Avulsed tooth is the tooth that has been totally displaced out of its socket
- Periodontal ligament (PDL) has a good choice of healing if the tooth is replanted soon
- Avulsed tooth should be bought immediately to maintain good root surface hold and proper PDL function
- Avulsed teeth should be stored in special media for tooth to avoid its property to get reattached when placed in socket
- Storage media used are:
  - Saline
  - Bovine milk
  - Hank's balancing solution
  - Patient saliva preferred location is buccal vestibule or under the tongue.

Intentional Replacement Technique

Factors affecting the procedure:
- Short time for out of socket tooth
- PDL cells on the root surface of the tooth should be kept moist either by media or saliva
- Reducing damage to cementum and PDL by gentle elevation and extraction of the tooth.

Steps in Replantation

- Before replantation endodontic treatment should be completed
- Pulp chamber should be restored
- Incision is made by no. 15 blade of the periodontal fibres and elevated to gain Class III mobility
- During extraction, forceps beak should be wrapped with gauge and is dipped in media, like saline and hanks bank solution to minimize cementum during the extraction process
- Root examination should be done with fibre optic illu-mination and magnification to evaluate Radicular defects, like resorption and perforation and also root fracture
- Root resection if required should be done with plain fissure bur in a high speed hand piece under irrigation constantly
- Following the repair, irrigation of the extraction socket is irrigated with saline. Any blood clot is removed by section and then the tooth is carefully placed in the socket

- A rolled gauze sponge is placed on the occlusal surface after the tooth has been inserted. The patient is told to bite down so that interocclusal force will make the tooth to seat into the socket
- The time period of this pressure should be approximately 5 minutes
- Stabilizing should be done by flexible wire with acid etching and bonding with composite resin with the adjacent tooth
- Patient is recalled after 7–14 days after replantation surgery to remove the stabilisation
- Postsurgical evaluation is done after:
  - 2 months
  - 6 months
  - 9 months
  - 12 months.

<hr>

Question 2

Write about indications and contraindications of periapical surgery. Write in detail about wound healing?

Answer

Periapical surgery: This surgery is performed to remove a portion of the root with undebrided canal space or to seal the canal apically when a complete seal cannot be accomplished with a non-surgical root canal treatment through the crown approach.

Indications

- Procedural accidents
- Horizontal apical fracture
- Anatomical problems
- Irretrievable material in root canal
- Biopsy and corrective surgery
- Symptomatic cases.

Contraindications

- An unidentified cause of treatment failure
- Anatomic factors
- Indiscriminate use of surgery
- Medical and systemic complications.

Assessment of Healing (Post-operative) by Andreasen and Rud (1972)

- Group 1: Complete healing
- Group 2: Incomplete healing (Scar tissue)
- Group 3: Uncertain healing
- Group 4: Unsatisfactory healing (failure).

Wound Healing (Post-periradicular Surgery)

Periradicular surgery facilitates regeneration of tissues rather than its repair, i.e. scar tissue formation.

The tissues included are:

- Free gingiva
- Attached gingiva
- Periosteum
- Alveolar mucosa
- Periodontal ligament (PDL).

Types of Healing

- Soft tissue healing
- Hard tissue healing.

Soft Tissue Healing

- Inflammatory phase
  - Clot formation
  - Early inflammation
  - Late inflammation.
- Proliferative phase
- Maturation phase.

- Inflammatory Phase:
  - Clot formation: Clot formation begins with three events:
    1. Blood vessel contraction
    2. Intravascular platelet aggregation
    3. Extrinsic and intrinsic clotting mechanism.
  - Early inflammation: Early inflammation is organised by PMNLs (polymorph nuclear leucocytes).
    - PMNLs enter wound site within 6 hours of clot stabilization by pavementing or emigration
    - The wound is decontaminated by phagocytosis
    - The number reaches peak at about 24–28 hours after injury and drops rapidly on 3rd day
    - PMNLs have short life span.
  - Late inflammation:
    - Macrophages enter the wound site by 48–96 hours after injury and reach peak concentration at 3rd–4th day
    - They remain in the wound until healing is done
    - Proliferative phase is initiated when cytokines are secreted
    - Macrophages initiates phagocytosis and digestion of microorganism and tissue debris
    - They ingest and process the antigens for presentation to T-lymphocytes which enters the wound after the macrophages.

❏ Proliferative Phase: Formation of granulation tissue can be seen. Cells that are involved are:
  ○ Fibroblasts (fibroplasias):
    ➤ They migrate to the wound site on the 3rd day after injury
    ➤ Granulation tissue formation happens on the 7th day
    ➤ Reconstruction is done by laying type III collagen and later type I collagen when maturation of wound happens
    ➤ Myofibroblast help in wound contraction mostly in incisional type wounds
    ➤ They align parallel with the wound surface and then contract, as the wound is drawn closer together at edges
    ➤ Elimination of cells happen by apoptosis when wound closure is finished.
  ○ Endothelial cells (angiogenesis):
    ➤ These cells form capillary buds from the blood vessels around the wound
    ➤ This happens with fibroblast. Proliferation and begins at 48–72 hours after the injury
    ➤ To have proper blood supply for active healing angiogenesis is required
    ➤ Stimulator of angiogenesis are:
      » Vascular endothelial growth factor (VEGF)
      » Basic fibroblast growth factor (BFGF)
      » Acidic fibroblast growth factor (AFGF)
      » Transforming growth factor O (TGFO)
      » TGF
      » Interleukin-1.
  ○ Epithelium:
    ➤ This helps in the epithelial seal formation on the fibrin clot surface
    ➤ This process begins at wound edge where basal and suprabasal prickle cells undergo rapid mitosis
    ➤ Cell migration across fibrin clot rate is 0.5–1 mm/day
    ➤ In wound healing, primary intention is the formation of epithelial seal. It takes 21–28 hours after reapproximation of wound margins.
❏ Maturation Phase
  ○ This phase begins at 5–7 days after the injury with a reduction in fibroblast, extracellular fluids and vascular channels
  ○ Wound matrix consists of fibronectin and hyaluronic acid
  ○ The collagen remodels and reorganise as the healing progresses. They decrease the cellularity and vascularity of the reparative tissue

○ As epithelial layer matures, it follows up the formation of epithelial seal
○ Mitosis and maturation happens when epithelial seal is differentiated to form a definitive layer of stratified squamous epithelium
○ The formation starts at 36–42 hours after suturing.
○ Hard tissue healing: The inflammatory and the proliferative phases are similar to soft tissue healing maturation phase happens with the cortical bone, cancellous bone, alveolar bone proper, endosteum, PDL, cementum, dentine and inner mucoperiosteal tissue.
○ Osteogenesis (osteoblasts): After haematoma formation in the bone crypt inflammation begins at the soft tissue and progresses with the proliferation of granulation tissue. It occurs between 2 and 4 days.
  ➤ Along with the cells in soft tissue healing, preosteoblasts and osteoblasts migrate into this region to form matrix vesicle based process and lamellar bone (osteoblast-secretion process)
  ➤ Osteoblasts help in mineralisation by secreting collagen rich ground substance along with alkaline phosphatase
  ➤ New bone formation takes place in about after 6 days
  ➤ The defect is filled in approximately 15–16 days.
○ Cemetogenesis (cementoblasts):
  ➤ It begins at 10–12 days after tooth resection
  ➤ Cementum covers the resected root end in 28 days to form a double seal (mechanical closure and cement closure at root)
  ➤ PDL fibres are arranged from cementum to the newly formed bone in about 8 weeks.

Question 3

Classify different flap designs used in surgical endodontics?

Answer

Classification of Surgical Flaps (According to Gutmann and Harrison)

❏ Full mucoperiosteal flaps (sulcular full thickness flap):
  ○ Triangular flaps (one vertical releasing incision)
  ○ Rectangular flaps (two vertical releasing incisions)
  ○ Trapezoidal flaps (broad-based rectangular) not used
  ○ Horizontal flaps (no vertical releasing incision).
❏ Limited mucoperiosteal flaps:
  ○ Submarginal curved (semilunar).
  ○ Submarginal scalloped rectangular (Luebke-Ochsenbein)
  ○ Free rectilinear submarginal flap (mucogingival flap).

Classification of Full Mucoperiosteal Flaps (According to Gutmann and Harrison)

Triangular Flap

It is formed by horizontal, intrasulcular incision and one vertical releasing incision.

Indications

- In periapical surgery
- Mandibular posterior tooth
- In mid root perforation repair and short roots.

Advantages

- It maintains the integrity of blood supply
- It can be easily repositioned and results in good wound healing.

Disadvantages

- In long roots it has limited access and visibility
- Vertical incision penetrates alveolar mucosa.

Rectangular Flap

It is formed by an intrasulcular, horizontal incision and two vertical releasing incisions.

Indications

- Periapical surgery
- In mandibular anterior teeth and in maxillary canines.

Advantage

Provides good access and visibility and less retraction tension.

Disadvantages

- Crestal bone loss
- Gingival recession
- Reduced blood supply to flap
- Difficult in suturing
- Increased incision and reflection time
- Not recommended for posterior teeth.

Trapezoidal Flap

It is similar to rectangle flap except there are two vertical releasing incisions that intersect the horizontal intrasulcular incision at an obtuse angle.

- This design provides better blood supply to the flapped tissues
- Blood vessels and collagen fibres are oriented in vertical direction in periosteal tissues; the vertical releasing incision that is angled will serve more of these vital structures
- This results in more bleeding and shrinkage of the tissue and hence, they are contraindicated in periradicular surgery.

Horizontal / Envelope Flap

This is obtained by horizontal, intrasulcular incision with no vertical releasing incisions.

It provides limited surgical access and hence limited applications.

Indications

- In hemisections and root amputation
- In repair of cervical defects, like resorption, root perforation and caries.

Limited Mucoperiosteal Flap

Semilunar Flap / Submarginal Curved Flap

- It is obtained by curved incision, beginning at the alveolar mucosa that extent into attached gingiva and then its curved back into alveolar mucosa
- Contraindicated in periradicular surgery.

Indications

- Trephination
- When aesthetic crowns are present.

Advantages

- Eliminates potential crestal bone loss
- Gingiva attachment integrity is maintained.

Disadvantages

- Crosses root eminencies
- Poor healing associated with scarring
- Limited access and visibility
- May not include the entire lesion
- Tendency for increased haemorrhage.

Luebke-Ochsenbein Flap/Submarginal Scalloped Rectangular Flap

- It is a modified rectangular flap
- The horizontal incision is given on buccal or labial attached gingiva and not on gingival sulcus
- The base of the incision should be wider
- The incision is scalloped and follows the contour of the marginal gingiva above free gingival groove.

Indications

- Periapical surgery
- Teeth with longer roots
- Presence of crowns
- Wide band of attached gingiva.

Advantages

- Ease in incision and reflection
- Prevents crestal bone loss
- Ease in repositioning

- Prevents gingival recession
- Ease in visibility.

Disadvantages

- Horizontal components disrupt the blood supply
- Hard to alter size of lesion.

Free-Form Rectilinear Submarginal Flap/ Mucogingival Flap

- This design is similar to luebke-ochsenbein design
- It has parallel vertical releasing incisions.

SHORT ESSAYS

Question 1

What is root resection?

Answer

Root resection is the removal of one or more roots of the molar.

Indications

- When endodontic treatment of one root is not possible or such kind of treatment fails
- Removal of root when there is untreatable furcation involvement to gain good oral hygiene in that area
- Endodontically non-treatable root perforation
- When there is root destruction by extensive decay
- Fractured root of an upper molar
- Extensive bone loss in maxillary molar.

Contraindication

- When bone loss involves more than one root and the remaining root has inadequate support
- When bridge spam time is long and when abutment tooth has inadequate support
- Fused roots.

Technique

- Local anaesthesia is administered and extent of outline is determined with probe of the alveolar bone destruction around the root to be removed
- Elevation of mucoperiosteal flap is done with contra angle hand piece and cross cut bur in the area where it joins the crown to remove the root
- Resected root and contour the tooth with a diamond or stone bur

- Root surface area is scaled and planed
- Replace the flap after the area is cleaned and a periodontal pack is given
- Suture the area
- Pack should be removed after 1 week.

Question 2

What is apicoectomy?

Answer

Apicoectomy is the surgical resection of the apex of the root.

Indications

- When anatomy of canal system has not been conductive to non-surgical treatment
- In case of deficient apical seal where root canal filling may extrude
- If root canal filling fails and retreatment cannot be effected by orthograde procedure
- In presence of necrotic material at the apex between the interface of root canal filling.

Steps

- Radiograph is taken to determine the root amputation
- Cleaning the area with antiseptic solution
- Local anaesthesia is administered
- The mucoperiosteal flap is raised to make an opening into the periapical region
- Extending is done in the labial plate to get good access
- Bone removal is done
- Root tip resection and curettage is done

- Retro preparation followed by retrograde filling is done to seal the root apex
- Debridement is done
- Suturing of mucoperiosteal flap is done and maintains firm pressure for 10 minutes
- Radiographic evaluation is done in follow up cases.

Post-operative Complications

- Excessive bone cutting causes mobility of the tooth
- Loss of bone structure in adjacent tooth
- Perforation in nasal cavity causing nasal fistula
- Damaging of mental nerve or the inferior alveolar canal if the tooth is near that region.

SHORT NOTES

Question 1

What is bicuspidisation?

Answer

It is a process where molar is cut into two separate mesial and distal portions without the removal of any part of the root or crown.

- This is done in mandibular molar which exhibit proper stability and anatomic features
- In the process, a tunnel-like effect of the furcation involvement is eliminated by creating two separate teeth from single molar
- In the end, the portion of tooth will require crown placement.

Question 2

What is semilunar incision?

Answer

Semilunar Incision

- In this process a, curved incision beginning in the alveolar mucosa which extends into the attached gingiva and then curves back into the alveolar mucosa
- It is contraindicated in periradicular surgery.

Indications

- In presence of aesthetic crowns
- In trephination.

Advantages

- It maintains integrity of gingival attachment
- Reduces the operating time with minimum incision
- Chances of potential crestal bone loss are eliminated.

Disadvantages

- It has limited access and visibility
- Predisposed to tearing and stretching.

Question 3

What is hemisection?

Answer

It is a procedure in which one root and its corresponding crown portion is cut and removed.

Indications

- When caries involved root portion
- When periodontal involvement in one of the root is severe
- Bone loss is very extensive in the furcation area.

Question 4

What is splinting?

Answer

Splinting is a device used to fasten teeth in the same dental arch to support them or to prevent or minimize its movement; it may connect natural teeth either directly or to a prosthesis.

- Physiological or semi-rigid splints are mostly used
- Time period is in between 7 and 10 days
- Splints used:
  - Acid etch resin
  - Soft arch wire
  - Orthodontic brackets
  - Ribbond fibre splint
  - Titanium splint.

Precautions

Patient is advised to eat soft diet and not to bite and put pressure on the splined tooth.

CHAPTER 23

Post-endodontic Restorations

Question 1

Write in detail about post and core. Discuss the technique for post and core?

Answer

Post: It is also known as dowel. It is a rigid restorative material placed in the root canal of a pulpless tooth or an endodontically treated tooth with reduced coronal tooth structure.

Core: It is a supragingival portion of restoration that replaces the bulk of lost coronal tooth structure for additional retention of crown.

Ideal Requisites of the Post

- To gain adequate retention within the root
- It should give the core and crown maximum retention
- It should protect the root by distributing the forces along the length of the root
- It should provide protection to crown margin cement seal
- It should be radiopaque
- It should be retrievable
- It should have good aesthetic in the anterior teeth
- It should be biocompatible
- It should possess required stiffness, flexibility and strength at the same time.

Uses

- It retains the restoration when there is no sufficient tooth structure
- By directing all the forces apically it protects the remaining tooth structure
- It provides rigidity under stress and load, and maintains marginal integrity.

Indications

- Roots having thin radicular dentine due to extensive caries
- Root with over instrumentation of walls
- It is indicated in teeth with less than 3–4 mm of vertical height
- Indicated in tooth with less than 25–30% tooth structure
- Non-rigid post is indicated when 25–30% tooth structure is remaining.

Armamentarium

- Endo-post:
  - Size: 70–140
  - Precious metal with high fusing point
  - They can be casted with gold or other metals.
- Endo-dowel:
  - Size: 80–140
  - Elastic plastic pins
  - They burn out of the investment and give rise to metal casting
  - Expensive.
- Para-post:
  - Standard size
  - No taper.

Canal preparation is done by:

- Hot pluggers
- Rotary drills
- Touch and heat 5004.
- H-files.

Tooth Preparation

Tooth preparation is done on the basis of amount of clinical crown present.

- Tooth preparation with an adequate clinical crown
- Tooth preparation with an inadequate clinical crown.

Tooth Preparation with Adequate Clinical Crown

For the better handling and casting purpose, the occlusal/incisal height is reduced. The core should be at least 2–5 mm long.

- The tooth that surrounds the canal should have sufficient bulk. So, it provides strong working purpose and avoids fracture of the preparation at the time of cementing
- Occlusal/incisal edges are given 45° tilt to avoid fracture from the lateral forces of mastication
- A fabricated full crown is finally placed over the cemented post and core.

Tooth Preparation with Inadequate Clinical Crown

- Retention is required if there is inadequate crown and also canal, pulp chamber and extra-coronal portion
- Old restorations, unsupported dentin and caries are removed
- The walls are made parallel to gain maximum retention
- Smoothing of internal design and rounding with soft dentine is included within the core
- To decrease the stress reverse bevel is used (Ferrule principle)
- To prevent twisting of the core grooves or key ways are made as anti-rotation device
- Aesthetically, the shoulder should always be carried subgingivally.

Impression for Post and Core

- Indirect technique
- Direct technique.

Indirect Technique

Canal enlarging instrument ends as a point, which is not flat for the post preparation:

- Post with bevel is used here
- This post should be seated to correct post length and should resist slight pressure
- Post is bent at the occlusal end and a lubricant is painted on the portion for the facilitation for its removal
- Gingival retraction is then done
- The material is placed using a rubber base impression material with a syringe and is placed at orifice around the preparation
- Regular tray material is used to make impression. The post is taken up along with the impression
- Opposite arch impression is taken
- Wax pattern is then made in the lab.

Direct Technique

Endo-post is used either as inlay wax or dipolymer acrylic resins for core pattern.

- The wall of the canal is lubricated, followed by wax/resin application to post and then the impression is taken
- Core built-up is done after that

- The portion of core that is protruded is used as a sprue
- Cast ring is used and then investing of cast is done
- Ring is allowed to cool after casting. Casting is then separated from the investment
- Core portion is polished after the excess post is cut and trimmed
- Placement of dry cotton is done in chamber after impression and temporary filling is given.

Cementation

- After temporary filling is removed, the preparation is dried using air or paper points
- Post/core is try-in. They should not be forced inside
- Clearance on the opposite side and laterally should be checked
- Cements used are:
  - Zinc phosphate
  - Zinc polycarboxylate
  - Glass ionomer cement (GIC)
  - Resin cements.
- Wall is coated with one of the cement and post and core is gently seated by hand pressure
- Grooves are made on the core for better retention
- The crown is then prepared on the core.

Question 2

Write about principles involved in selecting the restoration for endodontically treated teeth?

Answer

Principles involved are:
- Post design
- Post length
- Post diameter
- Number of posts
- Cement used.

Post Design

Custom Made

They are fabricated by either direct or indirect wax pattern:
- To produce negative replica of canal inlay wax or cold curve is used
- It is then processed in lab.

Advantages

- Better fit and no stress at the time of fitting
- It is preferred in severely flared canals
- It can be adapted in large, irregular canals and orifice
- Being a single metal they are stronger.

Disadvantages

- It acts as a wedge
- They are expensive
- Need more sittings and can be time consuming
- They need removal of additional tooth structure
- Porosity can lead to casting failure.

Prefabricated Posts

Types

- Parallel, tapered, parallel with tapered end
- Smooth surface, serrated, threaded hollow, solid, with and without vents.

Advantages

- Simple to use and is less time consuming
- It can be seated at only one appointment
- Cost effective
- It is stronger.

Disadvantages

- Chance of chemical reaction between post and core
- Removable prosthesis attachments cannot be fabricated
- If coronal structure is present post cannot be placed.

Parallel Posts

These posts are most retentive and can resist torque forces.
- The stress in them is distributed evenly along its length so there is less risk of dentin fracture

- The most stress area is the apex of preparation.

Disadvantages

- With the risk of perforation and weakening of dentinal walls they are not used in tapered roots
- They produce wedging effect as they are parallel with tapered ends
- They possess decreased retention and stress is mostly on coronal shoulder.

Post Length

- Post length should be 2/3 of the working length or the crown length
- Minimum of 4 mm of apical filling should be there
- Post length should be increased without change, without changing apical seal as increased post length increases retention
- It should be half of the bone supporting length of the root
- It should be along the axis of tooth.

Post Diameter

Average size of post = 1 mm. Increase diameter weakens the tooth structure.

Number of Posts

If there are multiple roots in the tooth, more than one post can be placed.

SHORT NOTES

Question 1

Write in short about core material?

Answer

Core material is a restorative material placed in the coronal area of a tooth which replaces carious, fractured or missing coronal structure and retains the final crown, i.e., amalgam, composite resin, glass ionomer resin, cast metal and ceramic.

Question 2

Name the types of post?

Answer

Posts are classified as:
- Prefabricated and cast post
- Metallic and non-metallic post
- Rigid and non-rigid post
- Aesthetic and non-aesthetic post.

Cement Type

Mostly cements used are:
- Zinc phosphate
- Zinc polycarboxylate
- Glass ionomer cement (GIC)
- Resin cements
- Restoration of tooth is done to protect it from fracture and to replace loss of tooth structure
- Restorations include:
  - Dowel
  - Core
  - Coronal restoration.
- Dowel increases retention and protects tooth by distributing forces along the root length.

CHAPTER 24

Endodontic Failures

LONG ESSAYS

Question 1

Write in detail about endodontic failures. How to overcome them?

Answer

Endodontic Failure

- Endodontic failure is the incomplete hard tissue healing with non-resolving post-treatment periapical radiolucency
- They can be symptomatic or asymptomatic
- Endodontic failures can be classified into:
  - Extra-radicular factors
  - Inter-radicular factors.

Extra-radicular Factors

- Microbial causes
  - Caused by bacteria and most common are *Actinomyces israelii* and *Propionibacterium propionicum*.
  - These bacteria are most commonly seen in conditions, like:
    - Abscessed periapical periodontitis
    - Over instrumentation
    - Infected periapical pocket cyst
    - Periapical actinomycosis.

Treatment: Surgical treatment is the choice of treatment in this condition (Apicoectomy).

- Non-microbial causes:
  - Foreign bodies: The foreign bodies can be
    - Gutta-percha (GP)
    - Cotton fibrils (cellulose granuloma)
    - Amalgam
    - Pulses (pulse granuloma).

  These foreign bodies causes chronic irritation when they reach the periapical region through root canal to form a granuloma.

  - Cholesterol crystals: They are formed from cholesterol released by
    - Macrophages
    - Plasma cells
    - Disintegrating erythrocytes
    - Circulating plasma lipids.

The crystals attract more macrophages and giant cells which don't degrade and results in apical periodontitis leading to stimulation of bone resorptive mediators.

Treatment: Granulomatous tissue removal by surgical procedure.

- True cyst:
  - Resolving of periapical radiolucency even after a good obturation is caused by the cyst
  - True cyst is not dependable on the pressure or absence of root canal infection.

Treatment: Enucleation of the cyst by surgical procedure.

  - Scar-tissue healing:
    - Presence and persistent periapical radiolucency even after few months of surgery suggest the lesion has heated with scar formation (without bone regeneration).

Diagnosis: Radiograph: It shows persisting radiolucency, in spite there is good orthograde obturation.

Inter-radicular Factors

Inter-radicular microorganisms that are reintroduced or persistent are the main causative factors for root canal failure.

- Microorganisms can be seen in iatrogenic mishaps, like ledges, perforations, separated instruments and improper cleaning and shaping
- Microorganisms are reintroduced due to improper apical as well as coronal seal

- These bacteria are predominantly gram positive anaerobes.
  Treatment:
  - When the cause is not definitive, no treatment is required
  - When the prognosis of the retreatment is poor, extraction is the choice of treatment
  - Surgical treatment
  - Non-surgical treatment
  - No surgical treatment and endodontic failure.

Pre-operative Factors

Due to misdiagnosis or not certain clinical or radiographical information.

Poor Case Selection

Predictable

- Non-negotiable canal
- Resorption
- Unrestorable tooth.

Unpredictable

- Occlusal trauma
- Transformation of apical abscess to cyst.

Poor Prognosis

- Avulsed tooth
- Lesions.

Operative

Failure to gain triological objectives.
- Improper removal of irritants from the canal
- Debris pushed beyond the apical foramen.

Prevention

- Avoiding over instrumentation
- Use of appropriate irrigants.

Failure

- Mishaps at the time of cavity preparation
- Mishaps during canal preparation
- Mishap during obturation
- Miscellaneous causes.

Missed Canals

Causes

- Lack of information and knowledge of anatomy, variations and pulp area
- Improper coronal access cavity preparation.

Identifying and Additional Canal

Additional canal is indicated when during the instrumentation the instrument is not centred in the root.

Additional Canal can be Pointed by Various Methods

- Magnification glasses
- Head lamps
- Transilluminating devices
- Horizontal angulating radiovisiography (RVG)
- Microscopes
- Endoscopes
- Dyes:
  - Ruddle's solution
  - Methylene blue
- Ultrasonic
- Sodium hypochlorite (NaOCl) (Champagne test).

Procedure

- After cleaning and shaping the pulp chamber is flooded with NaOCl which reacts with the residual pulp tissue
- If there is presence of canal that is missed it forms bubbles.

Prevention

- Good illumination
- RVG angulations
- Proper access preparation.

Prognosis

If two canals open into a single foramen the prognosis will be poor.

Supracrestal Perforation

The causes of supracrestal perforation can be:
- Post-space preparation
- Perforation during access cavity preparation
- While instrumentation.

Major Sites

- Just above the periodontal attachment
- In to periodontal ligament, e.g., furcation perforation.

Detecting the Perforation:

- Directly observed
- Unpleasant taste in mouth by the presence of leakage, seepage of saliva or NaOCl
- Bleeding in access cavity
- Radiograph.

Prevention

- ❑ Thorough knowledge of treatment and tooth anatomy
- ❑ Careful radiograph examination
- ❑ Access bur should be aligned along the long axis of tooth.

Crown Root Fracture

Causes

- ❑ Already existing infraction that becomes a true fracture
- ❑ It can be identified by:
  - ○ Transillumination
  - ○ Dyes.

Prevention

- ❑ De-occlusion of tooth before the working length is determined
- ❑ Using circumferential bands till the final restoration is done.

Management

- ❑ If fracture involves part of crown:
  - ○ Loose fragment are removed and treatment is done.
- ❑ More intense fracture:
  - ○ A non-restorable, extraction of the involved tooth is indicated.

Prognosis

Unpredictable because crown infraction may spread to the roots that can cause vertical fractures.

Ledge Formation

Causes

- ❑ Inadequate access: cavity preparation
- ❑ Using straight or large instruments with active cutting tip where the canals are curved.

Identifying

- ❑ When full working length is not reached by the instrument
- ❑ Loss of normal tactile sensation
- ❑ Radiographic evidence showing the instrument pointing away from the lumen of the canal.

Prevention

- ❑ Pre-curving the instrument
- ❑ Use of nickel-titanium (NiTi) files
- ❑ Canal should be irrigated and recapitulated frequently
- ❑ Use of stainless steel patency files for canal curvature determination
- ❑ Accurate radiographs interpretation.

Management

- ❑ Explore the canal by using a small pre-curved file (no-10/ls)
- ❑ The instrument curve should be pointed towards the wall opposite the ledge
- ❑ Greater taper NiTi file can be used
- ❑ The instrument is used in vaiven/watch winding motion, in the presence of lubricant or irrigant
- ❑ Ethylenediaminetetraacetic acid (EDTA) is avoided as chelation may lead to perforation.

Prognosis

Good prognosis, if ledge is bypassed and the canal is prepared to its full length.

Root Perforation

Classification

- ❑ Point perforation
- ❑ Strip perforation.

Sites

- ❑ Cervical
- ❑ Mid root
- ❑ Apical.

Causes

- ❑ Cervical third perforation occurs as a sequel to ledge formation
- ❑ Also by stripping of the inner curvature of the curved canal, like Gates-Glidden drills (GG), peizo reamers
- ❑ Mid root perforation occurs due to stripping, especially in distal wall
- ❑ Peizoo reamers if used, can increase the chance of perforation more
- ❑ Apical perforation occurs when the file is not negotiating the curved canal or if there is improper working length determination
- ❑ Perforation in curved canal is because of. ledge, apical transportation or apical zipping.

Identifying a Perforation

- ❑ Patient will suddenly complain of pain during treatment
- ❑ Sudden haemorrhage in previously dry canal
- ❑ Haemorrhage on a paper point placed in the canal
- ❑ Radiographs taken from different angles presence of periodontal pockets in cervical and mid root perforations
- ❑ Tactile resistance of canal space is lost.

Prevention

In cervical and mid root: When the root is curved filling should be done to avoid pressure of distal wall which is also called as "danger zone".

Management

Non-surgical procedures in the absence of periradicular periodontitis.

Material Used

- Geristore
- Mineral trioxide aggregate (MTA).

Obturation Related

Over/under extended root canal.

Under Obturation

- Due to loss of working length
- Improper master cone selection.

Over Obturation

By apical perforation.

Overfilling

When there is canal filled with excess obturating material.

Over Extension

When the canal is not filled properly and material extrudes beyond the apical foramen.

Diagnosis

- Radiographs
- Symptomatic tooth.

Management

- Semisolid (GP)
- Solids
- Pastes.

Removal of Gutta-percha without Core

Removal of GP depends on:
- Canal length
- Density of the filling
- Curvature of canal.

Technique

Gutta-percha is softened by:
- Heat
- Chemical.

Heat Softening

Rotary file is used in canal at speed of 1200–1500 rmp.
- Ultrasonic without coolant
- Controlled heating system, e.g., touch and heat
- Hand files that are heated over the flame.

Chemical Softening

The chemicals used are:
- Methyl chloroform (most common)
- Halothane
- Xylene
- Chloroform
- Eucalyptus oil.

Steps

The softened GP is removed with hand file and pitched with paper point.
- Negotiation of canal till apical constriction using pre-curved files and working is confirmed by radiographs.
- GP and sealers are removed using ultrasonics, while canal is irrigated with NaOCL
- Canal is overfilled and GP is removed till middle third using rotary file with solvent H-file is heated and inserted into the GP
- File is withdrawn gently after the GP cools which brings overextended GP along with it.

Miscellaneous

Irrigant Related

- All irrigant used are tissue irritants, if they extrude into the periradicular tissue
- They can cause inflammation reaction followed by tissue destruction.

Tissue Reaction Depends on

- Concentration
- Amount of exposure.

Prevention

- Use of needles with closed end and lateral vents
- Needle should not bind to the canal
- Using a monoject needle. The tip of needle should be 1–2 mm short of the apex.

Treatment

- Antibiotics, analgesics and antihistamine should be prescribed to stop infection
- Ice pack should be placed initially followed by saline soaks next day to decrease swelling

- In rare cases, steroids are given and hospitalisation may be needed
- If NaOCl is injected at maxillary sinus 30 mL of sterile water or saline should be injected to prevent damage to the sinus.

Tissue Emphysema

- It is the collection of gas or air in tissue spaces/facial planes
- This occurs during apical surgery. The air from high speed drill is directed towards the exposed soft tissue
- This causes:
  - Swelling
  - Erythema
  - Crepitus.

Treatment

Antibiotic therapy.

Prevention

- Direct air periapically is avoided
- During surgery low speed and minor high speed hand piece is used.

Post-operative Causes

- Trauma
- Fracture
- Super imposed non-endodontic lesion poor final restoration.

SHORT ESSAYS

Question 1

What is management of separated instruments within the root canal?

Answer

Instrument breakage is common problem in endodontic treatment.

Factors Influencing Broken Instrument Removal

- Cross sectional diameter of canal
- Curvature of canal
- General rule is that 1/3rd of the overall length of an obstruction can be exposed, which can be usually removed.

Surgical Indications

- Broken file is behind the curve
- File fragment is not visible because of curved roots
- Instrument is in the apical part of canal which is hard to retrieve.

Surgical Grasping Devices

- Indoor residual spraying (IRS) option
- Masserann kit
- End-excavator
- Wire loop technique.

Technique

- Patient should be informed about the mishap
- Radiograph is taken for proper treatment
- Use operating microscope.

Procedure

- Coronal access is done using high speed friction grip
- Radicular access is gained using rotary or hand files
- Gates-Glidden drill is used like "brushes" to create space and visibility
- Large GG are stopped out of the canal to create smooth flowing funnel that is largest at orifice
- Staging platform is made by selecting a GG with max, cross sectional diameter
- Before the radicular removal, cotton pellets over the other canal orifice to prevent re-entry of fragment into nearby canal system
- Ultrasonic instrument is used
- Airstream is applied
- CPR is moved in counter clockwise direction
- This loosens the instrument
- Wedging of energized tip between tapered file and canal wall cause the broken instrument to "jump out" of the canal.

CHAPTER 25

Tooth Discolouration and Its Management

Question 1

Write in detail about bleaching of vital teeth?

Answer

Bleaching of Vital Teeth

- In-office bleaching/power bleaching
- Outside the office bleaching
- Over the counter bleaching.

In-office Bleaching

- Thermocatalytic using light/heat procedure:
  - Placement of rubber dam
  - Teeth are then covered with 35% hydrogen peroxide (H_2O_2) with gauze
  - Activation of peroxide solution is by light/heat
  - Light is kept 30 cm (13 inches) away from the teeth and the beam of light should be directed to the surface to be bleached at 115°–140°F
  - At the time when heat is used temperature range should be 46°–60°C
  - Bleaching agent should be kept in contact of light/heat for approximately 30 minutes
  - Gauze is kept wet with dispensing it with fresh bleaching solution
  - After gauze is removed it is washed with warm water and then polished
  - Repeat the procedure till the desired shape is attained
  - Neutralize the solution with 5.25% sodium hypochlorite (NaOCL).
- Mc Innes solution.

Procedure

- Application of rubber dam
- Paste is applied on the teeth for 5 minutes and repeat after 1 minute in level with cotton application
- Neutralize the old Mc Innes solution with baking soda
- Irrigation is done with warm water
- Polishing is done.

Self-activating Bleaching Agents

Composition:

35% H_2O_2	:	0.4 mL
CaO	:	0.12 g
Aerosil	:	0.32–0.64 gm

Night Guard Bleaching (10% Carbamide Peroxide)

- It is also called as patient administered technique
- Shade evaluation is done before the treatment
- It is advisable to bleach one arch at a time
- Primary impression is taken followed by pouring cast
- Using a vacuum form machine, polyresin tray is made
- Trimming of the tray is done and is extended 1 mm short of the gingival margin or at the labial aspect. It is done to avoid irritation of gingiva by the bleaching material
- Tray made is then tried in the patient's mouth, to check for the perfect fit
- Instructions and method is given to the patient for loading gel and mouth fitting the tray
- Gel is only applied at the labial aspect of the tray and should be worn at the time of sleep for approximately 6–7 hours for 2 weeks
- Tray should be immediately discontinued if patient feels sensitivity at teeth
- Patient should never bite the tray
- Mouth should be properly rinsed after tray is removed every morning
- A weekly check-up is required.

Advantages

- It has no chair side time
- Saves patients' and dentists' time

- Self-applicable
- Easy technique.

Disadvantages

- Have more lab procedure
- Patient can complain of gag reflex while inserting the tray
- Gingival irritation
- Tooth becomes sensitive, so potassium nitrate with fluoride tooth pastes are used to decrease the sensitivity
- Altered taste sensation.

Tray Design

Types of trays used:
- Full vestibule tray
- Trays with/without reservoirs
- Trays with/without windows
- Scalloped or non-scalloped
- Trays with shortened borders.

Full Vestibule Tray

It is created by covering the whole vestibule region.

Trays with/without Reservoirs

- Trays with reservoirs are made with voids or space created in a bleaching tray
- It helps to hold extra material near the surface
- A flowable light cured resin/composite is placed on the buccal surface 1 mm away from the gingival border on the plaster model.

Trays with/without Windows

Windows allow bleaching for a single tooth to be bleached.

Scalloped/Non-scalloped Trays

Scalloped trays:
- They follow the tooth-gingiva interface and allow minimal soft tissue contact and less gingival irritation
- To prevent gingiva impinged tray is cut back 1 mm.

Non-scalloped trays:

- These trays are cut 2 mm over the labial incisors
- They provide better border seal and are less traumatic.

Trays with shortened borders:

- They are mostly used in patient with high gingival recession or the patients who have tendency of gag reflex
- This is the least recommended method.

Question 2

Write in brief about non-vital bleaching?

Answer

Non-vital Bleaching

It is a procedure that involves the use of chemical agents within the coronal portion of an endodontically treated tooth to remove tooth discolouration.

Material Used

- Sodium perborate
- Sodium percarbonate.

Sodium Perborate

- Contains 95% perborate when fresh
- It is an oxidizing agent
- It decomposes into sodium metaborate with contact to acid
- To hydrogen peroxide (H_2O_2), when contacted with air and to oxygen when contacted with water
- Three types available which differ in the oxygen content which in turn determines their bleaching efficiency
- They are safer than concentrated H_2O_2 solutions.

Sodium Percarbonate

- 13% available oxygen, higher than sodium perborate
- In case of sodium perborate the stability of active is quite lower
- Sodium percarbonate bleaching when mixed with water is safer in intracoronal bleaching than sodium perborate walking bleach method.

Types of Non-vital Bleaching

- In-office bleaching
- Walking bleach (out of office bleaching).

In-office Bleaching

Procedure:
- Place the rubber dam over the area to be bleached
- Cotton fibres are filled loosely in the pulp chamber and labial surface is covered with few strands of cotton fibre to form a matrix so that it retains the bleaching solution
- 35% H_2O_2 is used for saturation of cotton which is inserted inside the pulp chamber and also on the labial surface
- The excess solution is wiped immediately to avoid soft tissue irritation
- A thin-tapered instrument is heated and inserted into the pulp chamber for 5 minutes
- A temperature of 73°–75°C can be withstand by non-vital tooth without causing any discomfort
- Use of H_2O_2 can be replaced by light and heat form a bleaching light

- Heat and light speed up the breakdown of H_2O_2, so this lightens up the teeth more rapidly
- 5 minutes exposure for the tooth by bleaching and also replenish the bleaching agent at frequent intervals
- The heating instruments and cotton can be removed and this process is repeated for 4–6 times or 20–30 minutes each time placing new fibre cotton
- This is done along with walking bleach
- Sodium perborate should be changed weekly
- When bleaching is done final finishing is done by:
  - Filling chamber to 2 mm of cavosurface margin, a paste consisting of calcium hydroxide powder in sterile saline
  - Resealing of access opening is done.
- After 2 weeks temporary seal is removed, calcium hydroxide is rinsed
- Final restoration is done by using composite.

Walking Bleach

It was proposed by Nutting and Poe in 1963.

Before Bleaching

- Well-condensed root canal filling. Radiopaque without voids and it should be well adapted to the root canals
- Gutta-percha fillings should replace any silver cones
- If silver cones replacement is not possible, cavit is used to obturate the orifice of the root canal to prevent percolation of the bleaching solution in the periradicular tissue.

Technique

- The enamel surface is polished with prophylaxis paste
- Re-establishing of access cavity is done
- Application of petroleum jelly on the gingival tissues around the tooth to be bleached
- Rubber dam is then adapted on the tooth to be bleached
- Any gutta-percha extending into pulp chamber is removed
- To prevent percolation of bleaching agent orifice of the root canal is sealed with protective barrier
- 25% solution of citric acid is used to remove smear layer. Pulp chamber is then flush with 95% alcohol
- Prepared pulp chamber is filled with bleaching solution mixed with a paste of 35% H_2O_2 and sodium perborate
- Cotton pellet moistened with superoxol is placed over bleaching paste
- The access cavity is sealed at first by cavit and later by glass ionomer cement or zinc phosphate cement
- The mechanism is that after the pulp chamber is sealed it oxidizes and discolours the stain slowly continuing for longer period of time
- Bleaching effect is seen at maximum after 24 hours
- A weekly routine check-up is required
- Addition bleaching is required if the shade is too dark.

SHORT ESSAYS

Question 1

What are whitening tooth pastes?

Answer

Haywood Classification 1996

- More abrasive than usual:
  - It works on the criteria that it removes the surface staining by "Sanding" the teeth.
- Chemical removal of surface pellicle:
  - This process removes the surface pellicle which houses the surface stain
  - Chemical contain T_1O_2 which penetrates the surface irregularities of the tooth and white teeth illusion can be seen.
- Toothpastes with peroxides:
  - This process removes the surface pellicle which houses the surface stain
  - Chemical contain T_1O_2 which penetrates the surface irregularities of the tooth and white teeth illusion can be seen.

- Prophylaxis paste containing hydrogen peroxide (H_2O_2):
  - These are pastes containing H_2O_2 and pumice
  - During the process of prophylaxis they are applied to lighten and clean the tooth.
- Toothpaste containing sodium bicarbonate ($NaHCO_3$):
  - $NaHCO_3$ with small particle size allows penetration into the enamel and cleans inaccessible areas
  - $NaHCO_3$ threshold concentration: 45%
  - With a 65% concentration it consists of other products, like sodium lauryl sulphate which removes stain by $NaHCO_3$.
- Tooth pastes containing enzymes:
  - Enzymes, like bromelain and papain removes pellicle layer
  - This also inhibits development of plaque on the surface layer.
- Toothpastes with multicomponent:
  - Toothpastes that contain more than one component in the above mentioned are used as separate paste.

CHAPTER 26

Treatment of Traumatised Teeth

Question 1

Classify and write about traumatic injuries? Write in brief about avulsed tooth?

Answers

Classification of Traumatic Injuries

According to Ellis and Davey's

- **Class I:** Simple fracture of crown involving little or no dentin
- **Class II:** Extensive fracture of crown, with considerable amount of dentin involved but no pulp exposure
- **Class III:** Extensive fracture of crown, with considerable amount of dentin involved with pulp exposure
- **Class IV:** Traumatized tooth becomes non vital (with or without loss of crown structure)
- **Class V:** Tooth lost due to trauma
- **Class VI:** Fracture of root with or without loss of crown structure
- **Class VII:** Displacement of tooth without root or crown fracture
- **Class VIII:** Fracture of crown
- **Class IX:** Fracture of deciduous teeth.

Modification of Ellis and Davey

- **Class I:** Simple fracture of crown involving little or no dentin
- **Class II:** Extensive fracture, the crown involving considerable dentin, but not the dental pulp
- **Class III:** Extensive fracture of crown involving considerable dentin and the dental pulp
- **Class IV:** Loss of the entire crown.

Classification based on Endodontic Treatment

- Fracture of enamel
- Fracture of crown with indirect pulp exposure their dentin
- Fracture of crown with direct pulp exposure.

According to Robin Witch

He classified injuries of the primary teeth:
- Fracture of enamel slightly into dentin
- Fracture into dentin
- Fracture into pulp
- Fracture of the root
- Comminuted fracture
- Displaced teeth.

According to Garcia Godoy

- Enamel crack
- Enamel fracture
- Enamel, dentin fracture with out pulp exposure
- Enamel, dentin fracture with pulp exposure
- Enamel, dentin, cementum fracture without pulp exposure
- Enamel, dentin, cementum fracture with pulp exposure
- Root fracture
- Concussion
- Luxation
- Lateral displacement
- Intrusion
- Extrusion
- Avulsion.

According to Andreasen

Based on a system adopted by WHO in its application of the international classification of disease to dentistry and stomatology certain trauma entities were not defined and included in the WHO system.

The following classification includes injuries to teeth, supporting structures, gingiva and oral mucosa and is based on anatomical therapeutic and prognostic considerations.

This classification can be applied to both primary and permanent dentition.

A. Injuries to hard dental tissues and pulp

1. Crown infraction N 873.60: Incomplete fracture (Crack) of the enamel without loss of tooth substance
2. Uncomplicated crown fracture: A fracture contained to enamel (N 873.60) or involving enamel and dentin, but not exposing the pulp (N 873.61)
3. Complicated crown fracture N 873.62: Fracture involving enamel and dentin exposing pulp
4. Uncomplicated crown root fracture N 873.69: Fracture Involving enamel, dentin and cementum but not involving
5. Complicated crown root fracture N 873.64: Fracture involving enamel, dentin and cementum and exposing pulp
6. Root fracture N 873.63: Fracture Involving dentin, cementum and pulp.

B. Injuries to the periodontal tissues

1. Concussion N 873.66: Injuries to tooth supporting structures without (mobility) abnormal loosening or displacement of tooth, but with marked reaction to percussion
2. Subluxation N 873.66: Injury to tooth supporting structures with abnormal loosening but without displacement of tooth
3. Intrusive Luxation N 873.67: Displacement of tooth into alveolar bone accompanied by commination or fracture of alveolar Socket
4. Extrusive luxation N 873.66: Partial displacement of tooth out of its socket
5. Lateral luxation N 873.66: Displacement of tooth in a direction other than axially accompanied by communication or fracture of alveolar socket
6. Exarticulation (Complete avulsion) N 873.68: Complete displacement of the tooth out of its socket.

C. Injuries of the Supporting bone

1. Communication of alveolar socket:
   a. Mandible N 802.20
   b. Maxilla N 802.40.
   Crushing and compression of alveolar socket with intrusive and lateral luxation.
2. Fracture of alveolar socket wall:
   a. Mandible N 802.20
   b. Maxilla N 802.40.
   Fracture contained to the facial and lingual socket wall.
3. Fracture of the alveolar process:
   a. Mandible N 802.20
   b. Maxilla N 802.40.
   Fracture of alveolar process which may or may not involve the alveolar socket

4. Fracture of mandible and maxilla:
   a. Mandible N 802.21
   b. Maxilla N 802.42.
   Fracture involving base of mandibula or maxilla and often the alveolar process may or may not involve alveolar socket.

D. Injuries to gingiva or oral mucosa

1. Laceration of gingiva or oral mucosa N 873.69: Shallow or deep wound in mucosa resulting from a tear and usually produced by sharp object
2. Contusion of gingiva or oral mucosa N 902.00: Bruise usually produced by an impact from a blunt object and not accompanied by a break of continuity in the mucosa, causing submucosal haemorrhage
3. Abrasion of gingiva or oral mucosa N 910.00: Superficial wound produced by rubbing or scraping of mucosa leaving a raw bleeding surface.

According to Borum and Andreasen of Injuries to Primary Teeth

- ❑ Crown infraction
- ❑ Crown fracture (with and without pulp exposure)
- ❑ Crown and root fracture
- ❑ Root fracture.

Injuries to periodontal attachment:

- ❑ Concussion
- ❑ Subluxation
- ❑ Extrusion
- ❑ Lateral luxation
- ❑ Intrusion
- ❑ Avulsion.

Fracture of crown:

- ❑ Enamel
- ❑ Dentin with or without pulp exposure.

Root-fracture.

Crown-root fracture.

Question 2

Classify traumatic injuries of the anterior teeth. How will you manage Ellis Class III fracture in maxillary central incisors?

Answers

Classification of Traumatic Injuries

According to Ellis and Davey's

- ❑ **Class I:** Simple fracture of crown involving little or no dentin

- **Class II:** Extensive fracture of crown, with considerable amount of dentin involved but do pulp exposure
- **Class III:** Extensive fracture of crown, with considerable amount of dentin involved with pulp exposure
- **Class IV:** Traumatized tooth becomes non vital (with or without loss of crown structure)
- **Class V:** Tooth lost due to trauma
- **Class VI:** Fracture of root with or without loss of crown structure
- **Class VII:** Displacement of tooth without root or crown fracture
- **Class VIII:** Fracture of crown
- **Class IX:** Fracture of deciduous teeth.

Ellis Class III Fracture

- Crown fractures involving enamel, dentine and pulp are called complicated crown fractures
- The diagnosis depend on
- Patients history.
  - Clinical examination
  - Radiographs
  - Vitality tests.

Choice of treatment in Ellis Class III depends hugely upon certain factors:

- Stage of the tooth development: Treatment for the crown fracture is different in the developing stage of the tooth.
  - *Vital tooth*: Tooth is restored without vital pulp therapy, like pulpotomy or pulp capping because the apex formation is incomplete
  - *Immature non-vital tooth*: Apexification is done using calcium hydroxide or mineral trioxide aggregate (MTA) which is followed by obturation
  - In mature tooth, root canal therapy (RCT) is done.
- Time between the accident and treatment process:
  - Pulp exposure less than 48 hours: pulpotomy
  - Pulp exposure for more than 48 hours: pulpectomy or RCT.
- Restorative treatment plan:
  - While the composite restoration process partial pulpotomy is required
  - While in complex restoration process pulpectomy is needed.
- Associated periodontal injury:
  - When the surrounding periodontium is damaged and there is a nutritional supply damage, pulpectomy is always the treatment of choice.

Treatment for Vital Pulp for Young Permanent Tooth

Apexogenesis is a root induction procedure done for the young permanent molars where the apex and the roots are not completely formed

It is a form of vital pulp therapy thereby known as apexogenesis.

Indications

- Normal radiographic appearance
- Absence of sensitivity to percussion
- No abnormal response to thermal stimuli
- Little if any evidence of intracoronal abscess formation
- Lack of excessive hemorrhage
- No evidence of foul odour.

Contraindications

- Clinical evidence of degenerative changes in radicular pulp
- Avulsed and replanted or severely luxated tooth
- Severe crown root fracture that requires intraradicular retention for restoration
- Tooth with an unfavorable horizontal root fracture (i.e., close to the gingival margin)
- Carious tooth that is un-restorable
- Pathological periapical changes in the tooth.

Prognosis

The prognosis is good when shallow pulpotomy (Cvek technique) is done correctly, following a traumatic exposure. Conventional pulpotomy is slightly less successful. Calcific metamorphosis is frequent.

Cvek Pulpotomy (Partial Pulpotomy)

Technique:
- After diagnosis is completed, the tooth is anaesthetized.
- Perform the pulpal procedures under rubber dam isolation and aseptic conditions
- Cvek has shown that with pulp exposures resulting from traumatic injuries are characterized by a proliferative response with inflammation into the pulp. When this inflamed tissue is removed, healthy pulp tissue is encountered.
- Use an abrasive diamond bur, using high-speed with adequate water-cooling for pulp amputation thereby creating least damage
- Remove all filaments of pulp tissue coronal to the amputation site

- The preparation is thoroughly washed with physiologic saline or sterile water to remove all debris; water is removed by vacuum and cotton pellets
- Hemorrhage is controlled by cotton pellets slightly moistened with saline (i.e., wetted and blotted almost dry) placed against pulp stumps
- Once controlled, calcium hydroxide is placed against pulp stump and tooth is sealed, and closely monitored for development of any pathologic conditions
- A permanent type of restoration should always be placed in the tooth to ensure the retention of the pulp-capping material. The material of choice is usually a bonded composite restoration or a crown.

Calcium Hydroxide Pulpotomy

- Teusher and Zander (1938) reported on the use of calcium hydroxide paste as a pulp dressing in pulpotomy of both primary and permanent teeth
- Their histologic studies showed that the tissues was first necrotized, with acute inflammatory changes in the immediate tissue beneath. After 4weeks, development of new odontoblastic layer at the wound site i.e., Dentin bridge
- Internal resorption with root destruction occurs in primary teeth. This may be due to over stimulation of the undifferentiated cells of the pulp by calcium hydroxide
- Calcium hydroxide has been most successful on young permanent teeth, especially traumatized incisors.

Procedure

- Local anesthesia is administered
- Rubber dam is applied and exposed teeth and surrounding area is cleansed with a suitable germicide
- Roof of pulp chamber is exposed widely using a sterile #557-fissure bur with coolant
- A sterile, sharp spoon excavator is used to extirpate the pulp as nearly as possible in one piece.
- A clean amputation to the orifices of canals is necessary.
- Pulp chamber is then irrigated and cleansed with sterile water and cotton.
- Hemorrhage is controlled by pressure from cotton pellets impregnated with calcium hydroxide.
- Cement base of zinc oxide eugenol is placed over calcium hydroxide to seal the crown.
- Finally, stainless steel crown restoration is desired, since the dentin and enamel get brittle and dehydrated after pulpotomy treatment
- Periodic checkup to evaluate the health of the treated tooth is necessary.

Absence of pain or discomfort should be noted. Radiographs must be utilized to determine changes in periapical tissue or signs of internal resorption.

Cervical Pulpotomy

Traumatic exposures after 72 hrs and carious exposure are two examples where it is indicated.

Technique

- Amputation of Coronal pulp
- Control of hemorrhage.

Hemorrhage controlled with chemicals (aluminum chloride) or other hemostatic agent.

- Calcium hydroxide placed on amputation site
- Use of hard setting material (Dycal) if pulp amputation is only a few mm deep
- In Deeper amputation, calcium hydroxide is carried in amalgam carrier. The carrier is tightly packed with powder than three fourth of pellet is expressed and discarded
- A base and an interim restoration are placed.

Apexification

Indications

- It is indicated when there is incomplete root formation and there is necrosed pulp in a devloping tooth
- It is indicated in open apices which have thin dentinal walls because by instrumentation it is difficult to open apices and create apical stop which may effect root canal obturation.

Materials Used

- Calcium hydroxide
- Tricalcium phosphate
- MTA
- Bone morphogenetic proteins.

Limitation

- It can facture dentinal wall that are thin and prone to fracture
- There can be leakage if the canals are under filled
- Extrusion of obturating material can happen because lack of apical stop.

Procedure

- Rubber dam isolation is done
- After the access opening is done, the remnants of the pulp are removed. Barbed broaches are used

- Working length is determined
- Irrigation of the canal is done by 0.5% sodium chloride (NaCl), paper points are used for drying the canal
- The canal is then disinfected with calcium hydroxide in creamy consistency which is placed using the gutta-percha points
- To give the canal a bacterial seal a 1 week recall is given. With the pluggers thin paste of calcium hydroxide mixed with saline is placed after the debridement process
- The access cavity is then restored with temporary filling
- A 3 month recall is given and hard tissue barrier formation is seen in the radiograph
- This process is repeated if there is no barrier formation
- "Swiss cheese" consistency is seen in the apical barrier
- A final obturation is done after the calcium hydroxide is removed using sodium hypochlorite (NaOCl).

Obturation in Apexification

- Inverted gutta-percha technique
- Roll cone technique
- Thermo plasticised gutta-percha.

Disadvantage of Calcium Hydroxide Apexification

- It takes multiple sittings and is time consuming
- Calcium hydroxide weakens the bone structure as it disrupts the bond between the hydroxyapatite and collagen
- Patient needs to be patient and cooperative.

Mineral Trioxide Aggregate Apexification

- MTA gives a hard tissue barrier against which obturation is completed
- When there is a recall visit the calcium hydroxide, which is pushed further and beyond the apex provides a resorbable barrier against which MTA is condensed

- MTA is condensed up to 3–4 mm into the apical area of the canal
- A wet cotton pellet is placed into the canal which facilitates the MTA setting
- After 6 hours cotton pellet is removed and obturation is done up to the marginal bone level and it is followed by the resin restoration.

Pulpectomy

Pulpectomy is defined as the complete removal of the pulp to the level of the apical foramen.

Indications

- It is done when pulp exposure is beyond 72 hours
- If pulp damage is beyond recovery
- If pulp is degenerated or the vitality of the tooth is questionable.

Procedure

- Isolation is done by using rubber dam for the affected tooth
- Access opening is done. A barbed broach is used to remove the pulpal remnants
- Working length is determined using file and radiograph
- Cleaning and shaping is done followed by irrigation of canal with NaOCl
- Canal is then dried using paper points
- Intracanal medicament is placed
- To give a bacterial tight seal the access cavity is restored with temporary filling.
- At a recall after 2–4 days the canal is explored for drainage
- The dry canal is then obturated completely and the access cavity is restored using resin restoration.

SHORT ESSAYS

Question 1

What are luxation injuries?

Answer

They are the injuries that cause trauma to supporting structures of teeth which can be from minor crushing of periodontal ligament to total displacement of the teeth.

They are mostly caused by sudden impact such as blow, fall or striking a hard object.

Types

- Concussion
- Subluxation
- Lateral luxation
- Extrusive luxation
- Intrusive luxation.

Concussion

- In this there is no displacement of the tooth
- Mobility is not seen

- Due to trauma to the periodontal ligament tooth is susceptible to tenderness on percussion
- No sign of pulp damage.

Subluxation

- There is presence of mobility
- There is tenderness on percussion
- Periodontal ligament is damaged
- Displacement of teeth does not happen.

Treatment

- Radiographs should be taken to see the extent of the injury
- Endodontic treatment should be processed
- Follow up after 3 weeks to see the tooth condition.

Lateral Luxation

- Tooth is displaced from its position
- Periodontal ligament is ruptured with sulcular bleeding
- Tenderness on percussion is present.

Extrusive Luxation

- Tooth is displaced
- Tooth can be felt mobile with the touch of fingers
- Periodontal damage.

Treatment of Lateral and Extrusive Luxation

- The treatment module is to replace the teeth into the original place so that there is constant healing with respect to its original position

- Regular radiographs should be taken to know the extent of recovery.

Clinical Repositioning of Laterally Luxated Tooth

- Anaesthesia is administered
- Less pressure is implied
- Tooth is taken out from labial cortical plate
- Tooth is coronally moved and then placed in the original place.

Clinical Repositioning of Extruded Tooth

- Coagulum formed between root of the apex and floor of the socket is displaced by slow pressure
- Tooth is placed in its original place
- Splinting is done for 2 weeks.

Intrusive Luxation

- Tooth is placed in its socket
- This damages the pulp and surrounding structures the most
- Ankylosis is seen
- The clinical feature to diagnose is the metallic sound that can be heard at the time of percussion.

Treatment

- In case of mixed dentition re eruption is usually seen
- In case of permanent dentition orthodontic appliance is administered.

SHORT NOTES

Question 1

What is HBSS?

Answer

Hank's balanced solution is a preserving fluid is best used with a trauma reducing suspension apparatus.

HBSS is biocompatible with the tooth periodontal ligament cells and can keep these cells viable for 24 hours because of its ideal pH and osmolality.

Composition

- Sodium chloride
- Potassium chloride
- Glucose
- Calcium chloride
- Magnesium chloride
- Sodium bicarbonate
- Sodium phosphate.

SECTION 3

RECENTLY ASKED QUESTIONS

CHAPTER 27

Recently Asked Questions

INTRODUCTION TO OPERATIVE DENTISTRY

Long Essays

1. Enumerate the various diagnostic aids on the field of operative dentistry and endodontics discuss in detail the importance of radiographic examination and its limitation. [GOA]
2. Discuss the importance of gingival tissue management in conservative dentistry. Describe the various techniques of managing the gingival tissue. [TN]
3. Discuss the importance of history taking, patient's assessment and treatment planning in conservative dentistry. [MUHS]

Short Essays

1. Anaesthetic test. [RGUHS]
2. Methods of diagnosis of proximal caries lesion. [RGUHS]
3. Affected and Infected dentine. [RGUHS]
4. Secondary dentine. [NTR-NR]
5. Transillumination in endodontics. [RGUHS]
6. Diagnosis of occlusal and proximal caries. [MUHS]
7. Cold test. [RGUHS]

8. Contact point at different types and its importance in restorative dentistry. [RGUHS]
9. Classify hand instruments. Add a note on nomenclature. [NTRUHS]

Short Notes

1. Test cavity. [RGUHS (OS); NTRUHS (OR)]
2. Percussion. [RGUHS]
3. Diagnosis of dental caries. [NTR]
4. Tetracycline stains. [NTR-NR]
5. Dentine hypersensitivity. [MUHS]
6. Cold testing for tooth vitality. [MUHS]
7. Diagnostic aids. [MUHS]
8. Uses of radiographs. [MUHS]
9. Secondary dentine. [NTR-NR]
10. Tertiary dentine. [NTRUHS]
11. Col. [NTRUHS]
12. Embrasures. [RGUHS]
13. F.D.A.S tooth numbering system. [MUHS]
14. RVG. [RGUHS]
15. Gingival tissue management. [GOA]

PRELIMINARY CONSIDERATIONS FOR OPERATIVE DENTISTRY

Long Essays

1. Discuss the various methods of gingival tissue management. [MUHS]
2. Discuss the importance of isolation and various methods used to achieve the same. [NTRUHS (NR)]
3. List the various methods of isolation and discuss rubber dam isolation in detail. [TN]
4. Enumerate methods to isolate the teeth. Describe rubber dam. [MUHS]

5. Discuss pain control during cavity preparation. [MUHS]
6. Describe the methods of isolation of the operating field. Add a note on sterilization of hand instruments. [RGUHS]
7. Discuss the importance of isolation of the operating field and various methods to achieve it in conservative dentistry. [NTR-NR]
8. What is the importance of 'moisture control in operative dentistry'? Give different methods of controlling moisture during operative procedures. [RGUHS; BUHS]

9. Enumerate methods of sterilization. Discuss the importance of sterilization of operative instrument. [RGUHS]
10. How will you avoid injury to the soft tissues and supporting structures of a tooth during cavity preparation? [MUHS]
11. Classify various methods of isolation and discuss rubber dam in detail. [NTRUHS]
12. Discuss the importance of isolation and various methods used to achieve the same. [NTRUHS]

Short Essays

1. Retraction chord. [NTR-NR]
2. Gingival marginal trimmer and enamel hatchet. [MUHS]
3. Gingival retraction. [NTR-OR]
4. Rubber dam. [NTR-OR; MUHS]
5. Management of rubber dam. [NTR-OR]
6. Moisture contamination of dental amalgam. [RGUHS (OS)]
7. Moisture control in operative dentistry. [RGUHS; BUHS]
8. Methods and importance of tooth isolation during operative procedures. [RGUHS]
9. Management of gingival tissues during operative procedures. [NTR-NR]
10. Describe components of rubber dam kit and advantages of rubber dam in endodontics. [RGUHS]
11. Endo-perio lesions. [RGUHS OR and NR]
12. Enumerate isolation methods and discuss rubber dam application. [RGUHS]
13. Describe infection control. [RGUHS]
14. Contraindications of rubber dam. [RGUHS]
15. Direct method of isolation. [RGUHS]
16. Pain control during operative procedures. [NTRUHS]
17. Rolled cone method. [RGUHS]

18. Write briefly on emergencies in endodontics and management. [GOA]
19. Describe components of rubber dam kit. [NTR-NR]

Short Notes

1. Disinfection of impressions. [RGUHS]
2. Hydrogen peroxide. [RGUHS]
3. Hot salt sterilizer. [NTRUHS]
4. Sprue former. [MUHS]
5. Rubber dam. [TN]
6. Iontophoresis. [RGUHS OR and NR]
7. Universal operating position. [NTRUHS]
8. Pain pathway. [NTRUHS]
9. Gingival retraction. [RGUHS; NTR-NR]
10. Barrier techniques in infection control. [TN]
11. Gingival retraction cord. [RGUHS]
12. Importance of isolation. [GOA]
13. Moisture control in operative procedures. [RGUHS]
14. Hot air oven. [NTRUHS]
15. Handpiece asepsis. [TN]
16. Gingival marginal trimmer. [MUHS]
17. Rapid separators. [MUHS]
18. Sterilization of high speed handpiece. [GOA]
19. Gingival tissue management in conservative dentistry. [TN]
20. Methods of sterilization. [RGUHS]
21. Rake angle. [NTRUHS]
22. Rubber dam. [NTRUHS; TN; RGUHS]
23. Autoclave. [TN]
24. Moisture control in operative dentistry. [TN]
25. Methods of isolation. [MUHS]
26. Rubber dam retainer (clamp). [MUHS]
27. Advantages off rubber dam. [NTR-NR]

CARIOLOGY

Long Essays

1. Classify pulpal lesions. Differentiate between reversible and irreversible pulpitis. [GOA]
2. What are the causes of dentinal hypersensitive? Describe the methods of its managements. [TN]
3. Discuss aetiology and management of hypersensitive dentine. [NTR-OR]
4. Describe in detail the prophylactic treatment of dental caries. [RGUHS]
5. Describe deep caries management. [TN]

6. Discuss dentine hypersensitivity, ninth emphasis on various theories. Also mention its management. [RGUHS]
7. Discuss the management of hypersensitive dentine. [RGUHS]
8. How do you diagnose dental caries? Add a note on aetiology and classification of dental caries. [GOA]
9. Define dental caries. Classify. Enumerate sequelae. Briefly write management of mesio-occlusal caries in a mandibular first molar tooth. [TN]

Short Essays

1. Phoenix abscess. [RGUHS]
2. Phoenix abscess-cause, symptoms and treatment. [RGUHS]
3. Annealing and compaction procedures in direct gold. [RGUHS]
4. Methods of diagnosis of proximal caries lesion. [RGUHS]
5. Mention causes of hypersensitivity and management of the same. [RGUHS]
6. Mention the aetiological factors of pulpal diseases. [RGUHS]
7. Diagnostic AIDS to detect caries. [RGUHS]
8. Pulp polyp. [RGUHS]
9. Hypersensitivity. [RGUHS]
10. Prophylactic odontotomy. [NTR-NR]
11. Theories of hypersensitivity. [BUHS]
12. Tooth hypersensitivity. [NTRUHS]
13. Define and classify caries add a note on diagnosis of caries. [NTRUHS]
14. Classify matrices. Write about auto matrix system. [RGUHS]
15. Define and classify dental caries. Write a note on secondary caries. [RGUHS]
16. Root surface caries. [RGUHS]
17. Management of hypersensitive dentine. [NTR-NR]

Short Notes

1. Infected dentine. [RGUHS]
2. Caries detecting dyes. [RGUHS (RS)]
3. Pink tooth. [NTRUHS]
4. Hypersensitivity. [TN; BUHS]
5. Microorganism responsible for root caries. [RGUHS]

6. Phoenix abscess. [RGUHS]
7. Dentine hypersensitivity. [TN]
8. Tooth separation in restorative dentistry. [RGUHS]
9. Various aids used for the diagnosis of caries. [RGUHS]
10. Disclosing solution. [TN]
11. Preventive measures of dental caries. [TN]
12. Methods of caries detection. [GOA; TN]
13. Pit and fissure sealants. [NTR-NR]
14. Define dental caries add a note on diagnosis of caries. [GOA]
15. Purpose of separation of teeth. [RGUHS]
16. Irreversible pulpitis. [RGUHS]
17. Methods of diagnosis of proximal caries lesion. [RGUHS]
18. Clinical diagnosis of cavitated and non-cavitated caries. [TN]
19. Fissure sealants. [RGUHS]
20. Treatment of hypersensitive dentine. [GOA]
21. Secondary dentine. [RGUHS]
22. Affected and Infected dentine. [RGUHS]
23. R.V.G. [RGUHS]
24. Microbiological flora of pulp space. [GOA]
25. Classification of dental caries. [NTR-NR]
26. Diagnosis of dental caries. [BUHS]
27. Define caries. Classify. [TN]
28. Cemental caries. [RGUHS]
29. Pulpal necrosis. [RGUHS]
30. Geriatric caries. [RGUHS]
31. Enumerate diagnostic tests for dental caries. [MUHS]
32. ART. [TN]
33. Cavity liner. [RGUHS]
34. Saliva tests for caries risk assessment. [GOA]
35. Caries activity tests. [NTR-NR]
36. Causes of dentine hypersensitivity. [NTR-NR]

INSTRUMENTS AND SEPARATION

Long Essays

1. Bur and bur design. [MUHS]
2. Define matrix. Describe the matrices and retainers used while restoring class II cavity. [RGUHS]
3. Contact point at different types and its importance in restorative dentistry. [RGUHS]
4. Cutting and finishing bur. [MUHS]
5. Gingival marginal trimmer and enamel hatchet. [MUHS]
6. Speeds in dentistry. [MUHS]
7. Classify and describe the various Hand cutting Instruments. [RGUHS]
8. Classify hand cutting instruments used in conservative dentistry. Elaborate on modified chisels and instrument formula. [GOA]
9. Discuss the disadvantages of using low speed and high speed in operative dentistry. [GOA]
10. Instrument formulae and instrument rule. [MUHS]
11. Define matrix. Describe the matrices and I refiners used while restoring class II cavity. [RGUHS]
12. Discuss the importance of isolation and various methods used to achieve the same. [RGUHS OR and NR]
13. Classify and write in detail about operative hand instruments. Add a not on instrument formula. [TN]

14. Classify and discuss hand cutting instruments and rotary instruments used in operative dentistry. [RGUHS]
15. How will you gain the active separation of teeth in Operative dentistry? [NTR-OR]
16. Enamel hatchet and hoes. [MUHS]
17. Classify speeds in dentistry. Write in detail the advantages of high-speed diagnosis ultra-high speed in Dental practice. [NTR-OR]
18. Mono-angled chisel and hoe. [MUHS]
19. What is high speed? Classify and describe its advantages and disadvantages. [BUHS]
20. What is high speed? Classify and describe its advantages and disadvantages? [RGUHS]
21. Classify hand instruments write a note on instrument formula and on each instruments. [GOA]

Short Essays

1. Discuss hand cutting instruments used in restorative dentistry. [NTRUHS]
2. Grasps used with hand instruments. [RGUHS]
3. Define matrix. Discuss different types of matrices. [NTRUHS]
4. Define matrix. Describe various matrices. [RGUHS]
5. Abrasion. [RGUHS]
6. Anatomic matrix. [RGUHS]
7. Instrument formula. [NTR-NR, NTR-OR; RGUHS; MUHS, MUHS; RGUHS]
8. Wedges. [NTRUHS]
9. Design of auto matrix. [NTRUHS]
10. Classification and principles of tooth separators. [RGUHS]
11. Fish's zone. [RGUHS]
12. Wedges-types and methods of wedging. [RGUHS]
13. Preparation of teeth. [RGUHS]
14. Bur Design. [NTR-NR; NTRUHS]
15. Bur blade design. [RGUHS (RS)]
16. Indications of separation of teeth. [RGUHS (RS)]
17. 4 unit Instrument formulae. [MUHS]
18. Separation of teeth. [NTR-OR; RGUHS (RS)]
19. Anatomic matrix. [RGUHS]
20. Matrix band and retainers used for restorations. [RGUHS]
21. Bums and diamonds points. [RGUHS]
22. Dental burs. [NTR-OR; NTR-NR; RGUHS]
23. Classify and describe various hand instruments used in conservative dentistry. [GOA]
24. Matrices and matrix retainers. [RGUHS]
25. Ultrasonic and sonic instruments. [RGUHS]
26. Rotatory cutting instrument. [NTR-NR]
27. Classify hand-cutting instruments. [RGUHS]
28. Diamond abrasives. [MUHS]
29. Finger rests and guards. [NTR-OR]
30. Separators. [NTR-OR, NTR-NR]
31. Matrices. [NTR-OR; NTR-NR]
32. Gingival marginal trimmer. [NTR-OR, NTR-NR]
33. Contacts and contours. [NTR-NR]
34. Matrices and retainers used in restorative dentistry. [NTR-NR]
35. Hatchet and Hoe. [NTR-NR]
36. Instrument formula for hand cutting instruments. [NTR-OR]
37. What is high speed? Classify and describe its advantages and disadvantages. [BUHS]
38. Marginal trimmers. [NTR-OR]
39. Mechanical separators. [NTR-OR]
40. Bur blade design. [RGUHS]
41. Tofflemire matrix retainers. [NTR-NR]
42. Mechanical separation, different types and advantages. [RGUHS]
43. Amalgam carver. [NTR-NR]
44. Angle former. [NTR-NR]
45. Classify and describe hand-cutting Instruments. [RGUHS]
46. Advantages and disadvantages of high speed. [NTR-OR, NTR-NR]
47. Enamel hatchet. [NTR-OR; MUHS]
48. Indications of separation of teeth. [RGUHS]
49. High speed. [NTR-OR; RGUHS]
50. 4 unit Instrument formulae. [MUHS]
51. Separation of teeth. [NTR-OR; RGUHS]
52. Hand cutting instruments. [RGUHS]
53. Rake Angle. [RGUHS]
54. Ultra speed. [NTR-NR]
55. Non-metallic Matrices. [RGUHS]
56. Define matrix. Describe the matrices and retainers used while restoring class II cavity. [RGUHS]
57. Define matrix. Describe the matrices and retainers used while restoring class II cavity. [RGUHS]

Short Notes

1. Functions of matrix retainer. [RGUHS OR and NR]
2. Giromatic handpiece. [RGUHS]
3. Exploring instruments. [RGUHS]
4. Wooden wedges. [RGUHS]
5. Gingival marginal trimmer. [RGUHS]
6. Apical matrix. [NTRUHS]
7. Rake angle. [RGUHS; TN]
8. Tofflemire retainers. [NTR-NR; GOA]

9. Balancing of the hand instrument. [RGUHS]
10. Wedelstaedt chisel. [RGUHS; TN]
11. Separators. [NTR-NR; RGUHS; GOA; TN]
12. Bur design. [NTR-NR; RGUHS]
13. Wedges used in dentistry. [RGUHS]
14. Wedges used in dentistry. [RGUHS]
15. Mechanical separators. [RGUHS; RGUHS]
16. Wedges. [RGUHS; RGUHS; TN]
17. Tooth separation. [TN]
18. Slow separators. [RGUHS]
19. Rake angle. [RGUHS OR and NR]
20. Instrument grasps. [TN]
21. Angle former. [RGUHS]
22. Sonic handpiece. [RGUHS]
23. 245 bur. [NTRUHS]
24. Spoon excavator. [NTRUHS; RGUHS (RS)]
25. Gingival marginal trimmer. [GOA; TN]
26. Instrument formula. [RGUHS; TN]
27. Retainers for Class-II amalgam restoration. [RGUHS]
28. S-shaped matrix. [RGUHS (RS)]
29. Copper band matrix. [RGUHS (RS)]
30. D-II instrument. [RGUHS (RS)]
31. Double wedging. [RGUHS (RS)]
32. Dental bur. [NTRUHS]
33. Speed. [TN]
34. Burs. [TN]
35. Speed in dentistry. [TN]
36. Gingival marginal trimmer. [RGUHS]
37. Balanced forces technique. [RGUHS]
38. Wedges. [RGUHS; TN]
39. Bur head design. [TN]
40. Dental bar. [RGUHS; TN]
41. Matrix retainers and bond. [TN]
42. Mouth mirror. [RGUHS]
43. Tofflemire universal matrix retainer. [RGUHS]
44. Hatchet. [RGUHS]
45. Matrices and retainers. [RGUHS]
46. Ultra speed. [RGUHS]
47. Universal matrix retainers. [RGUHS]
48. Sharpening of hand instruments. [BUHS]
49. Aerotar. [BUHS]
50. Matrices. [RGUHS]
51. Contacts and contours in restoration dentistry. [TN]
52. Significance of contacts and contours. [NTR-NR]
53. Advantages and disadvantages of dental bur. [RGUHS]
54. Slow speed. [NTR-NR]
55. Wedge. [NTR-NR]
56. Auto matrix. [RGUHS; BUHS; RGUHS]
57. Separation of teeth. [TN]
58. Burns and diamonds points. [TN]
59. Importance of contacts and contours. [TN]
60. Separation of teeth and mechanical separators. [GOA]
61. Matrix and the uses. [TN]
62. High speed. [RGUHS; TN]
63. Dental burs. [NTR-NR]
64. Purpose of separation of teeth. [RGUHS]
65. Embrasures. [NTR-NR]
66. Elliot separator. [NTR-NR]
67. Sonic instrument. [GOA]
68. Types and uses of wedges. [TN]
69. Chisel and its modifications. [TN]

FUNDAMENTALS IN TOOTH PREPARATION

Long Essays

1. Define retention form. Discuss methods of retention cavity preparation. [NTRUHS]
2. Define retention form. How is it achieved in amalgam restorations. [RGUHS (OS); RGUHS]
3. Describe the technique of class II cavity preparation amalgam on mandibular first molar. [RGUHS]
4. Define an inlay and onlay. Describe the cavity preparation for a class II mesio occlusal lesion in mandibular first right molar. [TN]
5. Classify and describe the various hand cutting Instruments. [RGUHS]
6. Cavity preparation for class III composites. [RGUHS]
7. Discuss cavity preparation and restoration of an MOD cavity in a lower first permanent molar for amalgam. [TN]
8. What are different between a class II amalgam and preparation. [TN]
9. Describe in detail cavity preparation for class II conventional design in the mandibular right 1st molar mesial aspect. [TN]
10. Principles of cavity preparation and describe the secondary retention form in a class II cavity for silver amalgam restoration. [RGUHS (OS)]
11. What is the management of cervical abrasion attrition erosion and abfraction lesion give the manipulation of the choice of material in detail. [GOA]

12. Discuss the various treatment modalities of cervically eroded lesion in a lower 1st permanent molar. [MUHS]
13. Describe the technique of restoring an abrasive lesion in an upper first premolar. [NTR-OR]
14. Describe the various concepts of cavity design for amalgam restorations. [RGUHS]
15. What is model amalgam restoration, Describe in detail class II preparation for silver amalgam in this context, and compare it with G.V. Black's design. [MUHS]
16. What do you mean by 'extension for prevention'? How this principle is applied during the cavity preparation of various classes. [MUHS]
17. Discuss the resistance and retention form in Blacks' class II restorations. [RGUHS]
18. Discuss pain control procedures during cavity preparation. [MUHS]
19. Compare the features of a class II preparation for a silver amalgam restoration and a gold inlay restoration. [TN]
20. Describe in detail, the tooth preparation for a mesio occlusal inlay on mandibular first molar. [TN]
21. Describe class II cavity preparation for silver amalgam with stress on modem concepts. [RGUHS]
22. Discuss the initial and final stages of tooth preparation, for class II amalgam restoration. [TN]
23. Define class II cavity. What is conventional and conservation cavity preparation. Describe cavity preparation for MO preparation in a mandibular molar using conventional design. [TN]
24. Define resistance form. Give the features of the same in the class II cavity. [MUHS]
25. Describe the techniques of restoring erosion lesions in a maxillary first premolar with glass ionomer cement. Add a note or advantages and disadvantages of glass ionomers. [RGUHS]
26. Describe the techniques of restoring erosion lesions in a maxillary first premolar with Glass ionomer cement. Add a note on advantages and disadvantages of glass ionomer. [RGUHS]
27. Discuss the characteristics of class II inlay preparation in posterior teeth and compare it with class II preparation of silver amalgam. [MUHS]
28. Give GV Black's classification of cavities. [NTR-OR]
29. What are the clinical Indications for glass ionomer cements. What do you understand by 'sandwich tech'. Write in detail tooth preparation and restoration of class V erosion lesion in a posterior tooth. [RGUHS]
30. Describe briefly modem method of class II cavity preparation. Please also mention modification in this from GV Black principles. [NTR-OR]

31. Write the composition of Glass ionomer cements. Describe the procedure of restoring abrasive defect (class V restoration). [RGUHS]
32. Enumerate principles of cavity preparation. Describe retention and resistance form of class II cavity prepared on mandibular 1st molar for dental amalgam restoration. [MUHS]
33. Compare and contrast cavity for class II amalgam and gold restorations. [GOA]
34. Define cavity. Define cavity preparation. What factors will you take into consideration while deciding outline form for class II cavity preparation for amalgam restoration. [MUHS]
35. Discuss the principles of cavity preparation as applicable to current restorative dentistry practise. [MUHS]

Short Essays

1. Non-carious destruction of teeth. [RGUHS]
2. Tooth separators. [RGUHS]
3. Circumferential tie. [RGUHS]
4. Management of deep and shallow cavity. [RGUHS]
5. Enamel bevels. [RGUHS]
6. Retention form for class II amalgam restorations. [RGUHS]
7. Outline form. [NTR-NR]
8. Micro abrasion. [NTR-NR]
9. Causes of wasting diseases of teeth. [NTR-NR]
10. Convenience form in cavity preparation for amalgam restoration. [MUHS]
11. Various cavity designs for class II amalgam restorations. [RGUHS]
12. Abrasion lesions. [RGUHS]
13. Bevels. [MUHS; RGUHS; NTRUHS; RGUHS]
14. Mention causes of Hypersensitivity and management of the same. [RGUHS]
15. Write briefly on the causative factors cervical erosive lesions. Discuss the different treatment modalities for cervically eroded lesions. [GOA]
16. Classification of cavities. [MUHS]
17. Obtaining retention form of class I, II amalgam and class I inlay. [MUHS]
18. Retention form. [NTR-OR]
19. Enameloplasty. [MUHS]
20. Reverse Class II amalgam restoration. [MUHS]
21. Theories of hypersensitivity. [NTRUHS]
22. Steps in cavity preparation. [NTRUHS]
23. Types of direct filling gold and condensation of gold foil. [RGUHS]
24. Trephination. [RGUHS]

25. Enumerate different bevels write about bevels used in cast restoration. [RGUHS]
26. Minimal intervention dentistry. [NTRUHS]
27. Cervical lesions. [NTRUHS]
28. Pit and fissure caries. [RGUHS]
29. Significance of gingival seat in class II cavity. [NTRUHS]
30. GV black's classification of cavity. [RGUHS]
31. Objectives of cavity preparation for restoration. [MUHS]
32. Rake angle. [RGUHS]
33. Classify and describe hand cutting Instruments. [RGUHS]

Short Notes

1. Cavity design for class II inlay. [TN]
2. Cavity class II. [RGUHS]
3. Retention form. [RGUHS; RGUHS]
4. Prophylactic odontomy. [RGUHS]
5. Cavosurface angle. [RGUHS]
6. Mat Gold. [NTRUHS]
7. Tarnish and corrosion. [NTRUHS]
8. Air abrasion. [NTRUHS; RGUHS]
9. Smear layer. [NTRUHS]
10. Cavity preparation. [RGUHS]
11. Electralloy. [RGUHS]
12. Differences between class II amalgam and inlay cavity preparation. [TN]
13. Microabrasion. [RGUHS]
14. Attrition, Abrasion and Erosion. [TN]
15. Air abrasion in operative dentistry. [RGUHS]
16. Reverse curve. [RGUHS; NTRUHS; RGUHS; RGUHS]
17. General features of an inlay cavity. [TN]
18. Isthmus. [MUHS]
19. External outline form. [NTR-NR]
20. Reverse curve. [NTR-NR]
21. Abrasion. [NTR-NR; TN]
22. Retention form in class II cavity for silver amalgam. [MUHS]
23. Convenience form. [RGUHS; NTR-NR]
24. Abfraction. [NTR-NR]
25. Gold foil. [RGUHS; RGUHS]
26. Reverse bevels. [MUHS; NTRUHS]
27. AB fraction. [NTRUHS]
28. Tunnel preparation. [RGUHS]
29. Cervical resorption. [RGUHS]
30. Mat gold. [RGUHS]
31. Hatchet. [RGUHS]
32. Bur design. [RGUHS]
33. Ultra speed. [RGUHS]
34. Angle former. [RGUHS]
35. Sharpening of hand instruments. [RGUHS]
36. Aerotar. [RGUHS]
37. Gingival marginal trimmer. [RGUHS]
38. Rake angle. [NTR-NR]
39. Hypersensitivity. [MUHS]
40. Pit and fissure sealants. [RGUHS]
41. Proximal box preparation in class II cavity. [TN]
42. Modified, cavity preparation in composite. [TN]
43. Retention, resistance forms. [TN]
44. Bevels. [MUHS; TN]
45. Trephination. [TN]
46. Bevels in cavity preparation. [TN]
47. Importance and types of bevels. [GOA]
48. Mouth mirror. [RGUHS]

BASIC CONCEPTS IN AESTHETIC DENTISTRY AND ADHESION TO TOOTH STRUCTURE

Long Essays

1. Discuss aesthetics in dentistry. Write in detail about colour interpretation and colour phenomenon. [GOA]
2. Classify endodontic instruments. Describe the rationale of endodontic therapy 6. Finishing and polishing procedures for posterior restorations. [RGUHS]
3. Write about various tooth colour filling materials used in the field of conservative dentistry. [RGUHS]
4. Write in detail the management of an adult central incisor with a fractured mesial angle and no pulpal involvement. [GOA]
5. Discuss various techniques of vital bleaching. [RGUHS]
6. Classify the polyacrylic acid bond cement and describe its mechanism of adhesion to enamel and dentine. [RGUHS, BUHS]
7. Management of discoloured teeth. [NTRUHS]
8. Classify stains. Discuss various techniques for vital bleaching. [NTRUHS]
9. Define contact area. Describe the importance of contact and contours in restorative dentistry. How would you get a good contact for various restorative materials? [GOA]
10. Mention various anterior restoration materials and describe a technique of restoring Class III cavity while using anyone of them. [RGUHS]

11. Define bleaching and various methods of bleaching and state the indication for bleaching. [RGUHS]
12. Discuss in detail the management of proximal caries in respect to upper anterior teeth. [RGUHS]
13. Discuss about the various tooth coloured restorative materials used in conservative dentistry. [TN]

Short Essays

1. Acid etching on enamel. [NTR-OR; RGUHS; MUHS]
2. Interim restoration. [NTRUHS]
3. Night guard bleaching. [RGUHS]
4. Resin cements. [RGUHS]
5. Vital bleaching. [NTRUHS; RGUHS]
6. Laminates and veneers. [RGUHS]
7. Composition and mechanism of action of dentine bonding agents. [RGUHS]
8. Acid etch technique. [RGUHS; NTR-OR; MUHS]
9. Walking bleach. [RGUHS]
10. Dentine bonding agents. [NTR-OR; NTRUHS; RGUHS]
11. Cavity liners. [NTR-OR; NTR-NR]
12. Bilayered technique. [NTR-NR]
13. Luting cements. [NTR-NR]
14. Uses of zinc oxide eugenol cement. [NTR-NR]
15. Veneering materials. [NTR-NR]
16. Modified zinc oxide eugenol cement. [NTR-OR]
17. Glass cerment cements. [NTR-OR]
18. Zinc phosphate cement. [NTR-OR]
19. Bonding agents. [RGUHS OR & NR]
20. Finishing and polishing of composite restorations. [RGUHS]
21. Uses of zinc oxide eugenol cement. [NTR-NR]
22. Veneers. [NTR-NR]
23. Acid etching. [NTR-OR]
24. Calcium hydroxide. [NTR-NR]
25. Discuss the various tooth coloured restorative materials used in conservative dentistry. [GOA]
26. EDTA [NTR-OR]
27. Zinc polycarboxylate cement. [NTR-OR]
28. Inactivators. [NTR-OR]
29. Intermediate restorative materials. [NTR-OR]
30. Silicate cement. [NTR-OR]
31. Contacts and contours. [NTRUHS]
32. Bonding agents. [NTR-OR; MUHS; RGUHS]
33. Dentine bonding. [NTR-NR; RGUHS]
34. Dental bonding agent. [RGUHS]
35. Bilayered restoration. [RGUHS]
36. Direct composite veneers. [NTR-NR]
37. Lasers in dentistry. [NTR-NR]
38. Write about various tooth colour filling materials used in the field of conservative dentistry. [RGUHS]

Short Notes

1. Dentine bonding agents. [GOA; TN]
2. Veneers. [RGUHS; RGUHS; TN]
3. Hue. [TN]
4. Acid resistant pulp protective. [TN]
5. IMR. [RGUHS]
6. Effects of acid etching on enamel and dentine. [NTRUHS]
7. Composition and uses of zinc phosphate cement. [TN]
8. Laminate veneers. [TN]
9. Define cavity sealer, liner and base. [RGUHS]
10. Temporary restorative materials. [RGUHS]
11. Cavity varnish. [RGUHS]
12. Vital tooth bleaching. [RGUHS]
13. Incisal lapping preparation for veneers. [RGUHS]
14. Types and definition of adhesion. [RUGHS]
15. Dentine bonding. [TN]
16. Biocompatible materials. [TN]
17. Thermal test for pulp vitality. [TN]
18. Types of veneers. [TN]
19. Contact and contours. [NTRUHS]
20. Suspension liners vs. solution liners. [TN]
21. Direct veneer. [RGUHS]
22. Calcium hydroxide. [NTRUHS]
23. Laminates and veneers. [RGUHS]
24. Bases and liners. [NTRUHS; TN]
25. Enumerate generations of bonding agents. [NTRUHS]
26. Ultrasonic endodontics. [MUHS]
27. K-file. [MUHS]
28. Walking bleach. [NTRUHS; GOA; RGUHS]
29. Colour and shade matching. [GOA]
30. EDTA. [RGUHS]
31. Adhesive cement. [MUHS]
32. Dentine adhesives. [RGUHS]
33. Lasers. [RGUHS; NTR-NR]
34. Causes of discoloured teeth and their management. [GOA]
35. Enumerate tooth coloured veneering material. [NTR- NR]
36. Cavity liners. [TN]
37. Miracle mixtures. [TN]
38. Hybrid layer in dentine bonding. [TN]
39. Smear layer. [NTR-NR]
40. Bonding agents. [RGUHS; MUHS; TN]
41. Fissure sealants. [RGUHS]
42. Cerestore. [NTR-NR]
43. Dentine bonding systems. [GOA]
44. Polyalkenoate cements. [TN]

COMPOSITE RESIN RESTORATIONS

Long Essays

1. Give indications for composite resins. Describe the procedure of restoring fractured incisal angle. [NTR-NR]
2. Give the indication and contraindication of composite resin restoration. Describe the procedure for a composite restoration of an incisal 1/3 rd fracture. [TN]
3. Define composite resin. Classify, give clinical management of angle fractures without pulp exposure. [MUHS]
4. What are the advantages of composite resin restoration materials? Describe the procedure for acid etching and restoring a cavity with composite resin. [RGUHS]
5. Discuss the important clinical aspects of composite resin in restorative practice. [MUHS]
6. Compare and contrast composite resins with silicate cement. [MUHS]
7. Describe in detail the extended use of composites in aesthetic restorations. [RGUHS, BUHS]
8. Mention inductions and contraindications for composite resins. Describe the procedure of restoring fractured incisal angle in a maxillary incisor tooth. [RGUHS]
9. Describe composite resin in detail. [TN]
10. Discuss in detail the materials and various steps involved in placing a composite resin restoration mesioincisally fractured upper central incisor. [TN]
11. Describe the composite resin restoration in a class II fracture maxillary central incisor. [TN]
12. Define composites. Classify and write its composition. How will you manage a mesio-angular fracture of an upper central right incisor not involving the pulp of a patient aged 14 years? [RGUHS]
13. Describe the technique of restoring a fractured mesioincisal angle of 11 using composite resin. [TN]
14. What are the advantages of composite resin restoration materials? Describe the procedure for acid etching and restoring a cavity with composite resin. [RGUHS]
15. Describe class III and class V cavity preparation for composites. Discuss in brief the steps for restoring the same. [MUHS]
16. Define dental composites, classify, enumerate various indications and contraindications. Describe the restoration of class III cavity using composite resin restoration. [TN]
17. What are the indications and contra-indications for use of composite restorative material? Describe the procedure for a composite restoration of an incisal I/3rd fracture. [TN]
18. Enumerate various tooth coloured restoration materials. Describe the restoration techniques for light cure composite resin restoration. [MUHS]
19. Define composite. Classify and write its composition. How will you manage a mesioangular fracture of an upper left central incisor not involving the pulp of a patient aged 14 years? [TN]
20. Describe the technique of restoring a fractured incisal angle with composite resin. Add a note on posterior composite. [GOA]
21. Enumerate various uses of dental composite resin. Describe the restoration of class III cavity using composite resin restoration. [RGUHS]
22. Discuss status of composite resins as a posterior restorative material. [NTR-NR]
23. Classify composites. Describe the step-by-step procedure for an incisal build up for a fractured incisor involving only enamel. [TN]
24. What are tooth coloured restorations? Describe the properties of management and clinical performance of composite resins. [GOA]

Short Essays

1. Posterior composites - advantages and disadvantages. [RGUHS]
2. Give indications for composite resins. Describe the procedure of restoring fractured incisal angle. [NTR- NR]
3. Composites. [NTRUHS]
4. Polymerisation shrinkage. [RGUHS]
5. Microfilled composites. [RGUHS]
6. Classify dental composites discuss the properties manipulation and clinical performance of microfilled resins. [GOA]
7. Classify composite resins. [MUHS]
8. Types of fillers used in composite resins. [NTR-OR]
9. What are the advantages of composite resin restoration materials? Describe the procedure for acid etching and restoring a cavity with composite resin. [BUHS; RGUHS]
10. Types of fillers used in composite resins. [NTR-OR]
11. Describe in detail the extended use of composites in aesthetic restorations. [BUHS]
12. Classify composite resins. Write a note on nano composites. [RGUHS]
13. Methods of curing composite. [RGUHS]
14. Posterior composites. [RGUHS]
15. Discuss status of composite resins as a posterior restorative material. [NTR-NR]

16. Visible light cured composites.   [NTR-NR]

Short Notes

1. Packable composites.   [RGUHS]
2. Failures in composite restorations.   [RGUHS; TN]
3. Acid-etch technique.   [MUHS]
4. Hybrid layer.   [RGUHS]
5. Filler in composites.   [RGUHS]
6. Hybridization.   [RGUHS]
7. Finishing and polishing of composite restorations.
                                                     [RGUHS]
8. Microfilled composites.   [RGUHS; TN]
9. Etching.   [MUHS]

10. Bonding.   [RGUHS]
11. Acid etch technique.   [RGUHS]
12. Composite restorative materials.   [RGUHS]
13. Self-etching primers.   [RGUHS]
14. Posterior composites.   [NTRUHS; TN]
15. Acid etching and conditioning.   [MUHS]
16. Compomers.   [RGUHS]
17. Resin matrix.   [MUHS]
18. Acid etching.   [GOA; TN]
19. Light cure composite.   [RGUHS]
20. Advantages of light cure composite resin.   [MUHS]
21. Fillers and their role in composite resin.   [GOA]
22. Classify composite resins.   [MUHS]

GLASS IONOMER RESTORATIONS

Long Essays

1. Classify cements depending on their uses in restorative dentistry. Write down the composition, classification, manipulation and properties of conventional glass ionomer cement.   [MUHS]
2. Classify dental cements. Give the composition, manipulation and uses of poly carboxylate cement.
                                                     [MUHS]
3. Give the composition, manipulation and uses of glass ionomer cement.   [MUHS]
4. Discuss various factors considered prior to selection of a restorative material.   [MUHS]
5. What are the clinical indications for glass ionomer cements? What do you understand by 'sandwich technique'? Write in detail tooth preparation and restoration of class V erosion lesion in a posterior tooth.
                                                     [BUHS]
6. Write the composition of glass ionomer cements. Describe the procedure of restoring abrasive defect (class V restoration).   [BUHS]
7. What are tooth coloured restorations? Discuss anyone in detail.   [MUHS]
8. What is the ideal requirement of an aesthetic restorative material? How far the 'type of composite resins' fulfill this requirement.   [MUHS]
9. Compare and contrast composite resins with silicate cement.   [MUHS]
10. Describe merits and demerits of glass ionomer cement diagnosis applications in restorative dentistry. [NTR-NR]
11. Describe the techniques of restoring erosion lesions in a maxillary first premolar with glass ionomer cement.

Add a note on advantages and disadvantages of glass ionomer in dentistry.   [NTR-NR; RGUHS]
12. What are poly acrylate cements? Write about extended uses of glass ionomer.   [RGUHS]

Short Essays

1. Hybrid ionomer.   [NTR-OR, NTR-NR]
2. Type II glass ionomer cement.   [NTR-OR]
3. Glass ionomer cement.   [NTR-OR; NTR-OR; MUHS]
4. Type I and II inlay casting wax.   [MUHS]
5. Glass ionomer cement.   [NTR-NR]
6. Cavity varnishes and liners.   [MUHS]
7. Classification of glass ionomers.   [RGUHS]
8. Uses of glass ionomers.   [RGUHS]
9. Hybrid glass ionomer.   [RGUHS]
10. Resin modified GIC.   [RGUHS]
11. Mention the uses of glass ionomer cement and a note on its biocompatibility.   [RGUHS]
12. Write briefly on the composition of glass ionomers. What are the clinical advantages of glass ionomer cements? Classify intracanal medicaments used in endodontics.
                                                     [GOA]
13. Microfilled resins.   [MUHS]

Short Notes

1. Glass ionomer cement.   [RGUHS; TN]
2. Bilayered restoration.   [TN; RGUHS]
3. Metal modified glass ionomer cement.   [TN]
4. Recent advances in glass ionomer cements. [RGUHS]
5. Resin modified glass ionomers.   [RGUHS]
6. Sandwich technique.   [NTRUHS]

7. Sandwich restoration. [TN]
8. Resin reinforced glass ionomer cement. [GOA]
9. Hybrid glass ionomer cement. [TN]
10. Biocompatibility of glass ionomer cements. [TN]
11. Glass ionomer. [GOA]
12. Pulp responses to glass ionomer cements. [RGUHS]
13. Composition of glass ionomer cement. [MUHS]
14. Composition of inlay wax. [MUHS]
15. What is the composition of dental porcelain? Mention difference of manipulation. [BUHS]
16. Advantages and disadvantages of conventional and metal banded porcelain. [RGUHS]
17. Blue inlay wax. [MUHS]
18. Acid etching. [TN]
19. Tarnish and corrosion. [MUHS]
20. Reinforced glass ionomer. [RGUHS]
21. Uses of glass ionomer cement. [TN]
22. Calcium hydroxide. [MUHS]
23. Glass ionomer cement. [MUHS]
24. Inlay casting wax. [MUHS]
25. Types of glass ionomer cements and uses. [MUHS]
26. Resin modified glass ionomers. [MUHS]
27. Cavity varnishes and cavity liners. [MUHS]

DENTAL CERAMIC RESTORATIONS

Long Essays

1. Describe merits and demerits of glass ionomer cement diaSnosis ^P^tions in restorative dentistry. [NTR-OR]
2. Types, composition role of ingredients, methods of firing and shrinking of ceramics. [TN]
3. What is the composition of dental porcelain? Mention difference of manipulation. [BUHS]
4. Advantages and disadvantages of conventional and metal banded porcelain. [RGUHS]
5. What are the advantages and disadvantages of porcelain? Describe how the firing shrinkage in porcelain is compensated. [RGUHS]

Short Essays

1. Aluminous porcelain. [BUHS]

2. Porcelain teeth. [NTR-OR]
3. Percolation. [NTR-OR]
4. Porcelain bonded to metal. [RGUHS]
5. Ceramics. [NTR-NR]
6. CAD-CAM. [NTR-NR]

Short Notes

1. Dicor. [RGUHS; NTR-NR; TN]
2. Porcelain laminates. [RGUHS]
3. Dental porcelain. [RGUHS]
4. Shade matching for ceramics. [TN]
5. Ceramics - composition and condensation. [RGUHS]
6. Inceram. [RGUHS]
7. CAD/CAM. [NTRUHS]
8. Castable ceramics. [RGUHS; RGUHS]

AMALGAM RESTORATIONS

Long Essays

1. How will you achieve separation of tooth in operative procedures. [MUHS]
2. Write in detail about class II cavity preparation for amalgam restoration in upper 1st molar. Discuss the metrics of high copper alloy. [TN]
3. Write differences in Class II cavity for silver amalgam and gold inlay? [NTR-NR]
4. Outline the cavity preparation for class II silver amalgam restoration. [RGUHS]
5. Define retention and resistance form Describe the technique of obtaining the same for the class II cavity for silver amalgam? [NTR-NR]
6. Outline the cavity preparation for class II silver amalgam restoration? [RGUHS]
7. Describe class II cavity preparation for silver amalgam with emphasis on modern concepts? [NTR-OR]
8. Describe the technique of class II cavity I preparation for silver amalgam in an upper first molar. Mention the advantages of high copper amalgam? [NTR-NR]
9. Composition of high copper amalgam? [RGUHS]

10. Define dental amalgam. Mention the advantages and disadvantages of dental amalgam enumerate the reasons for failure of amalgam restorations. [RGUHS]
11. Discuss in detail manipulation of silver amalgam. Add a note on high copper amalgam. [NTRUHS]
12. Discuss the step-wise clinical manipulation of silver amalgam. [RGUHS (RS)]
13. Describe the causes of failure of amalgam restorations. [RGUHS (OS)]
14. Finishing and polishing procedures for posterior rest orations. [RGUHS]
15. Write in detail classification and steps in manipulation of silver amalgam. [MUHS]
16. Define reinforced restorations. Give advantages and disadvantages of pins. Describe placement of times pins for amalgam restorations. [MUHS]
17. Write in detail the class II cavity preparation for silver amalgam restoration and a not a usage of Hand cutting instruments? [NTR-OR]
18. Describe indication, contraindications, advantages, disadvantages of pin retain amalgam restoration. [MUHS]
19. Discuss the various treatment modality of a cervically eroded lesions in a lower 1st permanent molar. [MUHS]
20. Discuss hypersensitive Dentine in relation to its mechanism and management. [MUHS]
21. Discuss pins in restorative dentistry. [MUHS]
22. Define contact area? Describe the importance of contact and contour in restorative dentistry. How would you get a good contact point for various restorative material? [MUHS]
23. Describe briefly the polishing procedure for amalgam? [BUHS]
24. Define cavity preparation. Describe the outline form for silver amalgam restoration? [NTR-OR]
25. Define cavity, cavity preparation and prepared cavity. Discuss preparation of class II M.O cavity on a permanent mandibular first molar for amalgam. [RGUHS]
26. Classify silver alloys. Discuss the properties and importance of admixed alloy. [MUHS]
27. Write causes of failures of Amalgam restoration and how will you manage them. [MUHS]
28. Describe the aetiology and treatment of pain in the tooth after placing restoration. [MUHS]
29. Describe the technique of class II cavity preparations for silver amalgam in mandibular 1st molar? [NTR-OR]
30. Define 'dental matrix' and classify various types of dental matrix and enumerate ideal properties of dental matrix. [MUHS]
31. What are the principles covering the restoration from endodontically treated teeth. Describe the restoration given for endodontically treated tooth. [MUHS]
32. Describe in detail conservative class II preparation in amalgam in maxillary molar tooth. [RGUHS]
33. Describe in detail the modern method of class II cavity preparation of silver amalgam restoration. [RGUHS]
34. Describe the features of a class II mesioocclusal and molar in a adult for dental amalgam restoration. [RGUHS]
35. Define dental matrix, classify matrices. How would you obtain an ideal contact and contour for. [MUHS]
    A. Class II amalgam restoration
    B. Cast gold inlay.

Short Essays

1. Mercury hygiene? [NTR-OR, NTR-NR; RGUHS]
2. High copper amalgam? [NTR-OR; NTR-NR]
3. Gamma-2 phase of amalgam? [RGUHS]
4. Delayed expansion. [MUHS]
5. Mercury toxicity? [NTR-NR]
6. Mercuroscopic expansion. [RGUHS OR & NR]
7. Casting defects. [RGUHS]
8. High copper amalgam composition, manipulation and setting reaction. [RGUHS]
9. Finishing and polishing of posterior restoration. [RGUHS]
10. Trituration and condensation of silver amalgam. [RGUHS]
11. Condensation of amalgam. [NTRUHS]
12. Retentive pins. [MUHS]
13. Objective and indications of separation. [MUHS]
14. How will you achieve slow separation. [MUHS]
15. List the advantages of high copper amalgam. Mention the basis rules for class II cavity preparation for silver amalgam restoration add a note on mercury hygiene. [GOA]
16. Delayed expansion of amalgam? [NTR-OR]
17. Retro-grade amalgam filling. [MUHS]
18. Describe the various concepts of cavity design for amalgam restorations? [BUHS]
19. Dental amalgam. [MUHS]
20. Corrosion. [MUHS]
21. Retention for silver amalgam? [NTR-OR]
22. Mercuroscopic expansion? [NTR-OR; MUHS]
23. Preamalgamated alloy. [MUHS]
24. What is modem amalgam restoration? [MUHS]
25. Tarnish and corrosion. [MUHS]
26. High Copper Amalgam alloys. [MUHS]
27. Marginal leakage. [MUHS]
28. Finishing and polishing of amalgam restoration? [NTR-NR; RGUHS]
29. Metallurgy of silver amalgam? [NTR-NR]
30. Composition of high copper amalgam. [RGUHS]

31. Retention and resistance form for class II cavity for amalgam. [RGUHS]
32. Advantages of High copper amalgam? [NTR-NR]
33. Discuss in detail about mercury hygiene and add a note on high copper alloys. [GOA]
35. Phases of amalgam reaction. [MUHS]
36. Classify silver alloys write in detail the procedure for a Cl.II silver amalgam restoration. [GOA]

Short Notes

1. Hygroscopic expansion. [RGUHS]
2. High copper Amalgam. [RGUHS; TN]
3. Delayed expansion. [RGUHS; NTRUHS; MUHS; TN]
4. Steps in manipulation of amalgam. [TN]
5. Zinc free amalgam. [NTRUHS]
6. High copper amalgam. [RGUHS, TN]
7. Dental amalgam-definition and classification. [RGUHS]
8. Eames technique? [NTR-NR; RGUHS]
9. Mulling. [RGUHS]
10. Resistance form in class II cavity for silver amalgam. [MUHS]
11. Original gamma phase. [RGUHS, BUHS]
12. Marginal leakage of restorations. [RGUHS; BUHS]
13. Finishing and polishing of silver amalgam. [NTR-OR]
14. Marginal integrity of restorations. [RGUHS, BUHS]
15. Causes of failure of amalgam restorations. [RGUHS]
16. Mercury hygiene. [GOA; TN]
17. Butt join in amalgam restorations. [NTRUHS]
18. Back pressure porosity. [RGUHS]
19. Trituration. [RGUHS]
20. Role of matrix and wedges. [MUHS]
21. Tarnishing and corrosion. [NTR-OR; NTRUHS; MUHS]
22. Reverse curve. [MUHS]
23. Reinforced amalgam restoration. [MUHS]
24. Functions of matrix band. [MUHS]
25. Micro leakage around restoration. [TN]
26. Causes of failure of silver amalgam restoration. [TN]
27. Hypersensitive dentine management. [MUHS]
28. Resin matrix. [MUHS]
29. Properties of high copper amalgam alloys. [MUHS]
30. Delayed expansion of dental amalgam. [MUHS]
31. Rapid separators. [MUHS]
32. Tarnish and corrosion in amalgam. [TN]
33. Delayed expansion. [RGUHS]
34. Retro-grade amalgam. [TN]
35. Finishing and polishing of amalgam restoration. [NTR-NR]
36. Non-gamma 2 amalgam. [TN]
37. Importance of buccal contours. [MUHS]
38. Mercury toxicity. [RGUHS]
39. Non-Gamma phase. [RGUHS, BUHS]
40. Mercuroscopic expansion. [MUHS; TN]
41. Finishing and polishing of posterior restoration. [RGUHS]
42. Mulling of amalgam. [RGUHS]
43. Matrices. [MUHS]
44. Composition of High copper amalgam. [RGUHS]
45. Classification of silver alloys. [MUHS]
46. Gamma-II phase. [RGUHS]
47. High copper alloy. [RGUHS; MUHS]
48. Cavity bevels. [MUHS]
49. Wedges. [MUHS]
50. Matrices / retainers. [MUHS]

PIN-RETAINED RESTORATIONS

1. Classify pins what factors will you consider before using pins for an amalgam restoration in a badly mutilated tooth? Describe procedure of fixing threaded pin. [RGUHS]
2. Classify pins. Write in detail self threaded pins. [TN]
3. Give indications for pins in restorations. Briefly describe the technique. [RGUHS]

Short Essays

1. Self shearing pins. [NTR-OR]
2. T.M.S pins. [NTR-OR]
3. Pins in amalgam restoration. [NTRUHS]
4. Pin retained restoration. [RGUHS]
5. Thread mate system pins. [RGUHS]
6. Core material. [RGUHS]
7. Classify pins discuss in detail the causes of failure of pin retained amalgam restorations. [GOA]

Short Notes

1. Self treading pins. [TN]
2. Types of pin in amalgam restoration. [RGUHS; TN]
3. Pin retained restoration. [TN]
4. Post and core. [RGUHS]
5. Self shearing pin. [RGUHS; NTR-NR]
6. Retention pins. [TN]
7. Pin amalgam. [RGUHS]
8. Classifications of pins. [TN]
9. Amalgapin. [RGUHS]
10. Friction lock pins. [RGUHS]
11. TMS pins. [GOA; GOA]

CAST METAL RESTORATIONS

Long Essays

1. What are the various methods of determining working length? Write in detail Ingle's method of determining working length. [RGUHS]
2. Define cast restoration. Mention indication, contraindications, advantages and disadvantages of a cast restoration. Outline the different between class II amalgam and inlay cavity preparation. [TN]
3. What is an inlay? Discuss in detail the differences in class II cavity preparation for an inlay and for a silver amalgam restoration. [RGUHS]
4. Define inlay. Mention indications contraindications and various designs for inlay cavity. Discuss box preparation in detail. [RGUHS]
5. Describe the cavity preparation for class II gold inlay in maxillary first permanent molar. [RGUHS]
6. Enumerate and describe casting defects. [MUHS]
7. Describe in detail the class II mesio-occlusal cavity preparation for a gold inlay on a mandibluar first molar tooth? [RGUHS]
8. What are the indications for gold inlay? Describe the cavity preparation for class II gold inlay in upper first molar? [NTR-NR]
9. Give indications for cast gold restoration. [MUHS]
10. Write differences in class II cavity for silver amalgam and gold inlay? [NTR-NR]
11. Give indication for gold inlay. Describe class II cavity preparation for gold inlay in a molar tooth? [RGUHS]
12. Discuss in detail the differences between cast gold inlay preparation and amalgam preparation. [GOA]
13. Classify sprue formers. Write in detail important considerations for the same in casting procedures. [MUHS]
14. Classify casting defects. Describe in detail the mesio occlusal cavity preparation for gold inlay on mandibular first molar tooth. [RGUHS]
15. Define an inlay. Write the differences between a class II inlay cavity preparation and a class II cavity preparation for a silver amalgam restoration. [TN]
16. What is an 'indirect' restoration? Describe the indication, contraindications, advantages and disadvantages of a cast gold restoration. How do you prepare a class 2 MO cavity for a gold inlay on maxillary first molar? [TN]
17. Describe the class II cavity preparation for gold inlay and preparation of direct wax pattern? [NTR-OR]
18. Discuss the different cavity design for class II cavities for cast gold restorations. [RGUHS]
19. Give induction for gold inlay. Describe the differences in cavity preparations between silver amalgam and gold inlay? [NTR-OR]
20. Define inlay how you will prepare an inlay for a class II cavity. Classify intracanal medicaments used in endodontics. [GOA]
21. What are the various modification in inlay preparation illustrated. Give their indication, advantages and disadvantages. [MUHS]
22. Define Inlay. Describe the indications, contraindications, advantages and disadvantages of cast gold restorations? [NTR-OR]
23. Write in detail the class II cavity preparation for gold inlay and how do you proceed to take direct wax pattern? [NTR-OR]
24. What is an 'Inlay'? How will you prepare a class II cavity on maxillary 1st molar, for cast gold restorations. [RGUHS]
25. Mention the various sectors that contribute for retention's of cast restorations. Describe the procedure of taking direct wax pattern after cavity preparation is completed. [RGUHS]
26. Write in detail the procedure of taking a direct wax pattern in a MOD cavity in tooth no. 26 after cavity preparation is complete. Mention the precautions to be taken in avoiding distortion of wax pattern. [RGUHS]
27. Mention the defects in cast Gold restorations and what precautions will you take to prevent the same. [RGUHS]
28. Describe various casting defects in cast restorations and measures to prevent the same. [RGUHS]
29. Discuss the different cavity design for class II cavities for cast gold restorations? [BUHS]
30. Enumerate casting defects and measures to overcome them. [MUHS]
31. Describe the preparation of class II cavity for cast gold inlay in a lower 1st molar. [MUHS]
32. What are the different cast restoration on molars fabricated? Briefly give their Indications give on account of defects while fabrication. [RGUHS]
33. Mention about coronal restorations and discuss the significance. [RGUHS]
34. Describe the cavity preparation for class II gold inlay. Give the requirement of proper sprue and investing of wax pattern. [MUHS]

Short Essays

1. Bevels in cavity preparation. [NTR-OR]
2. Bevelling. [NTR-OR]

3. Write briefly on casting defects. [RGUHS]
4. Casting shrinkage. [MUHS]
5. Cavity bevels. [NTR-OR]
6. Cast gold inlay. [MUHS]
7. Management of loss of contact in cast inlay. [BUHS]
8. Disadvantages of cast restorations. [BUHS]
9. Porosity in casting. [MUHS]
10. Indications for the gold inlay. [NTR-OR]
11. Pickling. [MUHS]
12. Degassing direct gold. [NTRUHS]
13. Types of flares in inlay preparation. [RGUHS]
14. Direct wax pattern. [RGUHS]
15. Types of bevels. [NTR-NR]
16. Porosities in Gold castings and how will you rectify. [RGUHS]
17. Indications for cast gold restoration. [MUHS]
18. Casting defects. [MUHS]
19. Bevels. [NTR-OR; NTR-NR]
20. Electroforming of dies. [RGUHS]

Short Notes

1. Blue inlay wax. [MUHS]

2. Definition indication and disadvantage of cast gold inlay. [GOA]
3. Metal ceramic restoration. [TN]
4. Reservoir. [MUHS]
5. Types of cast gold alloys. [RGUHS; RGUHS]
6. Bevel's in inlay. [MUHS]
7. Back pressure porosity. [RGUHS]
8. Onlay. [RGUHS]
9. Enumerate casting defect. [MUHS]
10. Sprues. [MUHS]
11. Composition of inlay wax. [MUHS]
12. CAD-CAM technique agent. [RGUHS]
13. Significance of reservoir. [RGUHS]
14. Casting shrinkage. [RGUHS]
15. Disadvantages of cast restorations. [RGUHS]
16. Casting defects. [RGYHS]
17. Indication and contraindications of inlay. [MUHS]
18. Back pressure porosities. [MUHS]
19. Finishing of gold inlay? [NTR-OR]
20. Phosphate bonded Investment. [RGUHS]
21. Pressure casting. [RGUHS]
22. Management of loss of contact in cast inlay. [RGUHS]

DENTAL CASTING PROCEDURES

Long Essays

1. Enumerate the casting defects and discuss in detail. [NTR-OR]
2. What are the different cast restorations on molars fabricated? Briefly give their indications give on account of defects while fabrication. [BUHS]
3. Describe various casting defects in cast restorations and measures to prevent the same. [BUHS]
4. Describe briefly the methods used in compensating casting shrinkage of gold in casting procedures. [NTR-OR]
5. Write in detail the procedure of taking a direct wax pattern in a MOD cavity in tooth no. 26 after cavity preparation is complete. Mention the precautions to be taken in avoiding distortion of wax pattern. [BUHS]
6. Mention the defects in cast gold restorations and what precautions will you take to prevent the same. [BUHS]
7. Discuss the causes of casting defects and their prevention. [RGUHS]
8. Classify casting defects. Describe in detail the mesio occlusal cavity preparation for gold inlay on mandibular first molar tooth. [RGUHS; RGUHS]

9. What are porosities in casting? How will you prevent them. [TN]
10. Classify dental investments write in detail about failures of casting. [GOA]

Short Essays

1. Porosities in Gold castings and how will you rectify? [RGUHS]
2. Electroforming of dies? [RGUHS]
3. Investment material? [NTR-OR]
4. Write briefly on casting defects. [RGUHS]
5. Inlay wax? [NTR-OR]
6. Advantages and disadvantages indirect wax pattern? [NTR-OR]
7. Sub surface porosity in gold alloy castings? [NTR-OR]
8. Gypsum bonded investment material? [NTR-OR]
9. Casting techniques? [NTR-OR]
10. Casting machines? [NTR-OR, NTR-NR]
11. Porosities in dental castings? [NTR-OR]
12. Sprue? [NTR-OR]
13. Casting defects. [RGUHS]
14. Suck back porosity. [RGUHS]
15. Porosities in castings. [NTR-OR; NTRUHS]

16. Die materials. [RGUHS]
17. Discuss the shortcoming of dental casting procedure in inlay preparation how will you overcome the same. [GOA]
18. Intracanal medicaments. [RGUHS]
19. Sprue and sprue former. [NTR-NR]
20. Sprue former? [NTR-NR]

Short Notes

1. Sprue. [TN]
2. Dies. [TN]
3. Inlay wax. [TN]
4. Casting shrinkage of cast gold alloy and its compensations. [TN]
5. Inlay wax pattern. [TN]
6. Sprue former. [NTRUHS; TN]
7. Annealing. [RGUHS]
8. Casting defects? [BUHS; TN]
9. Investment of casting. [TN]
10. Back pressure priority? [RGUHS; GOA; TN]

11. Investment material. [NTRUHS]
12. Porosity. [TN]
13. Direct wax pattern for inlay. [TN]
14. Onlay. [RGUHS]
15. Reservoir? [RGUHS; TN]
16. Phosphate bonded Investment? [RGUHS, BUHS]
17. Pressure casting? [RGUHS, BUHS]
18. Significance of reservoir? [RGUHS, BUHS]
19. Disadvantages of cast restorations. [RGUHS]
20. Investment procedure. [TN]
21. Pinhole porosity. [TN]
22. Casting shrinkage? [RGUHS, BUHS; TN]
23. Back pressure porosity in gold. [GOA]
24. Pickling. [TN]
25. Gypsum bonded investment. [TN]
26. Gutta-percha. [RGUHS]
27. Root canal sealer. [RGUHS]
28. Hydrogen peroxide. [RGUHS]
29. Types of cast Gold alloys. [RGUHS]

DIRECT FILLING GOLD RESTORATIONS

Long Essays

1. Indications for direct filling gold? [NTR-NR]
2. What are the types of direct filling gold? Describe compaction technique and its uses in dentistry. How is a gold foil restoration finished? [RGUHS]

Short Essays

1. Compaction of direct filling gold? [NTR-NR]
2. Thermoplasticized. [RGUHS]
3. Direct filling gold. [NTRUHS (OR)]

4. Indications for direct filling gold. [NTR-NR]
5. Annealing and compaction procedures in direct gold. [RGUHS]

Short Notes

1. Composition and properties of Type III Gold. [RGUHS, BUHS]
2. Direct filling gold. [BUHS, RGUHS]
3. Powdered gold. [RGUHS (RS)]
4. Annealing and compaction procedures in direct gold. [RGUHS]

MISCELLANEOUS

Long Essays

1. Enumerate the various teeth coloured restorative material. Give composition, manipulation, indications and advantages of silicate cement? [NTR-OR]
2. Mention about coronal restorations and discuss the significance? [BUHS]
3. Discuss control of pain during operative procedures. [NTR-NR]
4. State various morphological defects of tooth structure. How will you treat them. [NTR-NR]
5. Describe a method conservative restoration of fractured maxillary vital incisor teeth. [NTR-OR]

Short Essays

1. CAD-CAM. [NTR-NR]
2. Tissue conditioner. [NTR-NR]
3. Plunger cusp. [NTR-NR]
4. Tunnel preparation. [NTR-NR]
5. Disclosing solution. [NTR-NR]
6. Zinc polycarboxylate cement. [RGUHS OR & NR]
7. Implants. [NTR-NR]
8. Lasers in dentistry. [NTR-NR]
9. Luting cements. [NTR-NR]
10. Cavity varnish. [NTR-OR, NTR-NR]
11. Circumferential tie. [NTR-NR]

12. Bilayered technique. [NTR-NR]
13. Dentifrice. [NTR-NR]
14. Thermoplasticized gutta-percha. [NTR-OR]
15. Soldering. [NTR-OR]
16. Inactivators. [NTR-OR]
17. Desensitizing agents. [NTR-OR]
18. Cavity varnish and liners. [NTR-OR]
19. Slice preparation. [NTR-OR]
20. Tarnish and corrosion. [NTR-OR]
21. Cavity liners. [NTR-OR]
22. Surface hardness. [NTR-OR]

Short Notes

1. Embrasures I mention types in short. [MUHS]
2. Machined restoration. [TN]
3. Bilayered restoration. [RGUHS]
4. Indirect restorations. [RGUHS]
5. Post and core. [NTR-NR]
6. Disclosing agent. [RGUHS]
7. Phosphoric acid. [NTR-NR]
8. Modulus of elasticity. [RGUHS OR & NR]
9. Dowel. [RGUHS]
10. ART Technique. [MUHS]

CLINICAL DIAGNOSTIC AIDS IN ENDODONTICS

Long Essays

1. Discuss endodontics. [BUHS]
2. Discuss briefly the diagnostic tests used in endodontics. [RGUHS]
3. What are the diagnostic tests for assessing a tooth for endodontic treatment? Give a note on the role of radiographs in endodontics. [TN]
4. Enumerate the different diagnostic aids in endodontics. Write in detail the procedure of electrical pulp testing. Add a note on false responses. [TN]
5. Enumerate various diagnostic aids used in endodontics. Give importance of radiographs in endodontics. [MUHS]
6. Describe the methods available for testing the vitality of a tooth. Mention the situation when false negative responses occur while using the vitalometers. [RGUHS, BUHS]
7. Enumerate the various diagnostic aids in the field of operative dentistry and endodontics; discuss in detail the importance of radiographic examination and its limitation. [GOA]
8. Enumerate various diagnostic aids employed in vitality testing of the tooth discuss radiographs in detail. [RGUHS; GOA]
9. Discuss various diagnostic aids in endodontics. Add a note on limitation of the endodontic radiographs. [BUHS; TN]
10. Discuss in detail the various diagnostic methods used in endodontics. [RGUHS, BUHS]
11. Describe the various diagnostic aids employed in endodontic practice. [NTR-OR]
12. List out the various tests for determining the vitality of the teeth. Discuss in detail about thermal tests in their efficiency. [RGUHS, BUHS]
13. Discuss various diagnostic aids in endodontics. [NTRUHS]
14. Mention the various clinical diagnostic aids used in endodontics and write in detail the vitality tests. [TN]
15. Write briefly on diagnosis and treatment planning in endodontics and add a note on pulp testers. [GOA]

Short Essays

1. Limitations of radiographs. [RGUHS]
2. Thermal tests. [RGUHS]
3. Percussion test. [RGUHS]
4. Test cavity. [MUHS]
5. Endodontic steps. [BUHS]
6. Vitality tests. [RGUHS]
7. Glass bead sterilizer. [RGUHS]
8. Write in detail the various diagnostic tests for clinical diagnosis of pulpal pathology. [MUHS]
9. Indications for root canal treatment. [MUHS]
10. Diagnostic aids used in endodontia and describe electric pulp test. [RGUHS]
11. Endometer. [RGUHS]
12. Heat test. [RGUHS]
13. Radio visiography. [RGUHS]
14. Radiography in endodontic. [RGUHS]
15. Thermal vitality test. [RGUHS]
16. Pulp vitality test. [MUHS]
17. Thermal tooth vitality test. [RGUHS]
18. Electric pulp testing-false positive and false negative reading. [RGUHS]
19. Electric pulp tests. [RGUHS; RGUHS (RS2)]
20. Clarke's technique. [RGUHS]

Short Notes

1. Interpretation of intra oral radiographs. [MUHS]
2. Laser Doppler flowmetry. [GOA]

3. Radiovisiography. [RGUHS (OS); RGUHS]
4. Electric Pulp test. [NTR-OR; RGUHS (RS); TN]
5. Test cavity. [NTR-OR; RGUHS (OS)]
6. Bisecting angle testing. [TN]
7. Thermal diagnostic test. [RGUHS]
8. Heat test for tooth vitality. [RGUHS]
9. Diagnostic aids. [MUHS; TN]
10. RVG. [NTR-NR; TN]
11. Pulp vitality tests. [NTR-NR; TN]
12. Thermal test. [NTR-OR; TN]
13. Endosonics. [NTRUHS]
14. Endometric endodontics. [GOA; TN]
15. Different barrier techniques. [TN]
16. Pulpotomy. [TN]
17. Role of radiographs in endodontic practice. [NTR-NR]
18. Intra oral digital radiography. [GOA]
19. Pulp tests. [NTR-OR]

20. Percussion test. [BUHS]
21. Uses of radiographs. [MUHS]
22. Importance of buccal-object rule in radiographs. [NTR-NR]
23. Heat testing in endodontics. [TN]
24. Electrical pulp testing. [TN]
25. Radiography in endodontics. [GOA]
26. False positive and false negative responses to electric pulp tester. [NTR-NR]
27. Endodontic triad. [BUHS]
28. Radiographic examination in Endodontics. [NTR-OR]
29. Limitations of radiographs. [BUHS]
30. Thermal tooth vitality test. [RGUHS]
31. Diagnostic aids used in endodontics and describe electric pulp test. [RGUHS]
32. Thermal vitality test. [RGUHS]
33. Vitality tests. [NTR-OR; TN]

ENDODONTIC EMERGENCIES

Long Essays

1. Write clinical features of phoenix abscess and management. [RGUHS]
2. Classify endodontic emergencies and give in detail diagnosis, management and treatment of acute periapical abscess. [MUHS]
3. Enumerate the endodontic emergencies and discuss in detail and management. [RGUHS; GOA]
4. Classify the endodontic emergencies and write their effective methods of treatment. [TN]

Short Essays

1. Reversible pulpitis. [RGUHS (OR and NR)]
2. Phoenix abscess. [NTR-OR]
3. Enumerate endodontic emergencies elaborate on phoenix abscess. [GOA]
4. Discuss endodontic flare and their management. [MUHS]

Short Notes

1. Hyperemia of pulp. [RGUHS]
2. Phoenix abscess. [RGUHS, (OR and NR)]

DENTAL PULP AND THE PERIRADICULAR TISSUES: EMBRYOLOGY AND ANATOMY

Short Essays

1. Accessory canals. [RGUHS]
2. Nerve fibres of pulp. [NTRUHS]

DISEASES OF DENTAL PULP AND PERIRADICULAR TISSUES

Long Essays

1. Classify periradicular diseases. Write in detail the causes, symptoms, diagnosis, differential diagnosis, treatment and prognosis of Acute Alveolar Abscess. [MUHS]
2. Classify the pulp diseases. Give aetiology, signs and symptoms differential diagnosis and treatment of acute pulpitis. [MUHS; GOA]
3. Write clinical features of phoenix abscess and management. [RGUHS]

4. Describe pulpal necrosis and their management. [RGUHS]
5. Enumerate the various causes of pulp diseases and describe the clinical features and management of irreversible pulpitis. [RGUHS]
6. Write the different causes of pulpal diseases and describe in detail clinical features and management of irreversible pulpitis. [TN]
7. Write in detail about causes of diseases of dental pulp. In short explain reaction of dental pulp to bacterial involvement. Classify diseases of dental pulp. [MUHS]

Short Essays

1. Acute pulpitis. [MUHS]
2. Classification of pulp diseases. [MUHS]
3. Reversible pulpitis. [NTR-OR]
4. Diagnosis and treatment of apical periodontitis. [MUHS]
5. Anachoresis. [NTR-OR]
6. Internal resorption. [NTR-NR; RGUHS (OS); RGUHS]
7. Balanced force technique. [NTRUHS]
8. Irreversible pulpitis. [NTR-OR; NTRUHS; RGUHS]
9. Acute reversible pulpitis. [RGUHS]
10. Acute reriapical abscess. [NTR-NR]
11. Resorption. [RGUHS]
12. Barodontalgia. [MUHS]
13. Phoenix abscess. [NTR-OR, NTR- NR]

14. Cracked tooth syndromes. [MUHS]
15. Classify resorption. Write about internal resorption. [RGUHS]
16. Pink tooth. [NTR-NR]

Short Notes

1. Weeping canal. [RGUHS]
2. Root resorption. [NTRUHS]
3. Diagnosis of chronic irreversible pulpitis. [NTRUHS]
4. Internal root resorption. [RGUHS]
5. Barodontalgia. [RGUHS]
6. Classify periradicular diseases. [RGUHS]
7. Root resorption-diagnosis and treatment planning. [RGUHS]
8. Irreversible pulpitis. [TN]
9. Hyperemia of pulp. [BUHS]
10. Pulpitis. [RGUHS]
11. Acute apical periodontitis. [RGUHS]
12. Internal resorption. [NTR-NR]
13. Atrophy and fibrosis of pulp. [NTR-NR]
14. Calcific metamorphosis of pulp. [NTR-NR]
15. Periapical cyst. [RGUHS]
16. Phoenix abscess. [MUHS; TN]
17. Fish concept. [GOA]
18. Clinical management of apical granuloma. [TN]

PRINCIPLES AND RATIONALE OF ENDODONTIC TREATMENT

Long Essays

1. Describe rationale and principles of endodontic treatment. [NTR-OR]
2. Describe the rationale and principles of Endodontic treatment. [NTR-OR]
3. Describe various procedures to maintain tooth vitality. [RGUHS]
4. Role of calcium hydroxide and hydrocortisone in pulp therapy. [MUHS]
5. Describe in Detail rational of endodontic treatment. [NTR-OR]
6. Discuss sterilization in endodontics. [RGUHS]
7. Classify endodontic instruments. Describe the rationale of endodontic therapy. [RGUHS]
8. Describe in detail the different techniques of pulp space therapy. [GOA]
9. Describe components of rubber dam and its advantages of rubber dam in endodontics. [RGUHS]
10. Define pulpotomy. Give indications and procedures of the same in a permanent lower first molar. [NTR-OR, RGUHS]

11. What is the rationale of endodontics. Give indication and contraindications of root canal treatment. [RGUHS, BUHS]
12. Explain a tooth badly carious, sensitive to both hot and cold. Periapical X-ray showing no periapical lesion but incompletely formed roots (apices) caries very nearer to pulp horn almost looking as if pulp is involved. Write in detail about various treatment modalities to be given importance in this case. [MUHS]

Short Essays

1. Inductions and contraindications of pulpotomy. [NTRUHS]
2. Chemical means of gingival retraction. [RGUHS]
3. Apexogenesis. [NTR-OR; RGUHS]
4. Pulpotomy. [NTR-OR; RGUHS]
5. Formocresol pulpotomy. [RGUHS]
6. Apexification and apicogenesis. [RGUHS; RGUHS]
7. Describe apexification and apexogenesis. [RGUHS]
8. Rational of endodontics. [NTR-NR; NTRUHS; RGUHS]
9. Pulp capping. [NTR-NR; MUHS; RGUHS]

10. Apexification and Apexogenesis. [NTR-NR; NTRUHS]
11. Mat gold. [RGUHS]
12. Write a short notes on rationale of endodontic therapy. [RGUHS]

Short Notes

1. Uses of calcium hydroxide in endodontics. [MUHS]
2. Uses of calcium hydroxide. [MUHS]
3. Anaesthetic techniques in endodontics. [TN]
4. Apexogenesis. [RGUHS]
5. Pulp capping. [MUHS; TN]
6. Indication and contraindications of pulp capping. [MUHS]
7. Irrigation in endodontics. [TN]

8. Indirect and direct pulp capping. [GOA]
9. Describe the Principles of Endodontic Treatment. [MUHS]
10. Rubber dam. [RGUHS, BUHS]
11. Pulp capping materials. [MUHS]
12. Pain control in endodontics. [TN]
13. Pulpotomy. [RGUHS; NTRUHS; TN]
14. Sterilization of root canal instruments. [RGUHS]
15. Retraction cord. [RGUHS]
16. Hot salt sterilizer. [RGUHS]
17. Rationale of endodontics. [GOA]
18. Apexification and apexogenesis. [GOA; TN]
19. Glass bead sterilizer. [RGUHS; NTRUHS]
20. Apexification. [RGUHS; NTRUHS; MUHS; TN]
21. Indirect pulp capping. [RGUHS]

ENDODONTIC INSTRUMENTS AND STERILIZATION

Long Essays

1. Discuss sterilization in endodontics. [BUHS]
2. Classify endodontics instruments. [RGUHS]
3. Classification of endodontic instruments. Describe the hand instruments used for canal preparation. [NTR-NR]
4. Discuss the various methods of sterilization of root canal instruments. [MUHS]
5. Classify endodontic instruments. Discuss cleaning and shaping of the root canal (BMP) by step-back, crown-down pressure less and balanced force techniques. [RGUHS]
6. Describe in detail about the methods of sterilization. [TN]
7. Classify endodontic instruments. Write about standardization. Describe the rationale of endodontic therapy. [TN]
8. Classify endodontics instrument. How are they standardized. Add a note on standardization of these instruments. [RGUHS]
9. Classify endodontic instruments and briefly describe the methods of sterilization of instrument? [NTR-OR]
10. Describe the rationale of endodontics therapy. [BUHS]
11. What are the differences between K-type reamer and AK-type file. Describe the preparation of an anterior root canal with hand instrument after access cavity is prepared. [BUHS]
12. Classify endodontics instruments. Describe standardization and sterilizing of these instruments. [RGUHS; RGUHS]

Short Essays

1. Endo Sonics. [NTR-OR]
2. Classification of endodontic instruments. [NTR-OR]
3. Hedstrom files. [NTR-OR]
4. Asepsis in endodontics. [NTR-OR]
5. Advantages and disadvantages of N ITI rotary endodontic instruments. [NTR-NR]
6. Sterilization of intracanal instruments. [NTR-OR]
7. Glass bead sterilizer. [NTR-NR; NTRUHS; RGUHS]
8. Endodontic instrument standardization. [RGUHS]
9. Hedstrom file. [RGUHS]
10. Classify endodontic instruments. Elaborate on standardization and sterilization of endodontic instruments. [GOA]
11. Gates-Glidden Drill. [NTR-OR]
12. Sterilization of endodontic instruments. [RGUHS]
13. Barbed broach. [NTR-OR]
14. Classify root canal instruments describe in detail standardization of root canal instrument. [BUHS]
15. Sterilization in endodontics. [MUHS]
16. Standardization of endodontics instruments and sterilization. [RGUHS]
17. Give classification standardization and sterilization of root canal instruments in detail. [GOA]
18. Endodontic files. [NTR-NR]
19. Hot salt sterilizer. [NTR-OR; MUHS]
20. Silicone stops. [RGUHS]
21. Apical matrix. [RGUHS]
22. Standardization of Root canal instruments. [RGUHS]

Short Notes

1.	Reamers and files.	[RGUHS; TN]
2.	Giromatic handpiece.	[GOA]
3.	Hedstrom files.	[RGUHS]
4.	Gingival retraction cord.	[TN]
5.	Endodontic spreads and pluggers.	[TN]
6.	Standardization of root canal instruments.	[TN]
7.	Lentulospiral.	[RGUHS]
8.	Cross-section of reamer and file.	[NTRUHS]
9.	Locators-generations and dentine.	[NTRUHS]
10.	Spiral root fillers.	[BUHS]
11.	Spreaders and plungers.	[RGUHS]
12.	Hot salt sterilizer.	[MUHS]
13.	Gates Glidden drills.	[NTR-NR]
14.	Sterilization of root canal instruments.	[BUHS; MUHS]
15.	Disinfection.	[NTR-NR]
16.	Flexible files.	[TN]
17.	Classification of endodontic instruments.	[TN]
18.	Standardization of endo instruments and their sterilization.	[TN]
19.	Chemic laving.	[NTR-NR]
20.	Barbed broaches.	[NTR-NR]
21.	Nitinol files.	[RGUHS]
22.	Standardization of endodontic instruments.	[TN]
23.	Apex locator.	[TN]
24.	Electronic apex locators.	[GOA]
25.	H-File.	[RGUHS]
26.	Sterilisation of high speed handpiece.	[GOA]
27.	Peeso reamers.	[NTR-NR; RGUHS]
28.	Endosonics.	[NTR-NR; TN]
29.	Glass bead sterilizer.	[RGUHS]
30.	Reamer.	[RGUHS; RGUHS; TN]

ENDODONTIC MICROBIOLOGY

Long Essays

1. Describe in detail the technique of culture examination and its importance in endodontic treatment. [RGUHS]

Short Essays

1. Culture in endodontics. [BUHS; RGUHS]
2. Endodontics microbiology. Add a note on culture techniques. [NTRUHS]
3. Culture media. [RGUHS]
4. Culture technique in endodontics. [NTR-OR]
5. Culture methods in endodontics. [NTR-NR; RGUHS]

Short Notes

1. Culture tests. [RGUHS; RGUHS]
2. False positive cultures. [GOA]
3. Microbial flora of the pulp space. [GOA]
4. Culture media used in endodontics. [NTR-NR, RGUHS]
5. Culture methods and reversal. [TN]
6. Root canal flora. [TN]
7. Negative culture. [RGUHS]
8. Culturing in endodontics. [RGUHS]

TOOTH MORPHOLOGY AND ACCESS CAVITIES

Long Essays

1. Write in detail the importance and procedures of root canal. [BUHS]
2. Inactivators in culture media. [MUHS]

Short Essays

1. Apical foramen. [RGUHS]
2. Poly antibiotic paste. [MUHS]

Short Notes

1. Apical constriction. [TN]
2. Lamina drug. [TN]
3. Accessory canals. [NTR-NR]
4. Anatomy of pulp cavity of maxillary first premolar. [TN]
5. Blunderbuss canal and its management. [TN]
6. C-shaped canal configuration. [NTR-NR]

ENDODONTIC AND BIOMECHANICAL PREPARATION AND WORKING LENGTH DETERMINATION

Long Essays

1. Describe the biomechanical preparation in endodontics. [NTR-OR]

2. Describe biomechanical preparation in endodontic practice. [BUHS]

3. Discuss in detail biomechanical preparation and the recent advances. [RGUHS]

4. What are the various methods of determining working length in endodontics. [NTR-OR]

5. Describe standardization of endodontic instruments. How the breakage of instrument inside the root canal is prevented. [MUHS]

6. What do you mean by cleaning and shaping. Describe in detail the step back preparation in a maxillary right central incisor. [TN]

7. What are the rules for cleaning and shaping the root canal. Enumerate the various biomechanical preparation techniques and discuss any one technique in detail. [TN]

8. What do you understand by term working length. Discuss the various methods of determining working length. [TN]

9. Discuss various methods of working length determination in endodontics. [MUHS]

10. What are the indications of pulpectomy. Describe the technique of pulpectomy. [MUHS]

11. Classify endodontics instrument. How are they standardized. Add a note on standardization of these instruments. [RGUHS]

12. Define working length how you will calculate the working length of a tooth. [RGUHS; BUHS]

13. Write in brief about the importance of the diagnostic phase, preparatory phase and obturation phase in success of endodontic therapy. [MUHS]

14. What do you understand by cleaning and shaping of root canal. Describe the instruments used for the same. [NTR-NR]

15. Mention the differences in structure and working of the root canal instruments such as: [MUHS]
    A. Barbed broach
    B. Reamer
    C. K-type File
    D. H-type File
    E. Endosonic diamond file.

16. Define working length. Write in detail one methods of working length determination. Discuss about step back method of preparation of root canal. [TN]

17. Give the classification, standardization and sterilization of root canal instruments. [MUHS]

18. Classify endodontic instruments. Discuss cleaning and shaping of the root canal (BMP) by step-back, crown-down pressure less and balanced force techniques. [RGUHS]

19. Mention the different types of root canal preparation and importance. Describe in detail about step back techniques. [TN]

20. Describe in detail cleaning and shaping of root canal. [RGUHS]

21. Define working length of root canal and enumerate different methods of determining working length and write one of the methods in detail. [MUHS]

22. Classify endodontics instruments. Describe the rationale of endodontics therapy. [RGUHS]

23. Discuss the methods of determining working length of the root canal. [TN]

24. Classify endodontics instruments. Describe standardization and sterilizing of these instruments. [RGUHS]

25. What are the complications encountered during routine endodontic treatment. Give aetiology and management of broken instrument in root canal. [MUHS]

26. Mention the various methods used to sterilize the root canal during root canal treatment. Describe anyone method in detail. [BUHS]

27. Discuss perforations as one of the major causes in failure of endodontics treatment. [RGUHS]

28. Write in detail the importance and procedures of root canal. [RGUHS]

29. Mention the common problems encountered during anterior root canal therapy and discuss their management. [RGUHS]

30. What are the differences between a k-type reamer and AK-type file. Describe the preparation of an anterior root canal with hand instrument after access cavity is prepared. [RGUHS]

31. Mention the various irrigants used in canal preparation. Discuss the use of intracanal medication in effecting sterilization of root canals. [RGUHS]

32. Discuss in detail biomechanical preparation and the recent advances. [BUHS]

33. Mention various irrigants used in endodontics. Describe ideal properties and techniques of irrigation. [BUHS]

34. What is biomechanical preparation. Describe various method of biomechanical preparation and discuss step back preparation. [MUHS]

35. Mention the various instruments used for root canal preparation. Describe in detail the procedure of your choice to ensure the rough canal preparation. [RGUHS]

36. Mention various methods to assess the length of root canal and describe anyone of the methods. [RGUHS, BUHS]

Short Essays

1. Irrigation in root canal therapy. [NTR-NR]
2. Step Back preparation. [NTR-OR, NTR-NR; NTRUHS]
3. Crown down pressure technique. [NTR-OR]
4. Root canal plugger and spreader. [MUHS]
5. Trephination. [NTR-OR]
6. Irrigation. [NTR-NR]
7. Mechanical instrumentation in endodontic field. [RGUHS]
8. Step back method. [RGUHS]
9. Ingle's method of determining working length. [NTR- NR]
10. Access cavity. [NTR-NR]
11. Classify endodontic instruments. [MUHS]
12. Reverse curve. [MUHS]
13. Chemical preparation of root canal. [MUHS]
14. Root canal irrigants. [RGUHS]
15. RVG in endodontics. [NTR-NR]
16. H-File. [MUHS]
17. Goldman's irrigating needle. [MUHS]
18. Access cavities in lower and upper molars. [NTR-OR]
19. Importance of determining the working length of a tooth during root canal treatment. [BUHS]
20. Mention the various methods used to sterilize the root canal during root canal treatment? Describe anyone method in detail. [RGUHS]
21. Classify root canal instruments describe in detail standardization of root canal instrument. [RGUHS]
22. Irrigation of root canals. [MUHS]
23. Apical dentine plug. [RGUHS]
24. Various methods of determining the root length. [RGUHS]
25. Standardization of endodontics instruments and sterilization. [RGUHS]
26. Use of chelating agents in endodontics. [MUHS]
27. Ideal requirement of irrigants. Mention various irrigants used during root canal treatment. [RGUHS]
28. Endodontic file and reamer. [MUHS]

Short Notes

1. EDTA. [RGUHS]
2. Standardization of root canal instruments. [MUHS]
3. Radiovisiography. [BUHS]
4. Access opening. [NTR-NR]
5. Apex locators. [NTR-NR]
6. Disinfection. [NTR-NR]
7. Nitinol files. [RGUHS]
8. Gates Glidden drill. [MUHS]
9. Root canal irrigants. [MUHS]
10. Standardization of endodontics instruments. [RGUHS]
11. Giromaticus. [RGUHS]
12. Importance of determining the working length of a tooth during root canal treatment. [RGUHS]
13. Endosonics. [RGUHS]
14. Formocresol. [MUHS]
15. K files. [MUHS]
16. RVG. [NTR-NR]
17. Endodontic files. [RGUHS]
18. Peeso reamers. [RGUHS]
19. Recapitulation. [NTR-NR; MUHS; RGUHS]
20. Root canal file. [MUHS]
21. Spiral root fillers. [RGUHS]
22. Endodontic steps. [RGUHS]
23. Glutaraldehyde. [RGUHS]
24. Reamers and files. [RGUHS]
25. Intrapulpal injection. [RGUHS]
26. Spreaders and plungers. [RGUHS]
27. Root canal plugger. [MUHS]
28. Different methods for root canal length determination. [GOA]
29. Barbed broaches, sodium hypochlorite. [RGUHS]
30. Measurement of working length. [TN]
31. Sodium Hypochlorite. [MUHS]
32. Zipping. [NTRUHS]
33. Working length determination. [TN]
34. Step back technique. [RGUHS; TN]
35. Working length in endodontics. [TN]
36. Ultrasonic endodontics. [MUHS]
37. RC preparation. [RGUHS, BUHS]
38. Access cavity. [RGUHS]
39. Crown down technique. [GOA]

MATERIALS IN ENDODONTICS

Long Essays

1. Root canal sealers. [NTRUHS]
2. Describe in detail intracanal irrigants and medi cements. [TN]
3. Describe zinc oxide eugenol containing root canal sealers. [RGUHS]
4. What is the ideal requirement of irrigants. Describe in detail the various irrigants used during root canal treatment. [GOA]
5. What are the ideal requirements of an irrigant used during root canal therapy. Describe the various irrigants used. [TN]
6. What are various root canal irrigants. Write in detail requirement and technique of irrigation. [NTRUHS]
7. What are requirements of ideal root canal filling material. What are the various obturation tech-niques? Discuss any one in detail. [RGUHS]
8. What is various root canal irrigants. Write in detail ideal requirements and techniques of irrigation. [RGUHS]
9. Classify obturating materials and sealers used in root canal treatment. [RGUHS]
10. Classify and describe the various intracanal medicaments in root canal treatment. [NTR-NR]
11. Mention the various irritants used in endodontics. Describe ideal properties and techniques of irrigation. [NTR-OR]
12. Mention the various irrigants used in canal preparation. Discuss the use of intracanal medication in affecting sterilization of root canal. [BUHS]
13. Classify intercanal medicaments used in endodontics. [GOA]
14. Write about various methods of disinfecting a root canal. [TN]
15. Classify and describe the obturation materials and sealers used in root canal treatment. [NTR-NR]
16. Enumerate various intracanal medicaments and explain in detail mechanism of action of calcium hydroxide in detail. [TN]
17. Give the complete list of root canal filling materials. Describe the technique of vertical condensation. [RGUHS]

Short Essays

1. Mineral trioxide aggregate. [GOA]
2. Pulp capping agents. [NTR-OR, NTR-NR]
3. MTA. [NTR-NR]
4. CMCP. [NTR-OR]
5. Thermoplasticized gutta-percha. [NTR-OR; RGUHS]
6. Retrograde filling materials. [NTRUHS; RGUHS]
7. Bleaching agents. [NTR-OR]
8. Gutta-percha. [NTR-OR, NTR-NR; NTRUHS]
9. Intracanal irrigants in endodontics. [RGUHS]
10. Roots end filling materials. [RGUHS]
11. Inter canal medicaments. [NTRUHS]
12. Reservoir. [RGUHS]
13. Obturating materials for primary teeth. [NTR-NR]
14. Ideal requirements of root canal sealers. [NTR-NR]
15. Poly-antibiotic pastes. [NTR-OR]
16. Chelating agents used in endodontics. [RGUHS]
17. Medicaments used in endodontics. [NTRUHS]
18. Importance of irrigation. [RGUHS]
19. RC PREP. [RGUHS]
20. Sodium hypochlorite. [NTR-OR, NTR-NR; NTRUHS]
21. Calcium hydroxide. [NTR-OR]
22. EDTA. [NTR-OR]
23. Intracanal medicaments. [NTR-OR]
24. Pulpotomy medicaments. [NTR-OR]
25. Root canal irrigants. [NTR-OR]
26. Uses of calcium hydroxide in endodontics. [NTR-OR]
27. Ideal requirement of irrigants. Mention various irrigants used during root canal treatment. [BUHS]
28. Root canal seals. [BUHS, RGUHS]
29. Use of sodium hypochlorite in endodontic. [RGUHS]

Short Notes

1. Tubliseal. [RGUHS]
2. Calcium hydroxide. [TN]
3. Endodontic irrigants. [TN]
4. Ledermix. [RGUHS]
5. H-files. [NTRUHS]
6. Hank balanced salt solution. [NTRUHS]
7. Carbamide peroxide. [NTR-NR; NTRUHS]
8. Core materials for obturation. [TN]
9. Sodium hypochlorite. [NTR-NR; RGUHS; MUHS; TN]
10. Uses of $Ca(OH)_2$ in endodontics. [NTR-NR]
11. Bleaching agents. [NTR-NR]
12. Role of $Ca(OH)_2$ in endodontics. [NTR-NR]
13. Uses of MTA in endodontics. [NTR-NR]
14. Poly antibiotic paste. [MUHS; RGUHS]
15. Hydrogen peroxide. [RGUHS, (OR and NR); TN]
16. Thermo plasticized gutta-percha. [GOA]
17. Thermo elasticized Gutta-percha. [NTR-OR]
18. Sodium hypochlorite solution. [NTR-OR]

19. R.C. prep. [BUHS]
20. Gross man's sealers. [NTR-NR; BUHS]
21. Non-eugenol sealers. [RGUHS]
22. Composition of Grossman's sealer. [NTRUHS]
23. Mineral trioxide aggregate. [RGUHS; GOA]
24. Calcium hydroxide cement. [TN]
25. MTA. [TN]
26. Idea requirements of irrigants. [RGUHS]
27. Diaket. [RGUHS]
28. Thermoplasticized gutta-percha. [NTRUHS]
29. Glutaraldehyde. [NTR-NR; RGUHS; MUHS]
30. Intracanal medicaments. [TN]
31. Root canal irrigants. [TN]
33. Sealants in endodontics. [TN]
34. Silver points. [RGUHS]
35. Hermetic seal of root canal. [TN]
36. Gelfoam. [RGUHS]
37. Gutta-percha. [NTR-OR; NTR-NR; RGUHS]
38. EDTA in endodontics. [NTR-NR; MUHS]
39. Pulpdent. [RGUHS]
40. Sub surface porosity. [RGUHS]
41. Roots end filling materials. [TN]
42. Root canal sealers. [TN]
43. Isopropyl alcohol. [RGUHS]
44. Intracanal medicaments. [TN]
45. Irrigating solution used during pulp space therapy. [GOA]
46. Formocresol. [TN]
47. Ca(OH)2 based root canal sealer. [NTR-NR]
48. Role of irrigants in endodontics. [TN]

OBTURATION OF ROOT CANAL

Long Essays

1. Describe the failures of root canal treatment and how will you overcome them. [MUHS]
2. Classify root canal give the method of obturation for each one of them. [MUHS]
3. Classify and describe the obturation materials and sealers used in root canal treatment. [NTR-OR]
4. Enumerate the clinical steps to be followed during root canal obturation with reasons. [MUHS]
5. Describe the various obturation technique of root canal? [RGUHS, BUHS]
6. Define obturation. When is the root canal ready for obturation. Describe in detail the thermoplasticized gutta-percha technique for obturation. [TN]
7. Give the list of root canal obturating materials and discuss lateral condensation technique. [RGUHS]
8. Enumerate the various obturating materials used for root canal treatment. Describe the technique of lateral condensation. [RGUHS, TN]
9. Percha technique. [RGUHS]
10. Discuss the various methods of root canal obturation. [RGUHS]
11. Enumerate the technique obturation of the root canal system. Describe vertical condensation in detail. [TN]
12. How do you know that the root canal system is ready for obturation. Discuss lateral condensation technique. [NTR-NR]
13. Enumerate various methods of obturations of root canal system. Describe lateral condensation method. [MUHS]
14. Define obturation. Describe in detail lateral condensation method. [MUHS]
15. Classify obturating materials. Describe lateral condensation method of obturation of root canal. [NTR-NR]
16. Enumerate the ideal requirements for a root canal filling material. [MUHS]
17. Describe the various methods of obturating the root canal. When is the canal ready for obturation. Write briefly on thermoplastic gutta-percha technique. [TN]
18. Classify root canal sealers. Describe zinc-oxide/eugenol containing sealers. [MUHS]
19. Enumerate various diagnostic aids in endodontics discuss in detail the importance of radiographic examination and give its limitations. [GOA]
20. Enumerate various methods of obturation of Root Canal. Describes vertical condensation method. [MUHS]
21. Describe the indication, contraindication, advantages and disadvantages of gutta-percha points as a root canal filling material. [MUHS]
22. List the various methods of root canal obtrusion and describe one technique, which you use in the clinic. [RGUHS, BUHS]
23. Describe in detail any good technique to obtain satisfactory optical seal of root canal. [RGUHS, BUHS]
24. Enumerate the various obturating materials used for root canal treatment. Describe the technique of lateral condensation. [RGUHS]
25. How would you know that root canal is ready for obturation of root canal. [MUHS]

26. Describe in detail lateral condensation technique of root canal obturation. [NTR-OR]
27. Enumerate various methods of obturations of root canal system with gutta-percha and explain anyone method in detail. [MUHS]
28. Enumerate the obturation methods in endodontic therapy. Write in detail about lateral molar using conventional design. [TN]
29. Write in detail about obturation techniques of root canal treatment including the latest methods. [RGUHS, BUHS]

Short Essays

1. Compactor method of obturation. [RGUHS]
2. Thermoplasticized gutta-percha technique. [NTR-OR]
3. Classification of endodontic instrument. [MUHS]
4. Hydrogen peroxide. [MUHS]
5. Describe in detail vertical condensation method. [MUHS]
6. Classification of root canal obturating materials. [MUHS]
7. Inverted cone method. [RGUHS]
8. Enumerate the various obturating used for curved root canals describe thermoplasticized gutta-percha technique. [GOA]
9. Thermoplasticized obturation. [RGUHS (OR and NR)]
10. McSpadden technique and obtura III system. [RGUHS]
11. Intra oral digital radiography. [GOA]
12. Lateral condensation technique. [N'TRUHS]
13. Sectional method of obturation. [RGUHS]
14. Lateral condensation. [RGUHS]

15. Warm gutta-percha technique. [NTR-NR]
16. When is root canal ready to receive filling. [MUHS]
17. Crown down-pressure less technique. [NTR-OR]
18. How will you sterilize a root canal and know it is ready for obturation mention different obturation methods. [GOA]

Short Notes

1. Lateral condensation. [RGUHS]
2. Gutta-percha. [MUHS]
3. Thermoplasticized gutta-percha techniques. [TN]
4. Thermoplasticized gutta-percha. [RGUHS]
5. Sectional method of obturation. [MUHS]
6. Cold lateral condensation. [TN]
7. Endodontic sealer. [MUHS]
8. When to obturate the root canal. [RGUHS]
9. Later condensation technique. [RGUHS]
10. Root canal seals. [RGUHS]
11. Composition of Gutta-percha cone. [MUHS]
12. Section technique of obturation. [TN]
13. Silver points. [RGUHS]
14. McSpadden technique. [RGUHS]
15. Various obturation techniques and their advantages. [MUHS]
16. Schilder's technique. [NTR-NR]
17. McSpadden compaction. [RGUHS, BUHS, RGUHS]
18. Enumerate various methods of obturations of root canal system. [MUHS]

POSTENDODONTIC RESTORATIONS

Long Essays

1. Enumerate indications, contraindications and technique of post and core. [NTR-NR]

Short Essays

1. Management of perforations. [NTRUHS]

2. Management of separated instruments within root canal. [RGUHS]
3. Post and Core. [RGUHS]

Short Notes

1. Core material. [RGUHS]
2. Post endodontic restoration. [TN]

MISHAPS AND FAILURES OF ENDODONTIC TREATMENTS

Long Essays

1. What are the procedural problems during endodontic therapy. Discuss their management. [GOA]
2. Discuss perforations as one of the major causes in failure of endodontic treatment. [BUHS]

3. Discuss in detail the sequelae and treatment of incomplete root canal filling. [NTR-OR]
4. Write various endodontic failures. How will you overcome them. [NTR-NR]

Short Essays

1. Problems arising during endodontic treatment. [RGUHS]

Short Notes

1. Ledge formation. [RGUHS]
2. Management of separated instruments within the root canal. [TN]

TREATMENTS OF TRAUMATIZED TEETH

Long Essays

1. Give step by step management of traumatically fractured central incisor in a 9-year-old child. [MUHS]
2. A boy, aged 8 years, comes to your clinic with a fractured central incisor due to sports injury. Outline and describe your line of treatment. [TN; RGUHS, BUHS]
3. How will you treat a young boy of 14 years coming to you with a recently fractured central incisor involving pulp. [RGUHS, BUHS]
4. An 18-year-old patient reports to the clinic with a fracture of maxillary central incisor involving dentine. Trauma happened one month back, discuss your treatment options. [RGUHS (OR and NR)]
5. Classify traumatic injuries. Write about management of avulsed upper incisor tooth in a 10-years-old patient. [RGUHS]
6. Classify traumatic injuries of anterior teeth. How will you manage Ellis class III fracture in maxillary central incisor. [TN]

Short Essays

1. Classification of injuries of teeth. [RGUHS]
2. Vertical root fractures. [NTRUHS]
3. Management of avulsed tooth. [RGUHS]
4. Types of root fracture and management. [RGUHS]

Short Notes

1. Management of avulsed tooth. [TN]
2. Classify traumatic injuries of anterior tooth. [TN]
3. Perio endodontics therapy. [BUHS]
4. Apexogenesis. [RGUHS (OR and NR)]
5. Avulsion. [RGUHS]
6. Ellis classification of fractured teeth. [RGUHS]
7. Resorption. [TN]
8. Methods of immobilization of traumatized teeth. [TN]
9. Luebke-Ochsenbein flap design. [RGUHS]
10. Replacement resorption. [TN]
11. Sealants in endodontic. [TN]
12. Internal resorption. [TN]

ENDODONTIC SURGERY AND REPLANTATION AND TRANSPLANTATION

Long Essays

1. Mention the indication for periapical surgeries and add a note on wound closure. [RGUHS, BUHS]
2. What is intentional replantation. What are the indications for this procedure. Write briefly about the technique of intentional replantation. [RGUHS, BUHS]
3. Discuss the sequelae apicoectomy and the measures to overcome them. [MUHS]
4. What is Replantation. Write in detail intentional replantation. [NTR-OR]
5. Classify various periapical lesions. Discuss in detail about treatment of periapical cyst. [MUHS]
6. Enumerate the indication for apicoectomy. Describe the procedure of apicoectomy with retrograde filling in upper central incisor. [RGUHS, BUHS]
7. Mention the indication of apical surgery and describe in detail the procedure of apicoectomy in relation to maxillary central incisor. [RGUHS, BUHS]
8. Define intentional replantation, Write indications, contraindications and techniques of intentional replantation. [NTR-NR]
9. Describe the outline of technique for immediate root resection. [RGUHS]
10. Classify different flap designs used in surgical endodontics add a note on Luebke-Ochsenbein flap. [GOA]
11. What are indications for apical surgery? Describe the procedure for apicectomy. [TN]
12. Discuss the post-operative complication of apicoectomy describe the measure to overcome them. [GOA]

13. Give indication and contraindication of apical surgical procedures. List various apical surgical procedures. [MUHS]
14. Give indication, contraindications and discuss the procedure of apicoectomy after Root Canal Obturation. [MUHS]
15. Defined endodontic surgery. Mention indications and contra indication. Add a note on investigations. [NTRUHS]
16. Give list of apical surgeries. Give indications and contraindications of same. [RGUHS]
17. Describe the procedure of apicectomy of maxillary left central incisor. [TN]
18. What is re-plantation. What are the indications and contra indication for this procedure. Write briefly about the procedure of intentional re-plantation. [RGUHS]
19. Enumerate endodontic surgery. Give indication and contraindications of each. [MUHS]
20. Give indications, for periapical surgery. Describe briefly the procedure of apicoectomy in a maxillary central incisor. [NTR-OR]
21. Classify the tooth fracture. Discuss the treatment of Avulsed tooth. [MUHS]
22. Give indications and contraindications for periapical surgery. Write briefly on apicoectomy. [RGUHS, BUHS]

Short Essays

1. Intentional replantation. [NTR-OR, NTR-NR; RGUHS]
2. Root end resection and preparation. [NTRUHS]
3. Intrapulpal anaesthesia. [RGUHS]
4. Indications for periapical surgery and flap designs in endodontic surgeries. [RGUHS; NTRUHS]
5. Re-implantation. [NTRUHS]
6. Incision and drainage. [RGUHS]
7. Apicoectomy. [RGUHS]
8. Indications and contraindications for intentional reimplantation. [RGUHS]
9. Intentional replantation. [RGUHS]
10. Indications of periapical surgery. [MUHS]
11. Indications for periapical surgery and flap designs in Endodontic surgeries. [RGUHS]
12. Flap designs in apicoectomy. [RGUHS]
13. Replantation of avulsed tooth. [NTR-NR]
14. Flaps for endo surgery. [TN]

15. Contraindication of peripheral surgery. [MUHS]
16. Hemisection. [MUHS; TN]
17. Replantation. [NTR-OR; RGUHS]
18. Indications for endodontic surgeries. [RGUHS]
19. Flap designs in surgical endodontics. [NTR-NR]
20. Luebke-Ochsenbein flap design and advantages. [RGUHS]
21. Endodontic endosseous implants. [NTR-NR]
22. Hemisection. [NTR-OR, NTR-NR]
23. Luebke-Ochsenbein flap. [NTR-NR]
24. Flap design for endodontic surgeries. [NTR-NR]
25. MO. [RGUHS]
26. Indications for periapical surgery. [NTR-OR]
27. Radisection. [NTR-OR]
28. Flap designs for periapical surgery. [NTR-OR]
29. Intention replantation. [MUHS]

Short Notes

1. Endodontic implants. [RGUHS]
2. Splinting. [RGUHS]
3. Bicuspidization. [RGUHS]
4. Apicoectomy. [TN]
5. Intentional replantation. [RGUHS]
6. Endodontic endosseous implants. [RGUHS]
7. Flaps for endodontic surgery. [TN]
8. Flap design. [RGUHS; TN]
9. Indications for periapical surgery. [RGUHS]
10. Semi lunar incision. [RGUHS]
11. Masseners kit. [NTR-NR; RGUHS]
12. Indications and contraindications for periapical surgery. [TN]
13. Sequelae of replantation. [GOA]
14. Flap designs in endodontics surgery. [GOA; TN]
15. Periapical curettage. [RGUHS]
16. Trapezoidal flap. [RGUHS]
17. Bicuspidization. [RGUHS]
18. Hemisection. [NTRUHS; RGUHS; TN]
19. Retro grade fillings. [TN]
20. Luebke-Ochsenbein flap design. [RGUHS]
21. Replantation. [RGUHS; TN]
22. Incisions for apical surgery. [TN]
23. Root end closure-physiologic Vs induced. [GOA]

ENDODONTIC PERIODONTAL INTER-RELATIONSHIPS

Long Essays

1. Classification of endodontic periodontic lesions. Write in detail about hemisection and radisection. [TN]

Short Essays

1. Perio endodontics therapy. [TN]
2. Classification of endo-perio lesions. [RGUHS]

LASERS AND ENDODONTIC IMPLANTS

Short Essays

1. Microbiological flora of pulp space. [GOA]
2. Endodontic implants. [RGUHS; RGUHS]

Short Notes

1. Endo-osseous implants. [NTRUHS]

SINGLE VISIT ENDODONTICS

Short Essays

1. Enlist the rules for access cavity preparation. Write in detail about access cavity preparation for all maxillary right side teeth taking into consideration the anatomical variations. [GOA]

Short Notes

1. Access cavity preparation in mandibular molar. [TN]
2. Access cavity in mandibular permanent first molar. [NTRUHS]
3. Single visit endodontics. [TN]
4. Apical foramen. [NTRUHS]

BLEACHING OF DISCOLOURED TOOTH

Long Essays

1. Enumerate the cause of discolouration of tooth. Discuss the various methods of bleaching and procedure to prevent the recurrences of discolouration. [RGUHS; GOA]
2. What are the causes for discolouration of teeth? Describe walking bleach technique. [RGUHS]
3. Describe the causes of discolouration of anterior teeth. How will you proceed to restore the aesthetic of these teeth? [RGUHS, BUHS]
4. Give the treatment of discoloured pulp less central incisor. [MUHS]
5. Describe the rational of bleaching a discoloured non-vital tooth describe extra canal bleaching procedure in a tetracycline stained tooth. [RGUHS, BUHS]
6. Discuss the management of a case with an injury to upper central incisor tooth without pulp exposure but with subsequent history of discolouration of the tooth. [MUHS]
7. Describe the procedure of bleaching of non-vital end-odontically treated tooth. [RGUHS, BUHS]
8. Describe in detail the classification and various treatment options of discoloured anterior teeth. [TN]
9. Classify the techniques for root canal preparation discuss crown down technique. [NTRUHS]
10. How will you manage a case of discoloured non-vital central incisor? [RGUHS]
11. What vitality tooth. How do you do it? What are the results? [TN]
12. Mention the various cases for discolouration of teeth. Describe the techniques of bleaching vital discoloured teeth. [NTR-NR]

Short Essays

1. Describe causes for discolouration of teeth. Mention the different methods of treatment. [RGUHS]
2. Walking bleach technique. [MUHS]
3. What are the causes of discolouration of teeth? Describe walking bleach technique. [RGUHS]
4. Describe causes for discolouration of teeth. Mention the different methods of treatment. [RGUHS]
5. Describe the management of discoloured inapt root canal treated teeth. [RGUHS, BUHS]
6. Bleaching of discoloured vital teeth. [NTR-OR]
7. Night Guard bleach. [NTR-OR]
8. Superoxol. [MUHS]
9. Walking bleach. [NTR-OR]
10. Bleaching of vital teeth. [RGUHS; NTRUHS]
11. Thermocatalytic technique of bleaching. [RGUHS (RS)]
12. Vital and non-vital bleaching techniques. [NTRUHS]

Short Notes

2. Discolourization. [RGUHS]
3. Hydrogen peroxide. [RGUHS]
4. Power bleaching. [TN]
5. Bleaching agents. [NTR-NR]
6. Management of tetracycline discoloured teeth. [TN]
7. Walking bleach. [TN]
8. Matrix bleaching. [TN]
9. Vital bleaching. [TN]
10. Non-vital bleaching. [TN]
11. Superoxol. [RGUHS]
12. Home bleaching. [TN]
13. Night guard bleach. [RGUHS]